The Role of Complement in Cancer Immunotherapy

The Role of Complement in Cancer Immunotherapy

Editor

Ronald P. Taylor

MDPI • Basel • Beijing • Wuhan • Barcelona • Belgrade • Manchester • Tokyo • Cluj • Tianjin

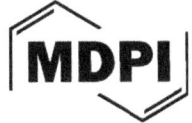

Editor
Ronald P. Taylor
Department of Biochemistry and
Molecular Genetics,
University of Virginia School of Medicine
USA

Editorial Office
MDPI
St. Alban-Anlage 66
4052 Basel, Switzerland

This is a reprint of articles from the Special Issue published online in the open access journal *Antibodies* (ISSN 2073-4468) (available at: https://www.mdpi.com/journal/antibodies/special_issues/Complement_Cancer_Immunotherapy).

For citation purposes, cite each article independently as indicated on the article page online and as indicated below:

LastName, A.A.; LastName, B.B.; LastName, C.C. Article Title. *Journal Name* **Year**, *Volume Number*, Page Range.

ISBN 978-3-0365-2938-7 (Hbk)
ISBN 978-3-0365-2939-4 (PDF)

© 2021 by the authors. Articles in this book are Open Access and distributed under the Creative Commons Attribution (CC BY) license, which allows users to download, copy and build upon published articles, as long as the author and publisher are properly credited, which ensures maximum dissemination and a wider impact of our publications.

The book as a whole is distributed by MDPI under the terms and conditions of the Creative Commons license CC BY-NC-ND.

Contents

About the Editor vii

Taylor, R.P.
Special Issue: The Role of Complement in Cancer Immunotherapy
Reprinted from: *Antibodies* 2021, 10, 29, doi:10.3390/10.3390/antib10030029 1

Margot Revel, Marie V. Daugan, Catherine Sautés-Fridman, Wolf H. Fridman and Lubka T. Roumenina
Complement System: Promoter or Suppressor of Cancer Progression?
Reprinted from: *Antibodies* 2020, 9, 57, doi:10.3390/10.3390/antib9040057 5

Clive S. Zent, Jonathan J. Pinney, Charles C. Chu and Michael R. Elliott
Complement Activation in the Treatment of B-Cell Malignancies
Reprinted from: *Antibodies* 2020, 9, 68, doi:10.3390/10.3390/antib9040068 27

Josée Golay and Ronald P. Taylor
The Role of Complement in the Mechanism of Action of Therapeutic Anti-Cancer mAbs
Reprinted from: *Antibodies* 2020, 9, 58, doi:10.3390/10.3390/antib9040058 41

Ronald P. Taylor and Margaret A. Lindorfer
How Do mAbs Make Use of Complement to Kill Cancer Cells? The Role of Ca^{2+}
Reprinted from: *Antibodies* 2020, 9, 45, doi:10.3390/10.3390/antib9030045 65

Maciej M. Markiewski, Elizabeth Daugherity, Britney Reese and Magdalena Karbowniczek
The Role of Complement in Angiogenesis
Reprinted from: *Antibodies* 2020, 9, 67, doi:10.3390/10.3390/antib9040067 91

Joshua M. Thurman, Jennifer Laskowski and Raphael A. Nemenoff
Complement and Cancer—A Dysfunctional Relationship?
Reprinted from: *Antibodies* 2020, 9, 61, doi:10.3390/10.3390/antib9040061 105

Fazrena Nadia Md Akhir, Mohd Hezmee Mohd Noor, Keith Weng Kit Leong, Jamileh A. Nabizadeh, Helga D. Manthey, Stefan E. Sonderegger, Jenny Nga Ting Fung, Crystal E. McGirr, Ian A. Shiels, Paul C. Mills, Trent M. Woodruff and Barbara E. Rolfe
An Immunoregulatory Role for Complement Receptors in Murine Models of Breast Cancer
Reprinted from: *Antibodies* 2021, 10, 2, doi:10.3390/10.3390/antib10010002 121

Ellinor I. Peerschke, Elisa de Stanchina, Qing Chang, Katia Manova-Todorova, Afsar Barlas, Anne G. Savitt, Brian V. Geisbrecht and Berhane Ghebrehiwet
Anti gC1qR/p32/HABP1 Antibody Therapy Decreases Tumor Growth in an Orthotopic Murine Xenotransplant Model of Triple Negative Breast Cancer
Reprinted from: *Antibodies* 2020, 9, 51, doi:10.3390/10.3390/antib9040051 133

Sophia Roßkopf, Klara Marie Eichholz, Dorothee Winterberg, Katarina Julia Diemer, Sebastian Lutz, Ira Alexandra Münnich, Katja Klausz, Thies Rösner, Thomas Valerius, Denis Martin Schewe, Andreas Humpe, Martin Gramatzki, Matthias Peipp and Christian Kellner
Enhancing CDC and ADCC of CD19 Antibodies by Combining Fc Protein-Engineering with Fc Glyco-Engineering
Reprinted from: *Antibodies* 2020, 9, 63, doi:10.3390/10.3390/antib9040063 145

Michelle Elvington, M. Kathryn Liszewski and John P. Atkinson
CD46 and Oncologic Interactions: Friendly Fire against Cancer
Reprinted from: *Antibodies* **2020**, *9*, 59, doi:10.3390/10.3390/antib9040059 . . . . **161**

About the Editor

Ronald P. Taylor is Professor Emeritus of Biochemistry and Molecular Genetics, University of Virginia. He completed his PhD in Chemistry at Princeton with Professor I. Kuntz, and he received training in protein chemistry from Professor R. Lumry, University of Minnesota. He joined the faculty at the University of Virginia, was promoted to Professor in 1983, and retired in 2016 after 43 years. His research has focused on complement and immunological bench to bedside investigations. He has published more than 220 papers, including 10 patents, several of which have been translated into ongoing clinical trials. He has served on the editorial boards of *Antibodies, Arthritis & Rheumatology, Haematologica, Leukemia Research,* and *The Journal of Immunology*. He is an Associate Editor of Immunopharmacology and Immunotoxicology. He is, to his knowledge, the only complementologist to have finished the Boston Marathon in under 3 hours (unofficially) and the New York City Marathon 59 seconds over 3 hours (officially).

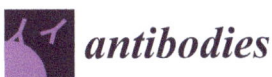

Editorial

Special Issue: The Role of Complement in Cancer Immunotherapy

Ronald P. Taylor

Department of Biochemistry and Molecular Genetics, University of Virginia School of Medicine, Charlottesville, VA 22908, USA; rpt@virginia.edu; Tel.: +1-434-987-1964

Citation: Taylor, R.P. Special Issue: The Role of Complement in Cancer Immunotherapy. *Antibodies* **2021**, *10*, 29. https://doi.org/10.3390/antib 10030029

Received: 30 June 2021
Accepted: 2 July 2021
Published: 23 July 2021

Publisher's Note: MDPI stays neutral with regard to jurisdictional claims in published maps and institutional affiliations.

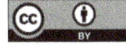

Copyright: © 2021 by the author. Licensee MDPI, Basel, Switzerland. This article is an open access article distributed under the terms and conditions of the Creative Commons Attribution (CC BY) license (https://creativecommons.org/licenses/by/4.0/).

The complement system plays an important role in critical aspects of immune defense and in the maintenance of homeostasis in the bloodstream, as well as in essentially all tissues and organs [1]. More than 100 years ago, Bordet was awarded the Nobel Prize for his discovery of complement. His work revealed that antibodies complexed with antigens activate complement and induce substantial inflammation, leading to cell and tissue destruction, and therefore it is not surprising that numerous clinical and basic science investigations have focused on "The Role of Complement in Cancer Immunotherapy", which is the topic of this Special Issue. Within the context of this title, the 10 articles in this issue examine a wide range of subjects, and this range illustrates the diverse and at times contradictory actions of complement in cancer.

The development of mAb technologies and the application of mAbs in cancer immunotherapy has led to a continuing and exponential phase of investigation and initiation of clinical trials, first punctuated by FDA approval of CD20 mAb rituximab for the treatment of B-cell lymphomas [2,3]. Although the efficacy of rituximab was and is clearly demonstrable, its apparent mechanisms of action were the subject of considerable controversy; however, its putative "apoptotic induction" has been set aside, and its therapeutic action has been clearly demonstrated to require immune effector mechanisms, which include complement-dependent cytotoxicity (CDC) [2,3]. Moreover, the basic science studies of rituximab have led to findings that have been most immediately applicable to understanding how other tumor-specific mAbs function, and the outcome of the studies of rituximab have also set the stage for the development of much more effective second- and third-generation mAbs that target CD20 as well as other tumor-associated antigens [4].

In terms of maintaining homeostasis, complement promotes wound healing and angiogenesis (essential to cell growth) and there is a substantial literature that describes how complement can establish an environment that allows for growth of tumors. This is most evident when the tumors are *not* recognized as foreign, and therefore can take advantage of the "cell growth"-promoting action of complement [1,5]. The encyclopedic review of Revel and colleagues comprehensively describes complement pathways as well as the numerous cases in which specific complement components, especially C1q and C5a, play important roles both in promoting tumor growth and in generating an immunosuppressive environment [1]. Weak immune responses to the tumors (titers of IgG and IgM insufficient to mediate cell killing) appear to activate and recruit complement proteins to foster cell growth, and the complement components can be produced by the host or generated by the tumors themselves. Revel et al. also document in mouse models the roles that complement can play in suppressing or promoting tumor growth; this again illustrates the apparent and unresolved contradiction between "promotor or suppressor of cancer progression".

Thurman and colleagues also recognize the "dysfunctional relationship" between complement and cancer, and review their interesting and provocative findings which have demonstrated that inflammation associated with complement activation can induce downstream oxidative damage and transformation (but not killing) of cells which leads to malignancy [6]. They note that non-lethal complement activation within the tumor microenvironment (TME) also promotes angiogenesis, thereby providing a favorable niche for a growing tumor. Moreover, they review a voluminous literature documenting the increased expression of complement control proteins on cancer cells, which is clearly an additional defensive measure that cancer cells appear to have evolved to avoid potential lethal cytotoxic "side effects" of modest complement activation. They also cite the seminal studies of Markiewski and Lambris, who first demonstrated that the C5a produced by cancer cells can attract myeloid-derived suppressor cells (MDSC) to the TME, thus providing yet another "pro-tumor" defensive activity of complement.

The review by Markiewski and colleagues focuses on complement-mediated (neo)angiogenesis, which helps to provide a blood supply to the growing tumor [5]. They report that complement influences the generation of the "Premetastatic Niche" in which, due to the action of C5a, MDSC are recruited before the arrival of tumor cells. These processes are described in exquisite detail, and the authors make clear that the factors mediating angiogenesis for tumors are also operative in other pathologies, including age-related macular degeneration (AMD). They note that targeting of certain complement factors including C5aR1 may be effective in the treatment of both cancer and AMD.

The role of complement and, in particular, complement receptors in mouse models of triple-negative breast cancer are examined in two particularly interesting and innovative articles [7,8]. This form of cancer lacks any of the common and targetable hormone receptors and is therefore particularly resistant to most conventional treatments. The groups of Woodruff and Rolfe examined the influence of the well-studied agent PMX53 (C5aR1 *antagonist*) as well as an *agonist* for both C3aR and C5aR1 (EP54), on the growth of syngeneic mammary carcinoma cell lines in mice [7]. The investigators report that in contrast to findings in several other mouse cancer models, PMX53 had no effect on tumor growth in this system. In most other models, the PMX53 suppressed tumor growth by interfering with "recruitment" of MDSC to the TME. On the other hand, while the EP54 agonist suppressed tumor growth, its actual mechanism of action was not clear, but was most likely due to enhancement of T-lymphocyte action in the TME. These findings once again emphasize the complex role of complement in cancer, and indicate that directed therapies based on complement must be carefully and specifically designed; it appears that there are few general rules that apply.

Teams led by Peerschke and Ghebrehiwet have been among the leading groups studying the biology and immunology of C1q and its receptors. In this issue, they have investigated how targeting the globular receptor to C1q (gC1qR) with a specific neutralizing mAb affects the growth of breast cancer cells in a mouse xenotranplant model of triple-negative breast cancer in which the gC1qR is upregulated on the tumor cells [8]. The investigators made use of a variety of elegant immunostaining techniques along with measures of tumor growth and report, for the first time, in vivo proof of principle for suppression of growth of triple-negative breast cancer cells accomplished by targeting gC1qR with a neutralizing mAb. Mechanisms of action of the mAb may include both induction of apoptosis of the tumor cells as well as inhibition of angiogenesis. Additional studies of these phenomena and possible translation to the clinic are anticipated.

Many of the key studies of the mechanisms of CD20 mAb-mediated killing of primary tumor cells (in most cases malignant B cells from patients with chronic lymphocytic leukemia (CLL)) have been reported by groups led by Golay or Zent [2,3]. The review by Golay and Taylor highlights the ex vivo studies in whole blood that were pioneered by Golay and Introna [3]. This work has clearly established that upon binding to CLL B cells, both rituximab and ofatumumab (but not obituzumab) make use of complement which most immediately kills B cells, and both groups have demonstrated that B cells opsonized with complement fragments can also be eliminated by immune cells that express receptors for both IgG (Fc receptors) and C3 fragments (such as CR3) in a synergistic process. Although these reactions are quite effective, they can be overwhelmed at high B-cell burdens, thus leading to exhaustion of complement, both in vivo and in vitro. Whether use of fresh frozen plasma as a complement source can effectively restore and or enhance the immediate action of these mAbs remains under investigation. Zent and colleagues have made use of a bedside to bench approach and find that phagocytosis of opsonized cells by macrophages appears to be the principal and most important mechanism by which B cells opsonized with rituximab or ofatumaub are eliminated [2]. Their work with primary CLL cells has definitively established that higher concentrations of mAbs (and therefore higher levels of opsonization of target cells) are required for CDC than for phagocytosis. Golay and Taylor also cite several bedside to bench investigations which indicate that upregulation of complement control proteins is *not* a mechanism of resistance employed by CLL cells to inhibit CDC mediated by rituximab or ofatumumab. Finally, both reviews discuss the important advance in the design of more effective complement-activating mAbs based on generating IgG molecules that more readily form hexamers upon binding to cells, thus allowing for more effective chelation of C1q [4]. The illustrations in both of these articles are elegant and informative.

Rosskopf and colleagues have made substantial advances in the area of IgG engineering by modifying mAbs to enhance their potential to more effectively target and destroy tumor cells [9]. They have made use of an FDA-approved CD19 mAb (tafasitamab) which has modest activity in inducing antibody-dependent cellular cytotoxicity (ADCC) but does not activate complement or induce CDC. They recognize that a key issue in engineering such IgG1 mAbs is that the C1q-binding regions and Fc-chelating sites on the mAbs are close together, thus presenting a challenge to generating a mAb with substantial levels of both activities. They found that by making directed changes in the amino acid sequence of the Fc region (EFTAE modification) along with expressing its afucosylated form, they were able to produce a mAb with considerably higher levels of both ADCC and CDC. The experimental methodologies used by the investigators encompass protein engineering, cellular binding assays of mAbs and C1q and functional CDC and ADCC assays, and are all elegant, rigorous and very well described. Their approaches provide a template for additional efforts in the optimization of mAbs for cancer immunotherapy.

The review by Taylor and Lindorfer examines in detail key steps in complement mediated lysis of B cells that are opsonized with highly effective complement-activating mAbs (hexamer-forming) specific for CD20 and CD37 [4]. There is indeed considerable co-localization of cell-bound mAb with C1q, and this is rapidly followed by "nearby" covalent deposition of C3b (colocalized with bound mAb), which is soon followed by assembly and deposition of the membrane attack complex (MAC, C5b-9) of complement. Ultimately the most direct cause of cell death is due to influx of lethal amounts of Ca^{2+} mediated by the MAC, and the entire process is complete in just a few minutes. One surprising outcome of these studies was the observation that CLL cells (not a cell line!) could indeed be killed by this mechanism *in the absence of C9*, thereby revealing that the Ca^{2+} influx mediated by the smaller C5b-8 pore was adequate to rapidly kill the cells. These observations can therefore set the standard for the generation and testing of future tumor-specific mAbs that make use of complement for cancer immunotherapy. It is most likely that as other highly effective complement fixing mAbs are developed, many of the phenomena described by Taylor and Lindorfer will be closely replicated with other cancer cells and their cognate mAbs. Whether CDC can be accomplished in the absence of C9 for these yet-to-be-developed mAbs is not clear, but based on the observations with the traditionally resistant CLL cells it is likely that C9 *will not* be required. Another lesson learned from these studies is that the action of mAbs that are particularly effective at activating complement exceeds the molecular thresholds for C1q binding and C3b deposition required for the generation of large quantities of the MAC, and therefore these mAbs are capable of overwhelming the natural defenses (including complement control proteins) expressed by tumor cells [4].

Elvington, Liszewski and Atkinson have written a comprehensive review on the complement control protein CD46, membrane cofactor protein (MCP), which was first described by the Atkinson lab more than 30 years ago [10]. Most research on this molecule has focused on human systems because CD46 is not expressed in mice. The protein is present on a wide variety of human cells and in addition to its many immunologic functions, it has been demonstrated to be the cell entry site of several viruses, including adenovirus and measles virus. Moreover, there is considerable evidence that CD46 is substantially overexpressed on tumor cells, and therefore it is under intense investigation as a prime target for cancer immunotherapy. These investigations include the use of CD46-directed mAb–drug conjugates; the CD46 mAb is specific for a conformational epitope expressed *only* on cancer cells. Other therapies under investigation make use of modified forms of measles virus or adenovirus that are engineered to only replicate in cancer cells (oncolytic viruses). As noted by the authors, the CD46 target is now the subject of more than 20 clinical trials in a variety of cancers, including melanoma and pancreatic cancer. Early on, it was discovered that CD46 protects cells from complement attack by serving as a co-factor for inactivation of deposited C3b and C4b. Therefore, it may be particularly interesting to examine the CDC activity against tumor cells by the cancer cell-specific CD46 mAb after it is engineered to form hexamers upon binding to cells. By specifically binding at high levels, only to CD46 expressed on the cancer cells, the hexamer-forming mAb may be quite effective at exceeding the molecular threshold for C3b deposition (see above) required for mediating downstream complement activation and cell lysis.

The paradoxical effects of the complement system in cancer will continue to present challenges in the development of effective mAbs for cancer immunotherapy. The 10 articles featured in this Special Issue should therefore be of considerable interest to basic scientists and to physician scientists investigating new approaches in the immunotherapy of cancer.

Funding: This research received no external funding.

Conflicts of Interest: The author declares no conflict of interest.

References

1. Revel, M.; Daugan, M.V.; Sautes-Fridman, C.; Fridman, W.H.; Roumenia, L.T. Complement system: Promoter or suppressor of cancer progression? *Antibodies* **2020**, *9*, 57. [CrossRef] [PubMed]
2. Zent, C.S.; .Pinney, J.J.; Chu, C.C.; Elliott, M.R. Complement activation in the treatmet of B-cell malignancies. *Antibodies* **2020**, *9*, 68. [CrossRef]
3. Golay, J.; Taylor, R.P. The role of complement in the mechanism of action of therapeutic anti-cancer mAbs. *Antibodies* **2020**, *9*, 58. [CrossRef] [PubMed]
4. Taylor, R.P.; Lindorfer, M.A. How do mAbs make use of complement to kill cancer cells: The role of Ca^{2+}. *Antibodies* **2020**, *9*, 45. [CrossRef]
5. Markiewski, M.M.; Daugherity, E.; Reese, B.; Karbowniczek, M. The role of complement in angiogenesis. *Antibodies* **2020**, *9*, 67. [CrossRef] [PubMed]
6. Thurman, J.M.; Laskowski, J.; Nemenoff, R.A. Complement and cancer—A dysfunctional relationship? *Antibodies* **2020**, *9*, 61. [CrossRef]
7. Akhir, F.N.M.; Noor, M.H.M.; Leong, K.W.K.; Nabizadeh, J.A.; Manthey, H.D.; Sonderegger, S.E.; Fung, J.N.T.; McGirr, C.E.; Shiels, I.A.; Mills, P.C.; et al. An immunoregulatory role for complement receptors in murine models of breast cancer. *Antibodies* **2021**, *10*, 2. [CrossRef] [PubMed]
8. Peerschke, E.I.; de Stanchina, E.; Chang, Q.; Manova-Todorova, K.; Barlas, A.; Savitt, A.G.; Geisbrecht, B.V.; Ghebrehiwet, B. Anti gC1qR/p32/HABP1 antibody therapy decreases tumor growth in an orthotopic muring xenotranplant model of triple negative breast cancer. *Antibodies* **2020**, *9*, 51. [CrossRef]
9. Roskopf, S.; Eichholz, K.M.; Winterberg, D.; Diemer, K.J.; Lutz, S.; Münnich, I.A.; Klausz, K.; Rösner, T.; Valerius, T.; Schewe, D.M.; et al. Enhancing CDC and ADCC of CD19 antibodies by combining Fc protein-engineering with Fc glyco-engineering. *Antibodies* **2020**, *9*, 63. [CrossRef]
10. Elvington, M.; Kiszewski, M.K.; Atkinson, J.P. CD46 and oncologic interactions: Friendly fire against cancer. *Antibodies* **2020**, *9*, 59. [CrossRef]

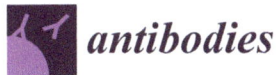

Review

Complement System: Promoter or Suppressor of Cancer Progression?

Margot Revel, Marie V. Daugan, Catherine Sautés-Fridman, Wolf H. Fridman and Lubka T. Roumenina *

Team Inflammation, Complement and Cancer, Centre de Recherche des Cordeliers, INSERM, Sorbonne Université, Université de Paris, F-75006 Paris, France; margot.revel@gmail.com (M.R.); dauganmarie7@hotmail.fr (M.V.D.); catherine.sautes-fridman@sorbonne-universite.fr (C.S.-F.); herve.fridman@crc.jussieu.fr (W.H.F.)
* Correspondence: lubka.roumenina@sorbonne-universite.fr; Tel.: +33-1-44-27-90-96; Fax: +33-1-40-51-04-20

Received: 13 August 2020; Accepted: 20 October 2020; Published: 25 October 2020

Abstract: Constituent of innate immunity, complement is present in the tumor microenvironment. The functions of complement include clearance of pathogens and maintenance of homeostasis, and as such could contribute to an anti-tumoral role in the context of certain cancers. However, multiple lines of evidence show that in many cancers, complement has pro-tumoral actions. The large number of complement molecules (over 30), the diversity of their functions (related or not to the complement cascade), and the variety of cancer types make the complement-cancer topic a very complex matter that has just started to be unraveled. With this review we highlight the context-dependent role of complement in cancer. Recent studies revealed that depending of the cancer type, complement can be pro or anti-tumoral and, even for the same type of cancer, different models presented opposite effects. We aim to clarify the current knowledge of the role of complement in human cancers and the insights from mouse models. Using our classification of human cancers based on the prognostic impact of the overexpression of complement genes, we emphasize the strong potential for therapeutic targeting the complement system in selected subgroups of cancer patients.

Keywords: complement system; cancer; immune infiltrate; tumor microenvironment; tumor growth; anaphylatoxins

1. Introduction

The 21st century was marked by a change in the paradigm of tumor perception. Scientists have established the important role of the immune system and inflammation in cancer development and especially the role of T cells. This concept was not only useful as an academic discovery but it also led to development of several novel treatments, as well as anti-immune checkpoint therapies (anti-PD1/PDL1, anti-CTLA4) that were rewarded by the Nobel prize of 2018. Immune cells have the ability to infiltrate tumors and form with other untransformed cells the tumor microenvironment (TME) [1]. The TME can impact positively or negatively the patient's outcome, depending on its composition [2]. The recruitment of immune cells inside the tumor is achieved thanks to the vascular network that also allows the recruitment of the components of the complement system. The complement system is often forgotten or underestimated, but it is a powerful inflammatory cascade and, as a part of innate immunity, it fully belongs to the TME [3]. The complement system is a set of more than thirty cell-bound or soluble proteins that can come inside the tumor via the circulation but also that can be produced by the tumor cells themselves and the infiltrated immune cells. The complement system is mostly described by its functions related to immunity but, recently, several papers attribute it non-immune functions as angiogenesis, organ development and regeneration or also neuroprotection [4,5].

In this review, we will focus on the different functions of this very complex system and how they can influence patient's outcome, depending of the cancer types or the pathway activated.

2. The Complement System

The first description of the complement system in 1890 assigned it antimicrobial functions [6]. However, due to its composition and the plurality of its actions, the complement system was very difficult to study and progress was dependent on the technologies available. Since the 1950s, with the development of protein chromatography and electrophoresis, data have never stopped to accumulate [7]. Complement is one of the first lines of defense against pathogens or stressed host cells, and can be triggered, depending on the activator, by three different pathways: classical, lectin and alternative. They lead to the formation of C3 and C5 convertases and the common terminal pathway (Figure 1). The complement proteins interact in a highly regulated proteolytic cascade to opsonize pathogens, induce inflammation, interact with cells of adaptive immunity, and maintain homeostasis [4]. The complexity of the complement system is not only due to its composition or its numerous functions (immune or non-immune) but also its ability to act extracellularly or intracellularly.

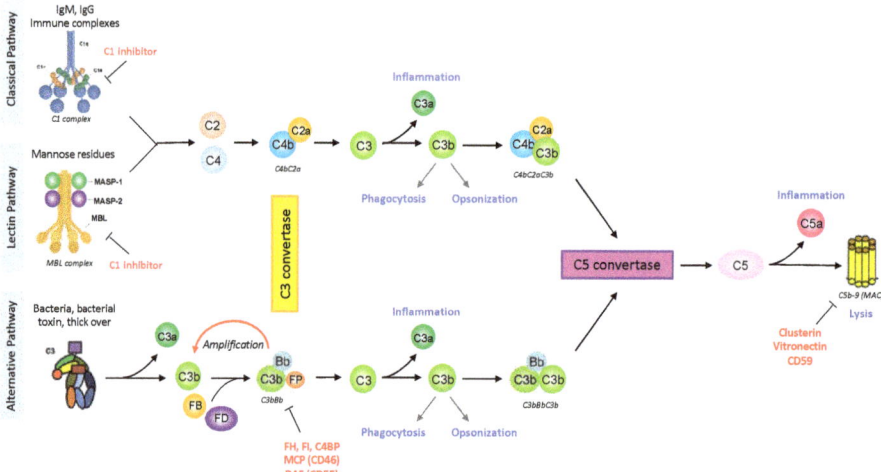

Figure 1. The complement system schematic summary. The classical pathway is activated by the binding of the C1 complex to immunoglobulins or endogenous ligand. The lectin pathway is analogous to the classical one but its activation is triggered by the fixation of the MBL-MASP complex to the pathogen surface. The alternative pathway is spontaneously initiated by the tick-over mechanism and can be amplified in case of recognition of an unprotected surface by complement regulators. These pathways will lead to the formation of the C3 convertase, an enzymatic complex able to cleave C3 into the anaphylatoxin C3a and C3b. The assemblage of a C3b molecule to the C3 convertase is at the origin of the C5 convertase. The C5 molecule can then be cleaved into the anaphylatoxin C5a and C5b, the latter initiating the terminal pathway. The complement cascade culminates with the formation of the multimeric Membrane Attack Complex (MAC, C5b-9) leading to cell activation or death. The complement system is very powerful in triggering inflammation, phagocytosis, opsonization or also lysis, therefore it is tightly regulated at each step by soluble regulators (C1 inhibitor, Factor I (FI), C4 Binding Protein (C4BP), Factor H (FH), Properdin (FP) clusterin, vitronectin) or membrane proteins (Complement Receptor 1 (CD35, CR1), Membrane Cofactor Protein (CD46, MCP), Decay acceleration Factor (CD55, DAF), CD59). The figure is created with BioRender.com.

2.1. Complement Activating Pathways

The classical pathway is activated after the binding of the C1 complex to its targets that can be an antigen-antibody (IgG or IgM) immune complex or an apoptotic cell. The C1 complex is composed of C1q molecules and two different serine protease C1r and C1s [8]. The hexagonal arrangement of the protein platforms (hexameric organization of the IgGs bound to an antigen, or the structure of IgM) is critical for the C1 complex activation [9,10]. The lectin pathway is activated by the recognition of sugar residues through a complex that is structurally and functionally very similar to the classical pathway [11]. The MBL molecule (mannan-binding-lectin), collectins or ficolins resemble C1q and are associated with several serine proteases (MASP1, MASP2 and MASP3), just like the C1 complex. These pathways will lead to the cleavage of C2 into C2a and C2b and C4 into C4a and C4b. C4b and C2a form the classical pathway C3 convertase (C4bC2a), an enzymatic complex able to cleave C3 into the anaphylatoxin C3a and C3b. The specificity of the alternative pathway, in physiology, is to be constitutively activated at low level, thanks to the tick-over mechanism: a spontaneous hydrolysis of a C3 molecule [12], used as a surveillance system. Although properdin could serve as alternative pathway initiator [13], this pathway usually does not need a trigger. This allows the formation of $C3(H_2O)$, a bio-active form of C3, structurally and functionally similar to C3b. $C3(H_2O)$ can bind Factor B (FB) that could be cleaved by Factor D (FD) into Bb and Ba fragments, forming the fluid phase alternative pathway C3 convertase: $C3(H_2O)Bb$, cleaving C3 into the anaphylatoxin C3a and opsonin C3b. In absence of activation the newly formed C3b will be hydrolyzed. In presence of an activating surface, C3b will bind covalently, recruit FB and FD, thereby forming the alternative C3 convertase (C3bBb). This mechanism allows the establishment of an amplification loop to increase the C3 cleavage and hence the C3b concentration at the target surface (pathogen or stressed cell).

2.2. Complement Effector Pathways

Covalent deposition of C3b on the target cell by any of the three pathways induces opsonization, allowing the elimination of the pathogen/stressed cell by phagocytosis [12]. When a certain density of C3b is reached, the molecule of C3b is assembled to the C3 convertase and leads to the formation of the C5 convertase (classical: C4bC2aC3b, or alternative: C3bBbC3b). This triggers the terminal pathway with the generation of the C5a and C5b fragments, and finally the last reaction with the formation of the membrane attack complex (MAC: composed by the molecules C5b, C6, C7, C8 and C9) [4].

Complement activation allows the formation of three different effectors: Opsonins (C3b, C4b and C1q) that can bind the target cell surface and promote its clearance. Anaphylatoxins (C3a and C5a) are released in the circulation and have an important role to induce inflammation and activate cells expressing anaphylatoxin receptors (C3aR, C5aR1/C5aR2). C5aR1 and C5aR2 seem to have opposite effects, especially in the tumor context [14]. MAC formed by the association of C5b molecule with C6 that acquire the ability to interact with lipid bilayer, the C7 and C8 molecules bind C5b and insert into lipid bilayer, then several molecules of C9 polymerize creating the lytic pore, causing membrane permeabilization, cell activation and/or the cell death [15].

2.3. Complement Regulators

Complement is a very powerful system that needs to be tightly regulated. To maintain the balance between complement activation on pathogens or altered host cells and inhibition on intact host cells, several regulators control each step of the proteolytic cascade (Table 1) [16].

Table 1. Complement regulators. The complement system is well regulated at different steps by various soluble or membranous proteins.

Regulated Steps	Regulators	Soluble or Membranous
C1 complex/MBL complex	C1 inhibitors	Soluble
	Factor H (FH)	Soluble
	CFHRs (1 to 5)	Soluble
	Properdin (FP)	Soluble
C3 convertases	C4 Binding Protein (C4BP)	Soluble
C5 convertases	Factor I (FI)	Soluble
	Membrane cofactor proteins (MCP/CD46)	Membranous
	Decay acceleration factor (DAF/CD55)	Membranous
	Complement receptor 1 (CR1)	Membranous
	CD59	Membranous
MAC	Clusterin	Soluble
	Vitronectin	Soluble

2.4. Complement Complexity

The complexity of complement is not only due to its composition or its numerous functions (immune or non-immune) but also due to its ability to act extracellularly or intracellularly. Indeed, although complement is often described as a set of plasma proteins mostly produced by the liver and working in the extracellular compartment, recent studies showed a potential intracellular role of its proteins, especially in T cells. In these cells, intracellular C3 and C5 can be cleaved into C3a and C5a, impacting cell metabolism and homeostasis, the induction of a Th1 and CTL response but the contraction of the T-cell response [17].

Furthermore, overactivation or deficiency of complement can trigger different pathologies, related to inflammation, coagulation, abnormal immune response, or abnormal cell clearance. A deficiency of some complement components can lead to an increased susceptibility to infections or auto-immune diseases [5]. Complement overactivation is classically associated with kidney diseases such as the atypical Hemolytic Uremic Syndrome (aHUS) and C3 Glomerulopathies [18], but also plays a role in pathologies such as multiple sclerosis [19], age-related macular degeneration [20], sickle cell disease [21], or schizophrenia [22], as well as with cancer [23].

3. Complement and Cancer

The complement components are mostly produced by the liver, but it is important to note that both tumor and stromal cells also have the ability to produce complement proteins. Thus, their concentration inside the tumor is both due to the contribution of the systemic compartment and the local production by the different cell types.

Analysis of complement gene expression in thirty different cancers revealed consistent patterns of expression: a high expression of genes coding for classical and alternative pathway; high expression of regulators and a low expression of the lectin pathway and the terminal pathway genes [3]. These data suggest that the tumor could benefit from the early complement proteins but then sets up brakes to avoid any deleterious effector functions. This study is in line with previous observations of an abnormal expression of complement proteins in different type of cancer, especially C1 complex [23], C3 [24], C4 [25], C5 [24], C3aR [24], C5aR1 [24], FB [26], FH [27], FI [28], CD46 [29], CD55 [30], CD59 [30]. Bioinformatic analysis of the prognostic impact of the complement genes allowed to classify cancers in four groups: protective complement (concomitant occurrence of favorable prognosis associated with high expression of complement genes), protective C3 (favorable prognosis found only for high C3 expression but not for the other genes), aggressive complement (concomitant occurrence of poor prognosis, associated with high expression of complement genes) and uncertain significance of complement (when no particular pattern is observed) [3] (Figure 2).

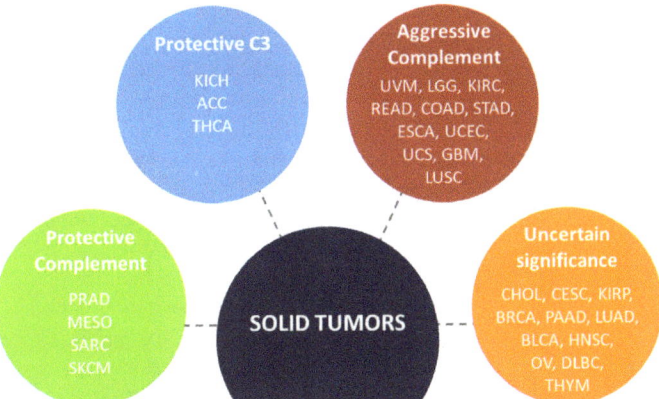

Figure 2. Impact of the complement gene expression on the survival of patients with solid tumors. ACC, adrenocortical carcinoma; BLCA, bladder carcinoma; BRCA, invasive breast carcinoma; CESC, cervical squamous carcinoma; CHOL, cholangiocarcinoma; COAD, colon adenocarcinoma; DLBC, diffuse large B cell lymphoma; ESCA, esophageal carcinoma; GBM, glioblastoma; HNSC, head and neck squamous cell carcinoma; KICH, kidney chromophobe carcinoma; KIRC, kidney renal clear cell carcinoma; KIRP, kidney renal papillary cell carcinoma; LGG, lower grade glioma; LUAD, lung adenocarcinoma; LUSC, lung squamous carcinoma; MESO, mesothelioma; OV, ovarian serous cystadenocarcinoma; PAAD, pancreatic adenocarcinoma; PRAD, prostate adenocarcinoma; READ, rectum adenocarcinoma; SARC, sarcoma; SKCM, skin cutaneous melanoma; STAD, stomach adenocarcinoma; THCA, thyroid carcinoma; THYM, thymoma; UCEC, uterine corpus endometrial carcinoma; UCS, uterine carcinosarcoma; UVM, uveal melanoma. The figure is created with BioRender.com.

It seems that it is not possible to reach a general conclusion as for the pro or anti-tumor role of the complement system. This context-dependent action is reflected by numerous studies, sometimes contradictory, about complement and cancer.

3.1. Activation of Complement in the Tumor Microenvironment

In a tumor context, it is not well understood how the complement system is activated, but several models show that the classical and alternative pathway components are found at a higher concentration in the tumor microenvironment [31]. The tumor cells develop the ability to produce a set of complement proteins and to hijack other proteins produced by host cells, to trigger the complement activation. In clear cell Renal Cell Carcinoma (ccRCC), tumor cells produce C1r and C1s and use C1q secreted by macrophages, in order to form a functional C1 complex and activate the classical pathway in IgG-containing deposits [23] or on cell-bound pentraxin 3 (PTX3) [32]. The hypothesis that the complement system could be activated by immunoglobulins is not new. In 1996, in thyroid carcinoma the presence of IgG, together with C4d, C3d and C5-positive staining suggested tumor-specific classical pathway activation [33]. In non-small cell lung cancer (NSCLC), IgM deposits are observed, pointing to a potential binding of the IgM to the neoantigens present at the tumor cell surface and a triggering of the classical pathway activation [34]. Furthermore, in human urothelial urinary bladder cancer, 50% of tumors with high levels of IgG antibodies also display C1q [35]. Interestingly, in this high IgG and C1q positive tumors, almost 40% also present membranous staining with an anti-C3a detecting antibody. This study suggests the possibility that the activation of the classical pathway could be favorable for the patient's survival [35]. However, recent studies revealed that in lung and renal cancers the activation of the classical pathway by intratumoral immunoglobulins is associated with poor prognosis [23,34]. Interestingly, C3aR and C5aR are likely expressed at the surface of most cell types in a tumor [36] suggesting that C3a and C5a could be used by the tumor cells to promote tumor growth. The activation of the complement system leads to the regulation of the immune system but also amplification of tumor cell invasiveness by acting on proliferation, migration, and epithelial-mesenchymal transition [37].

3.2. Role of Complement on Tumor Immunity

In the last decade, there was an increasing interest in the role of complement in cancer progression. Even if the classical functions of this system are to favor cell killing, its role in cancer appears to be mostly pro-tumoral. The first clue was the slower tumor growth in case of C3, C4 or C5aR deficiency in a TC1 cancer mouse model [38].

Mouse models were, and still are, very useful to study the mechanisms of action and impact of complement on immune cells in the case of cancer. Nevertheless, mouse models yielded some contradictory findings, stressing the context-dependent role of complement in cancer. C3 and C3a are reported to play an important role in cancer progression. Indeed, several studies using syngeneic mouse models (melanoma, breast, and colon cancer [39], or hepatocellular carcinoma [40]) go in the same direction. The C3 expressed notably by immune cells [41] enhances tumor growth by promoting an immunosuppressive environment. Its cleavage product C3a supports the recruitment of C3aR+ macrophages, and perturbation of C3a/C3aR axis disrupts immune infiltration, slowing tumor growth [41]. C3a also promotes T-cell apoptosis, inhibition of T-cell proliferation, inhibition of dendritic cell maturation, increasing of the macrophage and MDSC (myeloid-derived suppressor cells) recruitment, leading to a reduction in the number of CD8+ T cells [41]. A recent study suggests that C3b could impact tumorigenesis during chronic skin inflammation, in cutaneous squamous cell carcinoma (cSCC) model, but independently of C3aR or the terminal pathway (C5a/C5aR1/C5aR2 and MAC generation), likely by influencing tumor associated macrophages [42]. Another report suggests that in colorectal cancer, only the C5a/C5aR1 axis and not C3, could play an important role in the modulation of tumor immunity, by recruiting MDSC and promoting tumorigenesis [43]. Tumor cells can produce C3 molecules, and this production leads to PD-L1 antibody treatment resistance [44]. This mechanism is described in a colon cancer mouse model and goes through a modulation of the tumor associated macrophages response in order to repress anti-tumor immunity, via the C3a-C3aR-PI3Kγ way. These studies highlight again how the complement response can be context—dependent and even contradictory depending of the model and on the cancer types. The multitude of mechanisms by which C3 affects tumor growth is important and must be taken into consideration in the process of development of potential therapeutics [45].

The other anaphylatoxin, C5a, was largely studied too, for its role in tumor progression. Syngeneic mouse models (cervical cancer, lung cancer, or breast cancer) revealed that C5a and its receptor C5aR1 are involved in the recruitment of MDSC. C5a can amplify their capacities to produce reactive oxygen species (ROS) and reactive nitrogen species (RNS) creating an environment favorable for the suppression of the anti-tumor CD8+ T-cell mediated response [38]. In addition, the MDSC recruitment favors the generation of Treg and Th2 response that can suppress the anti-tumor CD8+ T cells [46], but also mediates production of the immunomodulators ARG1, CTLA-4, IL-6, IL-10, LAG3 and PDL1 [47].

An important regulator of the intratumoral levels of C5a is PTX3; this molecule interacts with C1q and FH to modulate the local complement activation. PTX3 is described as an oncosuppressor in mouse models, inhibiting complement activation via FH recruitment, limiting the production of C5a and CCL2 (a pro-inflammatory chemokine) and avoiding the recruitment of tumor-promoting macrophages. The PTX3 deficiency leads to a chronic complement-mediated inflammation, favoring spontaneous skin carcinoma development in a mice model [48]. On the other hand, in human cancer context (ccRCC), a high expression of PTX3 is associated with lower survival rates [32]. The authors explain it by the ability of PTX3 to activate the classical pathway, leading to the production of the pro-inflammatory C3a and C5a. The role of PTX3 as an anti- or pro-tumoral molecule is not yet well understood, but is context-dependent and may be different between mice and human. Interestingly, in ccRCC the complement system is activated via the classical pathway [23], but due to the presence of CD59 regulators [32], the activation is limited and does not go to the C5b-9 lytic pore formation. Therefore, tumor cells could benefit from a complement system activation, until a certain point.

This context-dependent role of the complement system is also true for the pro-inflammatory C3a and C5a molecules that can have anti-tumor functions and appear to be crucial for a good tumor response to radiotherapy [49]. In a carcinogen-induced cSCC model, C5a has an anti-tumoral impact [42], while in a virus-induced mouse model of cSCC, C5a has pro-tumoral impact, with the specificity to be generated independently of complement. The reason behind this phenomenon is unknown. One possible explanation could be linked to the level of locally generated C5a. Indeed, in a syngeneic lymphoma mouse model, the tumor cells producing low levels of C5a are more susceptible to apoptosis and less proliferative, leading to a smaller tumor size. These tumors are associated with an increase infiltration of granulocytes and macrophages and finally an increase IFNγ production by CD4+ and CD8+ T cells in lymph nodes and spleen [50]. However, tumors with high levels of C5a present an accelerated tumor growth with less CD4+ and CD8+ T cells, in the tumor, the spleen and the tumor-draingin lymph nodes. This concentration-dependent impact of C5a requires further exploration in different cancer contexts.

The complement system modulates the T-cell response in a tumor context but a role of complement proteins on the B cell response was also recently described. To be efficient, the chemotherapy has to induce a specific subset of B cells, the ICOS-L+ cells (Inducible T-cell Co-Stimulator Ligand) that express the Complement Receptor 2 (CR2). The interaction of C3 fragments with CR2 promotes the ICOS-L+ B cell generation. On the over hand, the over-expression of CD55 (a complement regulator) inhibits the complement activation and prevents the formation of ICOS-L+ B cell [51]. In this context, the activation of the classical pathway through the binding of the C1 complex and immunoglobulins produced by B cells, though, has not been investigated.

3.3. Impact of Complement on Tumor Cells

The tumor cells have the ability to produce complement proteins that can stimulate tumor growth directly, independently of the cascade activation. Tissue staining and transcriptomic analysis reveal that in many cancers types the presence of complement proteins is associated with a worse outcome for the patient.

3.3.1. Native Proteins

C1q is a multitasking protein that has a strong direct impact on tumor cells, positively and negatively affecting their biology. In human prostate, breast, cancer or neuroblastoma, anti-tumor role of C1q is described, as an apoptosis inducer. C1q activates WWOX, a tumor suppressor gene, then the phosphorylated form of WOX1 accumulates in nuclei and sends anti-proliferative and pro-apoptotic signals [52,53]. This function is also described in ovarian cancer. By using its globular domains, C1q induces apoptosis via TNF-α (Tumor Necrosis Factor) and Fas [54]. In contrast, in melanoma, C1q favors proliferation and migration of tumor cells, increases metastasis, and decreases survival [55]. These data on C1q highlight the possible context-dependent action in different types of cancer.

FH is mostly studied on lung and cSCC. In addition to protecting tumor cells from complement-mediated cytotoxicity, FH promotes cell migration [56]. However, FH deficient mice develop spontaneous hepatic tumors, suggesting an essential role of FH to control unwanted complement activation in the liver to avoid a complement-mediated chronic inflammation [57].

In cSCC, knock-down of C1s, C1r, FB, FH and FI exerts similar effects on the tumor growth. These proteins seem to be implicated in the promotion of the tumor cell proliferation, migration, and survival, via the activation of the signaling pathways PI3K and Erk 1/2 [28,56]. In ccRCC, tumor cells also produce a large spectrum of complement proteins [34], but whether they exert any function within the cells as for the cSCC remains unknown. Several types of tumors express complement proteins that seem to be produced by tumor cells, except for C1q (which usually comes from macrophages) [24].

The most logical suggestion is that complement proteins will be secreted in the tumor microenvironment and will activate the cascade, by hijacking C1q from the macrophages, as we found in ccRCC [23]. Nevertheless, another hypothesis is also possible: these proteins could remain within the cell and form an intracellular complement, or a "complosome" as suggested already for the T cells [58]. Although provocative and controversial [4,59], this hypothesis needs experimental verification, since compelling evidence suggests that at least C3 and C5 can be cleaved within the T cells, modulating their functions. If proven possible, intracellular and extracellular complements could act together to promote/control tumor growth. Moreover, some of the complement proteins are multitasking effectors, with functions outside of the complement cascade [55], which adds to the diversity of the complement proteins actions in cancer.

3.3.2. Activation Fragments

The recognition of the anaphylatoxins by their receptors (C3aR, C5aR1 and C5aR2) present at the surface of some tumor cells leads to the activation of the signaling pathways PI3K, Erk 1/2 and AKT. The activation of these pathways favors the proliferative, survival and invasive properties of tumor cell [60]. The ability of ovarian or lung tumor cells to produce these anaphylatoxins suggests a possible autocrine activation of the cells [61]. In addition to the impact in cell proliferation, an increase of the cell migration is also observed through the C3a-C3aR recognition in melanoma [39] or through the role of C5a in development of metastasis. Indeed, in mouse models, C5 deficiency drastically decreases the hepatic metastasis in colorectal cancer [62] and C5aR facilitates the lung metastasis in breast cancer [46]. This impact on cancer metastasis can be explained by another function of C5a. The C5a-C5aR axis directly impacts the tumor cell cytoskeleton, the cells gain in motility and release some metalloproteinases (MMP) [63]. The MMP are well known to contribute to the cell migration, invasion, and metastasis. Furthermore, MMP can activate the complement system by interaction with the globular domains of C1q [64].

The anaphylatoxins are not the only complement proteins involved in cancer progression. Most frequently in a tumor context, the complement activation is stopped before the formation of the MAC. Nevertheless, even when the lytic pore is assembled, the tumor cell could escape from the lysis by activating the PI3K, AKT, Erk1/2, p70 S6 kinase signaling pathways. This results in an inhibition of the apoptosis, and finally favors the tumor progression [65].

3.4. Role of the Complement on Angiogenesis

Neo-angiogenesis is critical for the tumor growth, by supplying tumor cells with oxygen and nutriments. This parameter is directly linked to the tumor aggressiveness [66]. Recently, a new role of C1q, independently of complement activation, was described. Subcutaneously injected cancer cells form tumors, which in the C1q deficient mice present a disrupted vasculature architecture that could be linked to VEGF-C (vascular endothelial growth factor C) expression [23,55]. This function is, though, also context-dependent, because in a spontaneous model of breast cancer, C1q-/- mice have enhanced neoangiogenesis and hence, bigger tumors [53]. These roles were recently described and still not well understood. The role of the anaphylatoxins C3a and C5a in angiogenesis is better characterized. In a mouse model, a C3 deficiency induces, just like C1q, an alteration of the vasculature architecture, in connection with VEGF expression [67]. Additionally, C5a promotes the migration, proliferation, and vessel formation by endothelial cells [68]. The pro or anti-angiogenic role of complement is controversial. Indeed a mouse model of mammary carcinoma, it was shown that C3 activation can impair the angiogenesis [69] as well as C1q [53].

To conclude, the complement system is involved in the key processes of the tumor progression: immunity, angiogenesis and tumor cell proliferation and spreading. Depending of the cancer types and the complement molecule, various pro- and anti-tumoral functions are described (Figure 3). This multitude of actions is a perfect example of the complexity of the complement system that we need to understand better.

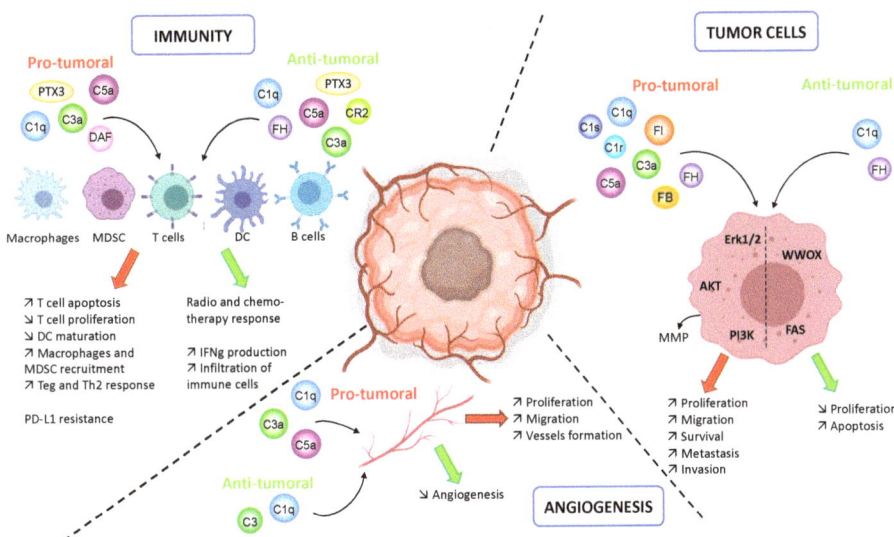

Figure 3. Overview of the complement functions in the context of cancer. In a tumor context, the complement system may impact the immunity, angiogenesis and the phenotype of the tumor cells. **Immunity**: the same complement proteins may impact several immune cells positively or negatively depending of the model or cancer type. The pro-tumoral activity is mostly involved in the recruitment of immune cells and in the suppression of their anti-tumoral response. The anti-tumoral activity is linked to an improvement of the response to therapy and an increase in the immune cells infiltration. **Angiogenesis**: depending on the model, the complement proteins may promote or hamper tumor growth by favoring or inhibiting the neoangiogenesis. **Tumor cells phenotype**: by modulating the signaling pathways Erk1/2, AKT and PI3K the complement proteins stimulate tumor growth. In other models, the modulation of other signaling pathway (WWOX and FAS) by complement proteins favor the apoptosis of tumor cells. The figure is created with BioRender.com.

3.5. Complement Biomarkers in Patients with Cancer

In cancer, complement components can be up-regulated or down-regulated (Table 2). Their overexpression is found at each step of the complement cascade: C1 complex (C1q, C1s), MBL complex (MBL, MASP2), alternative pathway (FH, C3), anaphylatoxins (C3a, C3a desArg, C5a, C3aR, C5aR1) and regulators (CD46, CD55, CD59). The down-regulation of complement proteins and particularly complement regulators is reported inside certain tumors, especially in ovarian cancer. Tumor cells develop several mechanisms to escape from MAC formation while benefiting from the complement activation (production of anaphylatoxins, C1q, etc.). Killing by MAC is prevented in general by overexpression of regulators and down-regulation of the terminal complement components, forming the C5b-9 complex. This appears as a general pattern, observed in transcriptomic profiles of numerous cancer types [3]. Indeed, the lack of terminal complement molecules (such as C7) would prevent the formation of the MAC [70]. MAC blockage can also be triggered by the Heat shock protein 90 (Hsp90). This protein directly interacts with the C9 molecules, are sequestered, preventing the polymerization and formation of the MAC [71].

Table 2. Overview of the different modifications of expression of complement proteins in a tumor context. The upper part of the table summarizes the overexpression of complement proteins described in different cancer types. The overexpression of complement proteins occurs at each step of the complement cascade: classical pathway, lectin pathway, alternative pathway, anaphylatoxins, MAC and regulators. The lower table summarizes the down-regulation of complement proteins described in the literature. The down-regulation of complement proteins involves the classical and alternative pathway, and complement regulators.

Overexpression			
Molecule	Type of Cancer	Mechanism of Action	Ref.
C1q	Glioblastoma	Plasma: increased C1q in the sera of patients in comparison with healthy controls.	[72]
C1s	Lung cancer	Plasma: increased levels of C1s in plasma of lung cancer patient in comparison with controls	[73]
	Prostate cancer	Tumor: Up-regulation of C1s expression in prostate tumors compared to matched normal prostate tissues	[74]
C4	Lung cancer	Plasma: elevated C4 levels in cancer patients in comparison to control group	[75]
C4a	Papillary thyroid cancer	Plasma: increased C4a in the sera of patients in comparison with healthy controls.	[76]
C4d	Lung cancer	Bronchial fluid: Higher levels of C4d in cancer patients than patients with control group.	[77]
	Lung cancer	Plasma: Higher levels of C4d in cancer patients than patients with benign nodules.	[25]
C3	Lung cancer	Plasma: elevated C3 levels in cancer patients in comparison to control group	[75]
	Neuroblastoma	Plasma: elevated C3 levels in cancer patients in comparison to healthy donors	[78]
	Pancreatic ductal adenocarcinoma	Tumor: Higher levels of C3 protein in cancerous tissues than in adjacent normal pancreatic tissues	[79]
	Pancreatic cancer	Tumor: Higher levels of C3 protein in cancerous tissues than in normal pancreatic tissues	[80]
C3a	Esophageal cancer	Plasma: Higher C3a levels in patients than healthy donors	[81]
C3a desArg	Breast cancer	Plasma: Higher C3a desArg level in patients than healthy donors	[82]
C5a	Non-small cell lung cancer	Plasma: Higher C3a levels in patients than healthy donors	[47]
C5aR1	Gastric cancer	Tumor: higher expression of C5aR1 in gastric tumoral tissues than in adjacent non-tumoral tissues	[83]
FH	Squamous lung cancer	Plasma: Up-regulation of FH in uranium exposed miners in comparison with exposed miners without lung disease	[84]
	Lung cancer	Bronchoalveolar lavage: Higher concentration of factor H in lung cancer patients than controls	[85]
	Cutaneous squamous cell carcinoma	Tumor: FH is more expressed in invasive cSCC than normal skin or in situ cSCC.	[56]
	Bladder cancer	Urines: FH and FH related protein are markers for bladder cancer	[86,87]
FI	Cutaneous squamous cell carcinoma	Tumor: FI is more expressed in invasive cSCC than normal skin or in situ cSCC.	[28]
C9	Squamous cell lung cancer	Plasma: C9 and its fucosylated form are significantly higher in SQLC patients, as compared to healthy control	[88]
CD46	Colon cancer	Tumor: CD46 is higher in colon cancer tissues compared with normal adjacent colon tissues	[89]
CD55	Colon cancer	Tumor: CD55 is higher in colon cancer tissues compared with normal adjacent colon tissues	[89]
CD59	Colon cancer	Tumor: CD59 is higher in colon cancer tissues compared with normal adjacent colon tissues	[89]
MASP2	Ovarian tumor	Tumor: MASP2 gene expression is higher with ovarian cancer compared with controls	[90]
MBL	Colon tumor	Plasma: MBL2 levels increases in patients compared to healthy blood donors.	[91]
	Ovarian tumor	Tumor: MBL2 gene expression is higher with ovarian cancer compared with controls	[90]

Table 2. *Cont.*

		Underexpression	
C1s	Ovarian cancer	Tumor: Down-regulation of C1s mRNA in ovarian tumor vs healthy control	[92]
	Ovarian cancer	Tumor: Down-regulation of C1s expression in stage III serous ovarian carcinoma compared to normal tissue	[93]
	Lung cancer	Tumor: decrease expression in lung tumor tissues in comparison with peritumoral tissues	[73]
C4BP	Ovarian cancer	Tumor: Down-regulation of C4BPA mRNA in ovarian tumor vs healthy control	[92]
C7	Ovarian cancer	Tumor: Down-regulation of C7 mRNA in ovarian tumor vs healthy control	[92]
FB	Glioblastoma	Plasma: decreased level of FB in GBM	[72]
FI	Gastric cancer	Plasma: FI is significantly lower in gastric cancer sera compared to normal sera. Declining expression with the advanced pTNM stage from stage I to IV of gastric cancer patients	[94]
FH	Colon cancer	Plasma: Decrease in FH protein level in the serum of colorectal cancer patients vs. normal control	[95]
	Ovarian cancer	Tumor: Down-regulation of FH mRNA in ovarian tumor vs healthy control	[92]
CD55	Ovarian cancer	Tumor: Lower expression of CD55 in ovarian cancer than in control	[30]

The modifications of expression are not only found locally inside the tumor but also in the systemic compartment. This characteristic is important for cancer patients and could be helpful in the future to classify the patient and adapt the treatment with a blood test. Even if this perspective is interesting, it is important to note that an increase or decrease of protein expression in the systemic compartment does not necessarily mean that a similar modification occurs locally inside the tumor. The correlation between the situation inside the tumor and in the plasmatic compartment has to be studied to better understand the actions of complement proteins in a tumor context.

4. Therapeutic Aspects

The bioinformatic analysis, even if it needs biological confirmation, shows us that the tumors are not all equal in the context of complement activation. This has to be considered for the development of new complement-affecting anti-cancer therapy [24].

4.1. Complement Inhibitors

Considering all the data, the complement inhibition and specifically the anaphylatoxins inhibition could be a promising treatment for patients with certain cancers. Currently, the only complement inhibitors approved are acting at the level of C5, such as Eculizumab [96]. It allows complement activation but without the formation of the C5a anaphylatoxin and the membrane attack complex. On the other hand, it appeared that to have an effective response to treatment like chemotherapy and radiotherapy, a low level of complement activation is needed [49,51]. Another complement blocking agent is PMX53 that can block the C5aR1 and allow a reduction of the tumor size, in lung and melanoma mouse models. This molecule also reduces the metastasis in pancreatic model. Nevertheless, these positive effects are not universal and are dependent on the cancer type [24]. As we discussed earlier, the complement activation sets an immunosuppressive microenvironment, so it will be interesting to combine anti-complement therapy with immune checkpoint inhibitors, to reverse this effect [97]. The involvement of C1q in several anti-tumor functions and the potential of the enhancement of the complement-mediated cytotoxicity (strong enough to form the MAC and to kill tumor cells) could be interesting for potential therapeutics. To improve the C1q activation, a new generation of therapeutic antibodies is currently being developed, as IgG hexamers [98].

4.2. Therapeutic Inhibition of C5aR1 on Tumor Cells Versus on Immune Cells

The anaphylatoxins receptors are present at the surface of the immune cells and at the surface of some tumor cells. C5a can interact with two different receptors, C5aR1 and C5aR2, with opposite functions. C5aR1 seems to have pro-tumoral role, whereas C5aR2 has more limited impact but tends to modulate the tumor growth [14].

A common mechanism of action of the C5a-C5aR1 axis is to induce an immunosuppressive microenvironment by recruiting cells that will inactivate the effector T cells. Even if the immune checkpoint inhibitors (anti-PD1/PD-L1) have the ability to reinvigorate the exhausted effector T cells, they cannot reverse the immunosuppressive environment set up, explaining why these drugs are not working equally between patients [99]. The positive effect of combined therapy was first confirmed in mouse lung, melanoma, and colon cancer models [97,100]. Since 2018, a clinical trial in lung and liver cancers using C5aR1 and PD-L1 inhibitors is in progress (Avdoralimab plus Durvalumab: STELLAR-001 clinical study, NCT03665129) [101]. The concept is to block C5aR1, expressed on subsets of MDSC and neutrophils, unleashing thus the anti-tumor activities of the T cells and NK cells. The first results of this clinical trial are encouraging [101]: reduction of the tumor growth, of the metastatic capacity and increase of patient's survival.

Even if C3aR and C5aR seem to be interesting targets for cancer treatment, it is important to recall that depending on the cancer their actions are not the same. Indeed, the study of the literature highlights cancer types with pro-tumor effects of C3aR/C5aR and others, with anti-tumor effects. The lung, colon, ovarian or breast cancer are often described as cancer with aggressive complement, implicated in the tumor development [102]. In parallel in these same cancers, the importance of a small amount of C3aR/C5aR seems to be necessary for a good response to radiotherapy [49]. Overall, for tumor cells C3aR/C5aR is needed for the growth, but these molecules are also needed for a good immune response as well as T-cell activation [103,104]. A treatment involving the C3aR/C5aR blocking must be well thought out, it is necessary to find an equilibrium between the positive impact that can have on tumor cells but without completely shutting down the T-cell response.

4.3. Complement Activation-Enhancing Therapeutic Antibodies

Monoclonal antibody (mAb)-based immunotherapy has shown promising results. Especially the anti-CD20 molecules in the context of hematological tumors. Their benefit is due in part to their ability to activate complement-dependent cytotoxicity through their Fc part [105]. In this review, we were focused on the impact of the complement system in solid tumors, but it is important to note that it plays also a role in hematological malignancies and especially on the response to therapy. The treatment of such tumors is with anti-CD20 [106], anti-CD52 [107] and anti-CD38 [108]. To be efficient these therapies are based on the mechanisms of complement-dependent cytotoxicity and complement-dependent cell-mediated phagocytosis [109]. However, in this type of cancers there often occurs complement deficiencies [110] with overexpression of complement regulators [111]. These data highlight one more time the high ability of the tumor cells to adapt their microenvironment for their development. In vitro, binding of submaximal C1q promotes complement-dependent cytotoxicity (CDC) of B cells opsonized with anti-CD20 mAbs Ofatumumab or Rituximab. Even if Rituximab allows complement activation via C1q binding, the amount of C3b deposition at the cell surface is not enough to generate the MAC, contrary to Ofatumumab, which is more effective to induce CDC [112].

It has been demonstrated that a single amino acid substitution in the IgG-Fc domain favors the formation of IgG hexamers, called HexaBodies [98]. These molecules bind more efficiently C1q [9], induce a strong complement activation and the CDC response even in presence of low level of C9 molecule [113]. Furthermore, very recent research showed that a hetero-hexamerization is possible, two m-Ab (anti-CD20 and anti-CD37) can cooperate to bind C1q and synergize their response to induce a superior CDC [114].

Another strategy is to use bi-specific antibodies. Such antibodies can recognize two different epitopes, for example one tumor-specific and the other one targeting complement membrane regulator.

Bi-specific antibodies were recently developed to induce the complement cytotoxicity, by the recognition of the properdin (the positive regulator of the alternative pathway, able to stabilize the C3 convertase at the cell surface) and the EGFR (Epidermal growth factor receptor) [115]. Even if this antibody induces an increase of C3b deposition, the large presence of complement inhibitors at the tumor cell surface protects the tumor cell against the complement cytotoxicity. Another bi-specific antibody was engineered to target HLA-class I and CD55and showed an increase of C3c deposition on colorectal cancer, compared to the antibody alone or a mix of the two [116]. This technology uses the properties of C1q to work more effectively when the density of epitope is higher. The bispecific Ab technology has led to several inventions as well as the creation of a modular bi-specific platform: one unique arm recruits C1q, associated with multiple other arms able to recognize B cells, T cells or also bacteria. This platform could be applicable for diverse pathologies (infection to cancer) [117].

These new ways to engineer antibodies open doors for very interesting combined therapies.

4.4. Activation Versus Inhibition of Complement in Cancer

The available data have to be taken with caution, as most of it comes from mouse models, which are not always in line with the human pathology. For example, mouse models of melanoma [39], sarcomas [48] and liver [57] cancer show that complement overactivation favors tumor growth, while the transcriptomic analysis of human cancers positions them in the group, where the complement activation is potentially anti-tumoral. Detailed studies in patient cohorts will be critical to resolve this contradiction.

It is very important to always evaluate the harm-benefit ratio. The different cancer types are not equivalent and, even inside the same type of cancer, the patients are not equal and a good treatment for one patient can be inefficient or even deleterious for others. The obvious risk of using complement inhibitors is that the killing of the tumor cells by the cascade, triggered by anti-tumor neoantigens antibodies, will be impaired. This mechanism could be operating in some contexts, such as the case of anti-FH antibodies in NSCLC [118]. Cancers, in which complement inhibition could be undesirable could be the ones with a positive correlation between the IgG and C1q deposits and a prolonged survival. It is likely that in these types of cancer C5b-9 deposits will be present and will be able to kill the tumor cell. This can be achieved either by the natural history of the tumor progression or after the action of certain drugs. Complement activating anti-tumor cells antibodies will be beneficial in such cancers as well. It is difficult to predict which patients could benefit from this approach. If our classification of the cancers based on the concomitant overexpression of complement genes and their correlation with prognosis is considered, the tumors in the complement protective group (Figure 2) should fall into this category. We still need experimental validation of this concept and staining for complement in these types of tumors. Interestingly, it is already known that in sarcoma and melanoma the presence of tertiary lymphoid structures, containing IgG-producing B cells, in the human tumors correlates with a favorable outcome and response to checkpoint inhibitors [119]. Whether complement plays a role in this process remains to be defined.

On the other part of the spectrum are the tumors in which complement overexpression correlates with poor prognosis [24], and in which complement activation was experimentally proven to be associated with poor prognosis, such as ccRCC [32], lung cancer [120] or potentially the gliomas. In these cases, complement inhibition may be beneficial for the patients. In these patients, application of therapeutic antibodies with enhanced complement activating capacity may be dangerous, because the cancer cells are very well adapted to resist to complement-mediated killing and benefit from the chronic inflammation. At least in ccRCC, the IgG deposits on tumor cells trigger the local complement activation without MAC formation.

The results of the STELLAR-001 clinical trial (anti-C5aR1 Avdoralimab + anti-PD-L1 Durvalumab) will be of great interest. Positive or negative results in lung and liver cancers may not necessarily be applicable to other cancers, for which separate studies have to be performed. Interestingly, liver cancer (HCC) belongs to the "Protective complement" group (in optimal cutoff) (Figure 2), where the concomitant overexpression of complement genes is rather associated with a favorable outcome, while in the NSCLC complement activation, measured at protein level, is associated with poor prognosis [120]. Staining for complement is needed in HCC in order to understand its mechanism of action in this type of cancer.

In any case, due to the pleiotropic effects of complement, it is complicated at present to predict whether and to what extend complement modulation will be beneficial or harmful in patients with cancer. This is, therefore, an exciting area of research with a great future potential.

5. Conclusions

Recent discoveries in the complement system are very challenging. The complement proteins act everywhere in the body, extracellularly and intracellularly, they have functions related to the complement activation or independent of it. This new understanding just adds to the already known complexity and plurality of this system. The actions of complement in the tumor context are diverse: action on the immune cells, on the cancer cells and also action on angiogenesis. What this review highlights is the complexity of these functions that can sometimes be opposite depending on the cancer type. It appears that the complement activation mostly has pro-tumor effects, but its complete inhibition may not be always desirable. Indeed, a good response to treatment (chemotherapy or radiotherapy) needs low level of complement activation for the setting of an anti-tumor immunity.

To conclude, it appears clear that the complement system has to be considered for the development of new therapies. However, a large spectrum of complement modulators are entering the market, opening numerous possibilities in cancer therapy [3].

Author Contributions: M.R. and L.T.R. proposed the outline of the review, M.R. wrote the first draft and prepared the figures; L.T.R., M.V.D., C.S.-F., W.H.F. discussed and edited the text. All authors have read and agreed to the published version of the manuscript.

Funding: This work was supported by grants from the Ligue Regionale Contre le Cancer and Fondation ARC Pour La Recherche Sur Le Cancer to LTR. This work was also supported also by grants from CARPEM (ExhauCRF program), INCa (HTE program), Canceropole Ile de France (R17054DD), Association pour la recherche en thérapeutiques innovantes en cancérologie (ARTIC) to CSF. The Labex Immuno-Oncology Excellence Program, INSERM, University of Paris and Sorbonne University also supported this work. MVD received a PhD fellowship from La Fondation ARC pour la recherche sur le cancer.

Conflicts of Interest: The authors declare no conflict of interest.

References

1. Fridman, W.H.; Pagès, F.; Sautès-Fridman, C.; Galon, J. The immune contexture in human tumours: Impact on clinical outcome. *Nat. Rev. Cancer* **2012**, *12*, 298–306. [CrossRef]
2. Fridman, W.H.; Zitvogel, L.; Sautès-Fridman, C.; Kroemer, G. The immune contexture in cancer prognosis and treatment. *Nat. Rev. Clin. Oncol.* **2017**, *14*, 717–734. [CrossRef] [PubMed]
3. Roumenina, L.T.; Daugan, M.V.; Petitprez, F.; Sautès-Fridman, C.; Fridman, W.H. Context-dependent roles of complement in cancer. *Nat. Rev. Cancer* **2019**, *19*, 698–715. [CrossRef] [PubMed]
4. Merle, N.S.; Church, S.E.; Fremeaux-Bacchi, V.; Roumenina, L.T. Complement System Part I—Molecular Mechanisms of Activation and Regulation. *Front. Immunol.* **2015**, *6*, 262. [CrossRef] [PubMed]
5. Merle, N.S.; Noe, R.; Halbwachs-Mecarelli, L.; Fremeaux-Bacchi, V.; Roumenina, L.T. Complement System Part II: Role in Immunity. *Front. Immunol.* **2015**, *6*, 257. [CrossRef]
6. Buchner: Zur Nomenklatur der schutzenden Eiweisskorper—Google Scholar. Available online: https://scholar.google.com/scholar_lookup?journal=Centr+Bakteriol+Parasitenk.&title=Zur+Nomenklatur+der+schutzenden+Eiweisskorper.&author=H+Buchner&volume=10&publication_year=1891&pages=699-701& (accessed on 7 September 2020).
7. Sim, R.B.; Schwaeble, W.; Fujita, T. Complement research in the 18th–21st centuries: Progress comes with new technology. *Immunobiology* **2016**, *221*, 1037–1045. [CrossRef]

8. Gaboriaud, C.; Thielens, N.M.; Gregory, L.A.; Rossi, V.; Fontecilla-Camps, J.C.; Arlaud, G.J. Structure and activation of the C1 complex of complement: Unraveling the puzzle. *Trends Immunol.* **2004**, *25*, 368–373. [CrossRef]
9. Sharp, T.H.; Boyle, A.L.; Diebolder, C.A.; Kros, A.; Koster, A.J.; Gros, P. Insights into IgM-mediated complement activation based on in situ structures of IgM-C1-C4b. *Proc. Natl. Acad. Sci. USA* **2019**, *116*, 11900–11905. [CrossRef]
10. Ugurlar, D.; Howes, S.C.; de Kreuk, B.-J.; Koning, R.I.; de Jong, R.N.; Beurskens, F.J.; Schuurman, J.; Koster, A.J.; Sharp, T.H.; Parren, P.W.H.I.; et al. Structures of C1-IgG1 provide insights into how danger pattern recognition activates complement. *Science* **2018**, *359*, 794–797. [CrossRef]
11. Garred, P.; Genster, N.; Pilely, K.; Bayarri-Olmos, R.; Rosbjerg, A.; Ma, Y.J.; Skjoedt, M.-O. A journey through the lectin pathway of complement-MBL and beyond. *Immunol. Rev.* **2016**, *274*, 74–97. [CrossRef]
12. Ricklin, D.; Reis, E.S.; Mastellos, D.C.; Gros, P.; Lambris, J.D. Complement component C3—The "Swiss Army Knife" of innate immunity and host defense. *Immunol. Rev.* **2016**, *274*, 33–58. [CrossRef] [PubMed]
13. Kemper, C.; Atkinson, J.P.; Hourcade, D.E. Properdin: Emerging roles of a pattern-recognition molecule. *Annu. Rev. Immunol.* **2010**, *28*, 131–155. [CrossRef] [PubMed]
14. Nabizadeh, J.A.; Manthey, H.D.; Panagides, N.; Steyn, F.J.; Lee, J.D.; Li, X.X.; Akhir, F.N.M.; Chen, W.; Boyle, G.M.; Taylor, S.M.; et al. C5a receptors C5aR1 and C5aR2 mediate opposing pathologies in a mouse model of melanoma. *FASEB J.* **2019**, *33*, 11060–11071. [CrossRef] [PubMed]
15. Tegla, C.A.; Cudrici, C.; Patel, S.; Trippe, R.; Rus, V.; Niculescu, F.; Rus, H. Membrane Attack by Complement: The Assembly and Biology of Terminal Complement Complexes. *Immunol. Res.* **2011**, *51*, 45–60. [CrossRef]
16. Noris, M.; Remuzzi, G. Overview of Complement Activation and Regulation. *Semin. Nephrol.* **2013**, *33*, 479–492. [CrossRef]
17. West, E.E.; Kunz, N.; Kemper, C. Complement and human T cell metabolism: Location, location, location. *Immunol. Rev.* **2020**, *295*, 68–81. [CrossRef]
18. Blanc, C.; Togarsimalemath, S.K.; Chauvet, S.; Le Quintrec, M.; Moulin, B.; Buchler, M.; Jokiranta, T.S.; Roumenina, L.T.; Fremeaux-Bacchi, V.; Dragon-Durey, M.-A. Anti-factor H autoantibodies in C3 glomerulopathies and in atypical hemolytic uremic syndrome: One target, two diseases. *J. Immunol.* **2015**, *194*, 5129–5138. [CrossRef]
19. Michailidou, I.; Willems, J.G.P.; Kooi, E.-J.; van Eden, C.; Gold, S.M.; Geurts, J.J.G.; Baas, F.; Huitinga, I.; Ramaglia, V. Complement C1q-C3-associated synaptic changes in multiple sclerosis hippocampus. *Ann. Neurol.* **2015**, *77*, 1007–1026. [CrossRef]
20. McHarg, S.; Clark, S.J.; Day, A.J.; Bishop, P.N. Age-related macular degeneration and the role of the complement system. *Mol. Immunol.* **2015**, *67*, 43–50. [CrossRef]
21. Merle, N.S.; Grunenwald, A.; Rajaratnam, H.; Gnemmi, V.; Frimat, M.; Figueres, M.-L.; Knockaert, S.; Bouzekri, S.; Charue, D.; Noe, R.; et al. Intravascular hemolysis activates complement via cell-free heme and heme-loaded microvesicles. *JCI Insight* **2018**, *3*. [CrossRef]
22. Sekar, A.; Bialas, A.R.; de Rivera, H.; Davis, A.; Hammond, T.R.; Kamitaki, N.; Tooley, K.; Presumey, J.; Baum, M.; Van Doren, V.; et al. Schizophrenia risk from complex variation of complement component 4. *Nature* **2016**, *530*, 177–183. [CrossRef]
23. Roumenina, L.T.; Daugan, M.V.; Noé, R.; Petitprez, F.; Vano, Y.A.; Sanchez-Salas, R.; Becht, E.; Meilleroux, J.; Clec'h, B.L.; Giraldo, N.A.; et al. Tumor Cells Hijack Macrophage-Produced Complement C1q to Promote Tumor Growth. *Cancer Immunol. Res.* **2019**, *7*, 1091–1105. [CrossRef] [PubMed]
24. Ajona, D.; Ortiz-Espinosa, S.; Pio, R. Complement anaphylatoxins C3a and C5a: Emerging roles in cancer progression and treatment. *Semin. Cell Dev. Biol.* **2019**, *85*, 153–163. [CrossRef] [PubMed]
25. Ajona, D.; Okrój, M.; Pajares, M.J.; Agorreta, J.; Lozano, M.D.; Zulueta, J.J.; Verri, C.; Roz, L.; Sozzi, G.; Pastorino, U.; et al. Complement C4d-specific antibodies for the diagnosis of lung cancer. *Oncotarget* **2018**, *9*, 6346–6355. [CrossRef]
26. Riihilä, P.; Nissinen, L.; Farshchian, M.; Kallajoki, M.; Kivisaari, A.; Meri, S.; Grénman, R.; Peltonen, S.; Peltonen, J.; Pihlajaniemi, T.; et al. Complement Component C3 and Complement Factor B Promote Growth of Cutaneous Squamous Cell Carcinoma. *Am. J. Pathol.* **2017**, *187*, 1186–1197. [CrossRef]
27. Ajona, D.; Castaño, Z.; Garayoa, M.; Zudaire, E.; Pajares, M.J.; Martinez, A.; Cuttitta, F.; Montuenga, L.M.; Pio, R. Expression of complement factor H by lung cancer cells: Effects on the activation of the alternative pathway of complement. *Cancer Res.* **2004**, *64*, 6310–6318. [CrossRef]

28. Riihilä, P.; Nissinen, L.; Farshchian, M.; Kivisaari, A.; Ala-Aho, R.; Kallajoki, M.; Grénman, R.; Meri, S.; Peltonen, S.; Peltonen, J.; et al. Complement factor I promotes progression of cutaneous squamous cell carcinoma. *J. Investig. Dermatol.* **2015**, *135*, 579–588. [CrossRef]
29. Ravindranath, N.M.H.; Shuler, C. Expression of complement restriction factors (CD46, CD55 & CD59) in head and neck squamous cell carcinomas. *J. Oral Pathol. Med.* **2006**, *35*, 560–567. [CrossRef]
30. Kapka-Skrzypczak, L.; Wolinska, E.; Szparecki, G.; Wilczynski, G.M.; Czajka, M.; Skrzypczak, M. CD55, CD59, factor H and factor H-like 1 gene expression analysis in tumors of the ovary and corpus uteri origin. *Immunol. Lett.* **2015**, *167*, 67–71. [CrossRef] [PubMed]
31. Pio, R.; Corrales, L.; Lambris, J.D. The role of complement in tumor growth. *Adv. Exp. Med. Biol.* **2014**, *772*, 229–262. [CrossRef] [PubMed]
32. Netti, G.S.; Lucarelli, G.; Spadaccino, F.; Castellano, G.; Gigante, M.; Divella, C.; Rocchetti, M.T.; Rascio, F.; Mancini, V.; Stallone, G.; et al. PTX3 modulates the immunoflogosis in tumor microenvironment and is a prognostic factor for patients with clear cell renal cell carcinoma. *Aging* **2020**, *12*, 7585–7602. [CrossRef] [PubMed]
33. Lucas, S.D.; Karlsson-Parra, A.; Nilsson, B.; Grimelius, L.; Akerström, G.; Rastad, J.; Juhlin, C. Tumor-specific deposition of immunoglobulin G and complement in papillary thyroid carcinoma. *Hum. Pathol.* **1996**, *27*, 1329–1335. [CrossRef]
34. Kwak, J.W.; Laskowski, J.; Li, H.Y.; McSharry, M.V.; Sippel, T.R.; Bullock, B.L.; Johnson, A.M.; Poczobutt, J.M.; Neuwelt, A.J.; Malkoski, S.P.; et al. Complement Activation via a C3a Receptor Pathway Alters CD4+ T Lymphocytes and Mediates Lung Cancer Progression. *Cancer Res.* **2018**, *78*, 143–156. [CrossRef] [PubMed]
35. Zirakzadeh, A.A.; Sherif, A.; Rosenblatt, R.; Ahlén Bergman, E.; Winerdal, M.; Yang, D.; Cederwall, J.; Jakobsson, V.; Hyllienmark, M.; Winqvist, O.; et al. Tumour-associated B cells in urothelial urinary bladder cancer. *Scand. J. Immunol.* **2020**, *91*, e12830. [CrossRef]
36. Wang, Y.; Zhang, H.; He, Y.-W. The Complement Receptors C3aR and C5aR Are a New Class of Immune Checkpoint Receptor in Cancer Immunotherapy. *Front. Immunol.* **2019**, *10*, 1574. [CrossRef]
37. Ajona, D.; Zandueta, C.; Corrales, L.; Moreno, H.; Pajares, M.J.; Ortiz-Espinosa, S.; Martínez-Terroba, E.; Perurena, N.; de Miguel, F.J.; Jantus-Lewintre, E.; et al. Blockade of the Complement C5a/C5aR1 Axis Impairs Lung Cancer Bone Metastasis by CXCL16-mediated Effects. *Am. J. Respir. Crit. Care Med.* **2018**, *197*, 1164–1176. [CrossRef]
38. Markiewski, M.M.; DeAngelis, R.A.; Benencia, F.; Ricklin-Lichtsteiner, S.K.; Koutoulaki, A.; Gerard, C.; Coukos, G.; Lambris, J.D. Modulation of the antitumor immune response by complement. *Nat. Immunol.* **2008**, *9*, 1225–1235. [CrossRef]
39. Nabizadeh, J.A.; Manthey, H.D.; Steyn, F.J.; Chen, W.; Widiapradja, A.; Md Akhir, F.N.; Boyle, G.M.; Taylor, S.M.; Woodruff, T.M.; Rolfe, B.E. The Complement C3a Receptor Contributes to Melanoma Tumorigenesis by Inhibiting Neutrophil and CD4+ T Cell Responses. *J. Immunol.* **2016**, *196*, 4783–4792. [CrossRef]
40. Xu, Y.; Huang, Y.; Xu, W.; Zheng, X.; Yi, X.; Huang, L.; Wang, Y.; Wu, K. Activated Hepatic Stellate Cells (HSCs) Exert Immunosuppressive Effects in Hepatocellular Carcinoma by Producing Complement C3. *OncoTargets Ther.* **2020**, *13*, 1497–1505. [CrossRef]
41. Davidson, S.; Efremova, M.; Riedel, A.; Mahata, B.; Pramanik, J.; Huuhtanen, J.; Kar, G.; Vento-Tormo, R.; Hagai, T.; Chen, X.; et al. Single-Cell RNA Sequencing Reveals a Dynamic Stromal Niche That Supports Tumor Growth. *Cell Rep.* **2020**, *31*, 107628. [CrossRef]
42. Jackson, W.D.; Gulino, A.; Fossati-Jimack, L.; Seoane, R.C.; Tian, K.; Best, K.; Köhl, J.; Belmonte, B.; Strid, J.; Botto, M. C3 Drives Inflammatory Skin Carcinogenesis Independently of C5. *J. Investig. Dermatol.* **2020**. [CrossRef] [PubMed]
43. Ding, P.; Li, L.; Li, L.; Lv, X.; Zhou, D.; Wang, Q.; Chen, J.; Yang, C.; Xu, E.; Dai, W.; et al. C5aR1 is a master regulator in Colorectal Tumorigenesis via Immune modulation. *Theranostics* **2020**, *10*, 8619–8632. [CrossRef] [PubMed]
44. Zha, H.; Wang, X.; Zhu, Y.; Chen, D.; Han, X.; Yang, F.; Gao, J.; Hu, C.; Shu, C.; Feng, Y.; et al. Intracellular Activation of Complement C3 Leads to PD-L1 Antibody Treatment Resistance by Modulating Tumor-Associated Macrophages. *Cancer Immunol. Res.* **2019**, *7*, 193–207. [CrossRef] [PubMed]

45. Janelle, V.; Langlois, M.-P.; Tarrab, E.; Lapierre, P.; Poliquin, L.; Lamarre, A. Transient complement inhibition promotes a tumor-specific immune response through the implication of natural killer cells. *Cancer Immunol. Res.* **2014**, *2*, 200–206. [CrossRef]
46. Vadrevu, S.K.; Chintala, N.K.; Sharma, S.K.; Sharma, P.; Cleveland, C.; Riediger, L.; Manne, S.; Fairlie, D.P.; Gorczyca, W.; Almanza, O.; et al. Complement C5a Receptor Facilitates Cancer Metastasis by Altering T-Cell Responses in the Metastatic Niche. *Cancer Res.* **2014**, *74*, 3454–3465. [CrossRef]
47. Corrales, L.; Ajona, D.; Rafail, S.; Lasarte, J.J.; Riezu-Boj, J.I.; Lambris, J.D.; Rouzaut, A.; Pajares, M.J.; Montuenga, L.M.; Pio, R. Anaphylatoxin C5a creates a favorable microenvironment for lung cancer progression. *J. Immunol.* **2012**, *189*, 4674–4683. [CrossRef]
48. Bonavita, E.; Gentile, S.; Rubino, M.; Maina, V.; Papait, R.; Kunderfranco, P.; Greco, C.; Feruglio, F.; Molgora, M.; Laface, I.; et al. PTX3 is an extrinsic oncosuppressor regulating complement-dependent inflammation in cancer. *Cell* **2015**, *160*, 700–714. [CrossRef]
49. Surace, L.; Lysenko, V.; Fontana, A.O.; Cecconi, V.; Janssen, H.; Bicvic, A.; Okoniewski, M.; Pruschy, M.; Dummer, R.; Neefjes, J.; et al. Complement is a central mediator of radiotherapy-induced tumor-specific immunity and clinical response. *Immunity* **2015**, *42*, 767–777. [CrossRef]
50. Gunn, L.; Ding, C.; Liu, M.; Ma, Y.; Qi, C.; Cai, Y.; Hu, X.; Aggarwal, D.; Zhang, H.-G.; Yan, J. Opposing roles for complement component C5a in tumor progression and the tumor microenvironment. *J. Immunol.* **2012**, *189*, 2985–2994. [CrossRef]
51. Lu, Y.; Zhao, Q.; Liao, J.-Y.; Song, E.; Xia, Q.; Pan, J.; Li, Y.; Li, J.; Zhou, B.; Ye, Y.; et al. Complement Signals Determine Opposite Effects of B Cells in Chemotherapy-Induced Immunity. *Cell* **2020**, *180*, 1081–1097. [CrossRef]
52. Hong, Q.; Sze, C.-I.; Lin, S.-R.; Lee, M.-H.; He, R.-Y.; Schultz, L.; Chang, J.-Y.; Chen, S.-J.; Boackle, R.J.; Hsu, L.-J.; et al. Complement C1q activates tumor suppressor WWOX to induce apoptosis in prostate cancer cells. *PLoS ONE* **2009**, *4*, e5755. [CrossRef] [PubMed]
53. Bandini, S.; Macagno, M.; Hysi, A.; Lanzardo, S.; Conti, L.; Bello, A.; Riccardo, F.; Ruiu, R.; Merighi, I.F.; Forni, G.; et al. The non-inflammatory role of C1q during Her2/neu-driven mammary carcinogenesis. *Oncoimmunology* **2016**, *5*. [CrossRef]
54. Kaur, A.; Sultan, S.H.A.; Murugaiah, V.; Pathan, A.A.; Alhamlan, F.S.; Karteris, E.; Kishore, U. Human C1q Induces Apoptosis in an Ovarian Cancer Cell Line via Tumor Necrosis Factor Pathway. *Front. Immunol.* **2016**, *7*, 599. [CrossRef]
55. Bulla, R.; Tripodo, C.; Rami, D.; Ling, G.S.; Agostinis, C.; Guarnotta, C.; Zorzet, S.; Durigutto, P.; Botto, M.; Tedesco, F. C1q acts in the tumour microenvironment as a cancer-promoting factor independently of complement activation. *Nat. Commun.* **2016**, *7*, 10346. [CrossRef] [PubMed]
56. Riihilä, P.M.; Nissinen, L.M.; Ala-Aho, R.; Kallajoki, M.; Grénman, R.; Meri, S.; Peltonen, S.; Peltonen, J.; Kähäri, V.-M. Complement factor H: A biomarker for progression of cutaneous squamous cell carcinoma. *J. Investig. Dermatol.* **2014**, *134*, 498–506. [CrossRef] [PubMed]
57. Laskowski, J.; Renner, B.; Pickering, M.C.; Serkova, N.J.; Smith-Jones, P.M.; Clambey, E.T.; Nemenoff, R.A.; Thurman, J.M. Complement factor H-deficient mice develop spontaneous hepatic tumors. *J. Clin. Investig.* **2020**. [CrossRef]
58. Arbore, G.; Kemper, C.; Kolev, M. Intracellular complement—The complosome—In immune cell regulation. *Mol. Immunol.* **2017**, *89*, 2–9. [CrossRef]
59. Ghebrehiwet, B. Complement proteins in unexpected places: Why we should be excited, not concerned! *F1000Research* **2020**, *9*. [CrossRef]
60. Lu, Y.; Hu, X.-B. C5a stimulates the proliferation of breast cancer cells via Akt-dependent RGC-32 gene activation. *Oncol. Rep.* **2014**, *32*, 2817–2823. [CrossRef]
61. Cho, M.S.; Vasquez, H.G.; Rupaimoole, R.; Pradeep, S.; Wu, S.; Zand, B.; Han, H.-D.; Rodriguez-Aguayo, C.; Bottsford-Miller, J.; Huang, J.; et al. Autocrine effects of tumor-derived complement. *Cell Rep.* **2014**, *6*, 1085–1095. [CrossRef]
62. Piao, C.; Cai, L.; Qiu, S.; Jia, L.; Song, W.; Du, J. Complement 5a Enhances Hepatic Metastases of Colon Cancer via Monocyte Chemoattractant Protein-1-mediated Inflammatory Cell Infiltration. *J. Biol. Chem.* **2015**, *290*, 10667–10676. [CrossRef]

63. Nitta, H.; Wada, Y.; Kawano, Y.; Murakami, Y.; Irie, A.; Taniguchi, K.; Kikuchi, K.; Yamada, G.; Suzuki, K.; Honda, J.; et al. Enhancement of human cancer cell motility and invasiveness by anaphylatoxin C5a via aberrantly expressed C5a receptor (CD88). *Clin. Cancer Res.* **2013**, *19*, 2004–2013. [CrossRef] [PubMed]
64. Rozanov, D.V.; Sikora, S.; Godzik, A.; Postnova, T.I.; Golubkov, V.; Savinov, A.; Tomlinson, S.; Strongin, A.Y. Non-proteolytic, receptor/ligand interactions associate cellular membrane type-1 matrix metalloproteinase with the complement component C1q. *J. Biol. Chem.* **2004**, *279*, 50321–50328. [CrossRef]
65. Vlaicu, S.I.; Tegla, C.A.; Cudrici, C.D.; Danoff, J.; Madani, H.; Sugarman, A.; Niculescu, F.; Mircea, P.A.; Rus, V.; Rus, H. Role of C5b-9 complement complex and response gene to complement-32 (RGC-32) in cancer. *Immunol. Res.* **2013**, *56*, 109–121. [CrossRef] [PubMed]
66. Carmeliet, P. Angiogenesis in health and disease. *Nat. Med.* **2003**, *9*, 653–660. [CrossRef] [PubMed]
67. Nunez-Cruz, S.; Gimotty, P.A.; Guerra, M.W.; Connolly, D.C.; Wu, Y.-Q.; DeAngelis, R.A.; Lambris, J.D.; Coukos, G.; Scholler, N. Genetic and pharmacologic inhibition of complement impairs endothelial cell function and ablates ovarian cancer neovascularization. *Neoplasia* **2012**, *14*, 994–1004. [CrossRef] [PubMed]
68. Kurihara, R.; Yamaoka, K.; Sawamukai, N.; Shimajiri, S.; Oshita, K.; Yukawa, S.; Tokunaga, M.; Iwata, S.; Saito, K.; Chiba, K.; et al. C5a promotes migration, proliferation, and vessel formation in endothelial cells. *Inflamm. Res.* **2010**, *59*, 659–666. [CrossRef]
69. Bandini, S.; Curcio, C.; Macagno, M.; Quaglino, E.; Arigoni, M.; Lanzardo, S.; Hysi, A.; Barutello, G.; Consolino, L.; Longo, D.L.; et al. Early onset and enhanced growth of autochthonous mammary carcinomas in C3-deficient Her2/neu transgenic mice. *Oncoimmunology* **2013**, *2*. [CrossRef]
70. Ying, L.; Zhang, F.; Pan, X.; Chen, K.; Zhang, N.; Jin, J.; Wu, J.; Feng, J.; Yu, H.; Jin, H.; et al. Complement component 7 (C7), a potential tumor suppressor, is correlated with tumor progression and prognosis. *Oncotarget* **2016**, *7*, 86536–86546. [CrossRef]
71. Rozenberg, P.; Ziporen, L.; Gancz, D.; Saar-Ray, M.; Fishelson, Z. Cooperation between Hsp90 and mortalin/GRP75 in resistance to cell death induced by complement C5b-9. *Cell Death Dis.* **2018**, *9*, 150. [CrossRef]
72. Bouwens, T.A.M.; Trouw, L.A.; Veerhuis, R.; Dirven, C.M.F.; Lamfers, M.L.M.; Al-Khawaja, H. Complement activation in Glioblastoma multiforme pathophysiology: Evidence from serum levels and presence of complement activation products in tumor tissue. *J. Neuroimmunol.* **2015**, *278*, 271–276. [CrossRef]
73. Zhao, P.; Wu, J.; Lu, F.; Peng, X.; Liu, C.; Zhou, N.; Ying, M. The imbalance in the complement system and its possible physiological mechanisms in patients with lung cancer. *BMC Cancer* **2019**, *19*, 201. [CrossRef] [PubMed]
74. Grzmil, M.; Voigt, S.; Thelen, P.; Hemmerlein, B.; Helmke, K.; Burfeind, P. Up-regulated expression of the MAT-8 gene in prostate cancer and its siRNA-mediated inhibition of expression induces a decrease in proliferation of human prostate carcinoma cells. *Int. J. Oncol.* **2004**, *24*, 97–105. [CrossRef] [PubMed]
75. Oner, F.; Savaş, I.; Numanoğlu, N. Immunoglobulins and complement components in patients with lung cancer. *Tuberk Toraks* **2004**, *52*, 19–23.
76. Lu, Z.-L.; Chen, Y.-J.; Jing, X.-Y.; Wang, N.-N.; Zhang, T.; Hu, C.-J. Detection and Identification of Serum Peptides Biomarker in Papillary Thyroid Cancer. *Med. Sci. Monit. Int. Med. J. Exp. Clin. Res.* **2018**, *24*, 1581–1587. [CrossRef]
77. Ajona, D.; Razquin, C.; Pastor, M.D.; Pajares, M.J.; Garcia, J.; Cardenal, F.; Fleischhacker, M.; Lozano, M.D.; Zulueta, J.J.; Schmidt, B.; et al. Elevated levels of the complement activation product C4d in bronchial fluids for the diagnosis of lung cancer. *PLoS ONE* **2015**, *10*, e0119878. [CrossRef] [PubMed]
78. Kim, P.Y.; Tan, O.; Diakiw, S.M.; Carter, D.; Sekerye, E.O.; Wasinger, V.C.; Liu, T.; Kavallaris, M.; Norris, M.D.; Haber, M.; et al. Identification of plasma complement C3 as a potential biomarker for neuroblastoma using a quantitative proteomic approach. *J. Proteom.* **2014**, *96*, 1–12. [CrossRef]
79. Chen, J.; Wu, W.; Chen, L.; Ma, X.; Zhao, Y.; Zhou, H.; Yang, R.; Hu, L. Expression and clinical significance of AHSG and complement C3 in pancreatic ductal adenocarcinoma. *Zhonghua Yi Xue Za Zhi* **2014**, *94*, 2175–2179.
80. Chen, J.; Wu, W.; Zhen, C.; Zhou, H.; Yang, R.; Chen, L.; Hu, L. Expression and clinical significance of complement C3, complement C4b1 and apolipoprotein E in pancreatic cancer. *Oncol. Lett.* **2013**, *6*, 43–48. [CrossRef]
81. Zhang, X.; Sun, L. Anaphylatoxin C3a: A potential biomarker for esophageal cancer diagnosis. *Mol. Clin. Oncol.* **2018**, *8*, 315–319. [CrossRef]

82. Chung, L.; Moore, K.; Phillips, L.; Boyle, F.M.; Marsh, D.J.; Baxter, R.C. Novel serum protein biomarker panel revealed by mass spectrometry and its prognostic value in breast cancer. *Breast Cancer Res. BCR* **2014**, *16*, R63. [CrossRef] [PubMed]
83. Chen, J.; Li, G.-Q.; Zhang, L.; Tang, M.; Cao, X.; Xu, G.-L.; Wu, Y.-Z. Complement C5a/C5aR pathway potentiates the pathogenesis of gastric cancer by down-regulating p21 expression. *Cancer Lett.* **2018**, *412*, 30–36. [CrossRef] [PubMed]
84. Helmig, S.; Lochnit, G.; Schneider, J. Comparative proteomic analysis in serum of former uranium miners with and without radon induced squamous lung cancer. *J. Occup. Med. Toxicol. Lond. Engl.* **2019**, *14*, 9. [CrossRef] [PubMed]
85. Pio, R.; Garcia, J.; Corrales, L.; Ajona, D.; Fleischhacker, M.; Pajares, M.J.; Cardenal, F.; Seijo, L.; Zulueta, J.J.; Nadal, E.; et al. Complement factor H is elevated in bronchoalveolar lavage fluid and sputum from patients with lung cancer. *Cancer Epidemiol. Biomark. Prev. Publ. Am. Assoc. Cancer Res. Cosponsored Am. Soc. Prev. Oncol.* **2010**, *19*, 2665–2672. [CrossRef]
86. Cheng, Z.-Z.; Corey, M.J.; Pärepalo, M.; Majno, S.; Hellwage, J.; Zipfel, P.F.; Kinders, R.J.; Raitanen, M.; Meri, S.; Jokiranta, T.S. Complement factor H as a marker for detection of bladder cancer. *Clin. Chem.* **2005**, *51*, 856–863. [CrossRef]
87. Heicappell, R.; Müller, M.; Fimmers, R.; Miller, K. Qualitative determination of urinary human complement factor H-related protein (hcfHrp) in patients with bladder cancer, healthy controls, and patients with benign urologic disease. *Urol. Int.* **2000**, *65*, 181–184. [CrossRef]
88. Narayanasamy, A.; Ahn, J.-M.; Sung, H.-J.; Kong, D.-H.; Ha, K.-S.; Lee, S.-Y.; Cho, J.-Y. Fucosylated glycoproteomic approach to identify a complement component 9 associated with squamous cell lung cancer (SQLC). *J. Proteom.* **2011**, *74*, 2948–2958. [CrossRef]
89. Shang, Y.; Chai, N.; Gu, Y.; Ding, L.; Yang, Y.; Zhou, J.; Ren, G.; Hao, X.; Fan, D.; Wu, K.; et al. Systematic immunohistochemical analysis of the expression of CD46, CD55, and CD59 in colon cancer. *Arch. Pathol. Lab. Med.* **2014**, *138*, 910–919. [CrossRef]
90. Swierzko, A.S.; Szala, A.; Sawicki, S.; Szemraj, J.; Sniadecki, M.; Sokolowska, A.; Kaluzynski, A.; Wydra, D.; Cedzynski, M. Mannose-Binding Lectin (MBL) and MBL-associated serine protease-2 (MASP-2) in women with malignant and benign ovarian tumours. *Cancer Immunol. Immunother. CII* **2014**, *63*, 1129–1140. [CrossRef]
91. Ytting, H.; Jensenius, J.C.; Christensen, I.J.; Thiel, S.; Nielsen, H.J. Increased activity of the mannan-binding lectin complement activation pathway in patients with colorectal cancer. *Scand. J. Gastroenterol.* **2004**, *39*, 674–679. [CrossRef]
92. Li, W.; Liu, Z.; Liang, B.; Chen, S.; Zhang, X.; Tong, X.; Lou, W.; Le, L.; Tang, X.; Fu, F. Identification of core genes in ovarian cancer by an integrative meta-analysis. *J. Ovarian Res.* **2018**, *11*, 94. [CrossRef]
93. Kim, Y.-S.; Hwan, J.D.; Bae, S.; Bae, D.-H.; Shick, W.A. Identification of differentially expressed genes using an annealing control primer system in stage III serous ovarian carcinoma. *BMC Cancer* **2010**, *10*, 576. [CrossRef] [PubMed]
94. Liu, W.; Liu, B.; Xin, L.; Zhang, Y.; Chen, X.; Zhu, Z.; Lin, Y. Down-regulated expression of complement factor I: A potential suppressive protein for gastric cancer identified by serum proteome analysis. *Clin. Chim. Acta Int. J. Clin. Chem.* **2007**, *377*, 119–126. [CrossRef]
95. Lim, L.C.; Looi, M.L.; Zakaria, S.Z.S.; Sagap, I.; Rose, I.M.; Chin, S.-F.; Jamal, R. Identification of Differentially Expressed Proteins in the Serum of Colorectal Cancer Patients Using 2D-DIGE Proteomics Analysis. *Pathol. Oncol. Res. POR* **2016**, *22*, 169–177. [CrossRef] [PubMed]
96. Ricklin, D.; Mastellos, D.C.; Reis, E.S.; Lambris, J.D. The renaissance of complement therapeutics. *Nat. Rev. Nephrol.* **2018**, *14*, 26–47. [CrossRef] [PubMed]
97. Ajona, D.; Ortiz-Espinosa, S.; Moreno, H.; Lozano, T.; Pajares, M.J.; Agorreta, J.; Bértolo, C.; Lasarte, J.J.; Vicent, S.; Hoehlig, K.; et al. A Combined PD-1/C5a Blockade Synergistically Protects against Lung Cancer Growth and Metastasis. *Cancer Discov.* **2017**, *7*, 694–703. [CrossRef] [PubMed]
98. Diebolder, C.A.; Beurskens, F.J.; de Jong, R.N.; Koning, R.I.; Strumane, K.; Lindorfer, M.A.; Voorhorst, M.; Ugurlar, D.; Rosati, S.; Heck, A.J.R.; et al. Complement is activated by IgG hexamers assembled at the cell surface. *Science* **2014**, *343*, 1260–1263. [CrossRef] [PubMed]

99. Brahmer, J.; Reckamp, K.L.; Baas, P.; Crinò, L.; Eberhardt, W.E.E.; Poddubskaya, E.; Antonia, S.; Pluzanski, A.; Vokes, E.E.; Holgado, E.; et al. Nivolumab versus Docetaxel in Advanced Squamous-Cell Non-Small-Cell Lung Cancer. *N. Engl. J. Med.* **2015**, *373*, 123–135. [CrossRef] [PubMed]
100. Zha, H.; Han, X.; Zhu, Y.; Yang, F.; Li, Y.; Li, Q.; Guo, B.; Zhu, B. Blocking C5aR signaling promotes the anti-tumor efficacy of PD-1/PD-L1 blockade. *Oncoimmunology* **2017**, *6*, e1349587. [CrossRef]
101. Massard, C.; Cassier, P.; Bendell, J.C.; Marie, D.B.; Blery, M.; Morehouse, C.; Ascierto, M.; Zerbib, R.; Mitry, E.; Tolcher, A.W. Preliminary results of STELLAR-001, a dose escalation phase I study of the anti-C5aR, IPH5401, in combination with durvalumab in advanced solid tumours. *Ann. Oncol.* **2019**, *30*, v492. [CrossRef]
102. Afshar-Kharghan, V. The role of the complement system in cancer. *J. Clin. Investig.* **2017**, *127*, 780–789. [CrossRef] [PubMed]
103. Zhang, R.; Liu, Q.; Li, T.; Liao, Q.; Zhao, Y. Role of the complement system in the tumor microenvironment. *Cancer Cell Int.* **2019**, *19*, 300. [CrossRef] [PubMed]
104. Arbore, G.; West, E.E.; Rahman, J.; Le Friec, G.; Niyonzima, N.; Pirooznia, M.; Tunc, I.; Pavlidis, P.; Powell, N.; Li, Y.; et al. Complement receptor CD46 co-stimulates optimal human CD8+ T cell effector function via fatty acid metabolism. *Nat. Commun.* **2018**, *9*, 4186. [CrossRef]
105. Taylor, R.P.; Lindorfer, M.A. Cytotoxic mechanisms of immunotherapy: Harnessing complement in the action of anti-tumor monoclonal antibodies. *Semin. Immunol.* **2016**, *28*, 309–316. [CrossRef] [PubMed]
106. Coiffier, B.; Haioun, C.; Ketterer, N.; Engert, A.; Tilly, H.; Ma, D.; Johnson, P.; Lister, A.; Feuring-Buske, M.; Radford, J.A.; et al. Rituximab (anti-CD20 monoclonal antibody) for the treatment of patients with relapsing or refractory aggressive lymphoma: A multicenter phase II study. *Blood* **1998**, *92*, 1927–1932.
107. Zent, C.S.; Secreto, C.R.; LaPlant, B.R.; Bone, N.D.; Call, T.G.; Shanafelt, T.D.; Jelinek, D.F.; Tschumper, R.C.; Kay, N.E. Direct and complement dependent cytotoxicity in CLL cells from patients with high-risk early-intermediate stage chronic lymphocytic leukemia (CLL) treated with alemtuzumab and rituximab. *Leuk. Res.* **2008**, *32*, 1849–1856. [CrossRef] [PubMed]
108. Van de Donk, N.W.C.J.; Janmaat, M.L.; Mutis, T.; Lammerts van Bueren, J.J.; Ahmadi, T.; Sasser, A.K.; Lokhorst, H.M.; Parren, P.W.H.I. Monoclonal antibodies targeting CD38 in hematological malignancies and beyond. *Immunol. Rev.* **2016**, *270*, 95–112. [CrossRef]
109. Lee, C.-H.; Romain, G.; Yan, W.; Watanabe, M.; Charab, W.; Todorova, B.; Lee, J.; Triplett, K.; Donkor, M.; Lungu, O.I.; et al. IgG Fc domains that bind C1q but not effector Fcγ receptors delineate the importance of complement-mediated effector functions. *Nat. Immunol.* **2017**, *18*, 889–898. [CrossRef]
110. Middleton, O.; Cosimo, E.; Dobbin, E.; McCaig, A.M.; Clarke, C.; Brant, A.M.; Leach, M.T.; Michie, A.M.; Wheadon, H. Complement deficiencies limit CD20 monoclonal antibody treatment efficacy in CLL. *Leukemia* **2015**, *29*, 107–114. [CrossRef]
111. Dzietcenia, J.; Wróbel, T.; Mazur, G.; Poreba, R.; Jaźwiec, B.; Kuliczkowski, K. Expression of complement regulatory proteins: CD46, CD55, and CD59 and response to rituximab in patients with CD20+ non-Hodgkin's lymphoma. *Med. Oncol. Northwood Lond. Engl.* **2010**, *27*, 743–746. [CrossRef]
112. Pawluczkowycz, A.W.; Beurskens, F.J.; Beum, P.V.; Lindorfer, M.A.; van de Winkel, J.G.J.; Parren, P.W.H.I.; Taylor, R.P. Binding of submaximal C1q promotes complement-dependent cytotoxicity (CDC) of B cells opsonized with anti-CD20 mAbs ofatumumab (OFA) or rituximab (RTX): Considerably higher levels of CDC are induced by OFA than by RTX. *J. Immunol.* **2009**, *183*, 749–758. [CrossRef] [PubMed]
113. Cook, E.M.; Lindorfer, M.A.; van der Horst, H.; Oostindie, S.; Beurskens, F.J.; Schuurman, J.; Zent, C.S.; Burack, R.; Parren, P.W.H.I.; Taylor, R.P. Antibodies That Efficiently Form Hexamers upon Antigen Binding Can Induce Complement-Dependent Cytotoxicity under Complement-Limiting Conditions. *J. Immunol.* **2016**, *197*, 1762–1775. [CrossRef]
114. Oostindie, S.C.; van der Horst, H.J.; Lindorfer, M.A.; Cook, E.M.; Tupitza, J.C.; Zent, C.S.; Burack, R.; VanDerMeid, K.R.; Strumane, K.; Chamuleau, M.E.D.; et al. CD20 and CD37 antibodies synergize to activate complement by Fc-mediated clustering. *Haematologica* **2019**, *104*, 1841–1852. [CrossRef] [PubMed]
115. Pedersen, D.V.; Rösner, T.; Hansen, A.G.; Andersen, K.R.; Thiel, S.; Andersen, G.R.; Valerius, T.; Laursen, N.S. Recruitment of properdin by bi-specific nanobodies activates the alternative pathway of complement. *Mol. Immunol.* **2020**, *124*, 200–210. [CrossRef] [PubMed]
116. Gelderman, K.A.; Lam, S.; Sier, C.F.; Gorter, A. Cross-linking tumor cells with effector cells via CD55 with a bispecific mAb induces beta-glucan-dependent CR3-dependent cellular cytotoxicity. *Eur. J. Immunol.* **2006**, *36*, 977–984. [CrossRef] [PubMed]

117. Cruz, J.W.; Damko, E.; Modi, B.; Tu, N.; Meagher, K.; Voronina, V.; Gartner, H.; Ehrlich, G.; Rafique, A.; Babb, R.; et al. A novel bispecific antibody platform to direct complement activity for efficient lysis of target cells. *Sci. Rep.* **2019**, *9*. [CrossRef]
118. Ajona, D.; Hsu, Y.-F.; Corrales, L.; Montuenga, L.M.; Pio, R. Down-regulation of human complement factor H sensitizes non-small cell lung cancer cells to complement attack and reduces in vivo tumor growth. *J. Immunol.* **2007**, *178*, 5991–5998. [CrossRef]
119. Petitprez, F.; de Reyniès, A.; Keung, E.Z.; Chen, T.W.-W.; Sun, C.-M.; Calderaro, J.; Jeng, Y.-M.; Hsiao, L.-P.; Lacroix, L.; Bougoüin, A.; et al. B cells are associated with survival and immunotherapy response in sarcoma. *Nature* **2020**, *577*, 556–560. [CrossRef]
120. Ajona, D.; Pajares, M.J.; Corrales, L.; Perez-Gracia, J.L.; Agorreta, J.; Lozano, M.D.; Torre, W.; Massion, P.P.; de-Torres, J.P.; Jantus-Lewintre, E.; et al. Investigation of complement activation product c4d as a diagnostic and prognostic biomarker for lung cancer. *J. Natl. Cancer Inst.* **2013**, *105*, 1385–1393. [CrossRef]

Publisher's Note: MDPI stays neutral with regard to jurisdictional claims in published maps and institutional affiliations.

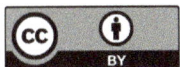

© 2020 by the authors. Licensee MDPI, Basel, Switzerland. This article is an open access article distributed under the terms and conditions of the Creative Commons Attribution (CC BY) license (http://creativecommons.org/licenses/by/4.0/).

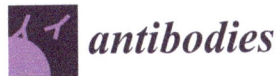

Review

Complement Activation in the Treatment of B-Cell Malignancies

Clive S. Zent [1,*], Jonathan J. Pinney [2,3], Charles C. Chu [1] and Michael R. Elliott [2,3]

1. Wilmot Cancer Institute and Department of Medicine, University of Rochester Medical Center, Rochester, NY 14642, USA; charles_chu@urmc.rochester.edu
2. Department of Microbiology, Immunology, and Cancer Biology, University of Virginia, Charlottesville, VA 22908, USA; jjp2xr@virginia.edu (J.J.P.); mre4n@virginia.edu (M.R.E.)
3. Center for Cell Clearance, University of Virginia, Charlottesville, VA 22908, USA
* Correspondence: clive_zent@urmc.rochester.edu; Tel.: +1-585-276-6891

Received: 15 September 2020; Accepted: 22 November 2020; Published: 1 December 2020

Abstract: Unconjugated monoclonal antibodies (mAb) have revolutionized the treatment of B-cell malignancies. These targeted drugs can activate innate immune cytotoxicity for therapeutic benefit. mAb activation of the complement cascade results in complement-dependent cytotoxicity (CDC) and complement receptor-mediated antibody-dependent cellular phagocytosis (cADCP). Clinical and laboratory studies have showed that CDC is therapeutically important. In contrast, the biological role and clinical effects of cADCP are less well understood. This review summarizes the available data on the role of complement activation in the treatment of mature B-cell malignancies and proposes future research directions that could be useful in optimizing the efficacy of this important class of drugs.

Keywords: complement; cytotoxicity; phagocytosis; monoclonal antibody; B-cell lymphoma; chronic lymphocytic leukemia (CLL)

1. Introduction

Unconjugated monoclonal antibodies (mAb) have an important clinical role in the management of mature B-cell malignancies [1–5]. The major mechanism of action of the mAbs targeting CD20, CD38, and CD52 surface antigens on B cells is activation of innate immune cytotoxicity. mAb-opsonized B cells can undergo Fc-induced cellular cytotoxicity by fixed macrophages via antibody-dependent cellular phagocytosis (ADCP) or by NK cells through antibody-dependent cellular cytotoxicity (ADCC), two of the major mechanisms of innate immune cytotoxicity [6–17]. A third major mechanism of innate immune cytotoxicity is mediated via activation of complement, thereby promoting complement-dependent cytotoxicity (CDC). In this proteolytic cascade [18,19], the lymphocytes are killed after downstream generation and binding of membrane attack complexes (MAC) which permeabilize the cell membrane. The details of these reactions can be found within this special issue, Figure 1 in the review by Golay and Taylor, and Figure 16 in the review by Taylor and Lindorfer. The B cells can also be killed via activation of ADCP by effector cells through complement receptors (CR) binding to C3-derived fragments covalently attached to the surface of target cells (cADCP) (Figure 1) [19–24].

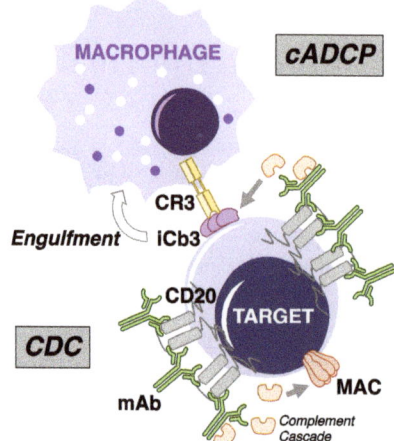

Figure 1. Overview of cytotoxic mechanisms underlying mAb-mediated complement fixation. Depiction of type I anti-CD20 mAb binding to surface of target cells. Complement-dependent cytotoxicity (CDC) occurs following formation and binding of multiple copies of the membrane attack complex (MAC) on the target cell surface downstream of mAb-induced initiation of the complement cascade. Target cell killing by complement receptor-mediated antibody-dependent cellular phagocytosis (cADCP) results from mAb-mediated deposition and covalent binding of C3 activation fragments to the cell surface, which are in turn recognized by complement receptors (CR3 is shown) which trigger activation of phagocytic pathways in phagocytes such as macrophages.

We will review the clinical data on the role of complement activation by mAb in the treatment of mature B-cell lymphoid malignancies and our current understanding of the role of activation of complement in killing malignant B lymphocytes.

2. Complement-Activating Therapeutic mAb

The development of rituximab, the prototype unconjugated chimeric (mouse Fab$_2$/human IgG1 Fc) anti-CD20 mAb, was the culmination of a multi-decade effort to utilize mAbs to treat malignancies of the immune system and autoimmune disease [25–27]. Use of rituximab for the treatment of mature B-cell lymphoid malignancies (FDA approval 1997) caused a paradigm shift in treatment of B-cell lymphomas [26]. Rituximab monotherapy was tolerable and achieved durable responses in the treatment of indolent B-cell lymphomas but was not curative. Combination of rituximab with standard chemotherapy regimens as chemoimmunotherapy (CIT) significantly improved treatment outcomes, including survival, in aggressive diffuse large B-cell lymphoma which is a potentially curable disease [1,2]. This success was followed by a plethora of concomitant and sequential mAb-containing treatment regimens, some of which have significantly improved treatment outcome and patient survival [3–5].

Next-generation anti-CD20 mAbs were developed to overcome the perceived limitations of rituximab. The fully human IgG1 wild-type Fc mAb ofatumumab (FDA approved 2009) was selected for improved CD20 binding properties (decreased off rate) and proximity of binding to the cell membrane, both of which increased complement activation [28,29]. In contrast, the development strategy for the humanized anti-CD20 mAb obinutuzumab (FDA approved 2013) was to optimize NK cell-mediated ADCC [30]. This was achieved through glycoengineering to defucosylate the human IgG1 Fc carbohydrate moiety, which substantially increased Fc receptor (FcR) affinity [30]. Obinutuzamab is not an efficient complement-activating mAb [30]. There is minimal published direct comparative data on the clinical efficacy of rituximab, ofatumumab and obinutuzumab as monotherapies, in CIT, or in combination with other targeted therapies.

Alemtuzumab (FDA approval 2001), a humanized rat anti-CD52 mAb utilizing wild-type human IgG1 Fc [31], is highly effective at killing circulating B and T lymphocytes by activation of both complement- [32] and cell-mediated cytotoxicity [13]. Alemtuzumab is an effective monotherapy for relapsed/refractory chronic lymphocytic leukemia/small lymphocytic lymphoma (CLL) patients [33,34]. Unfortunately clinical utility was limited by short durations of response and increased risk of opportunistic infections secondary to T cell depletion [35,36]. Alemtuzumab therapy of CLL has been largely superseded by targeted small molecule inhibitors but it remains an important treatment option for other rare B-cell malignancies such as B-cell prolymphocytic leukemia [37].

Daratumomab (multiple myeloma FDA approval 2015) is a fully human IgG1 mAb targeting CD38 that could have a role in treatment of other CD38-positive B-cell malignancies [38]. Daratumumab was selected because of its ability to activate complement [39]. In contrast, isatuximab, the second anti-CD38 mAb FDA approved for treatment of plasma cell diseases, does not appear to induce significant CDC in primary multiple myeloma cells [40].

mAbs are now an integral component of targeted therapy of B-cell malignancies based largely on very promising data from clinical trials. However, a better understanding of the mechanisms of action of these valuable drugs and the B-cell characteristics that determine sensitivity and resistance to mAb-mediated cytotoxicity is needed to continue to improve their efficacy. This knowledge should then allow for rational development of combination therapy with other drugs. These data will be critical for designing and testing regimens that can exploit orthogonal cytotoxic mechanisms so as to eliminate resistant subclones of malignant B cells and improve patient outcomes.

3. Mechanism of Action of mAb

Although mAb-containing treatment regimens are now standard of care for many diseases, their mechanisms of action and how pathological B cells evade their cytotoxic effects are not well defined. The mAb described above have limited or no direct cytotoxic effects and their therapeutic effects result primarily from activation of innate immune cytotoxicity [21,41–46].

Complement activation results in generation of MAC that can cause target cell lysis or necrosis. This has been demonstrated in vitro for mAb with wild-type IgG1 constant regions including rituximab, ofatumumab, alemtuzumab and daratumumab [21,28,39,45]. Although mAb-induced CDC can rapidly (within minutes) kill a large fraction of targeted B cells in vitro, the therapeutic significance of this mechanism in treatment of human lymphoid malignancies is not well defined [21]. There is circumstantial evidence that mAb-induced CDC is partially responsible for clearance of circulating B cells in patients with B-cell malignancies, but the role of complement activation and killing of malignant lymphocytes via generation of the MAC in lymphoid tissues is poorly understood.

Initial in vitro studies of rituximab-mediated cellular cytotoxicity demonstrated circulating human mononuclear cell-mediated ADCC of rituximab-opsonized B cells [47]. Subsequent studies showed that the primary mediators of this in vitro ADCC were NK cells [44]. A recently published study suggests that circulating NK cells have a low cytotoxic capacity and that NK cell ADCC is unlikely to be an important mechanism of mAb-induced clearance of circulating malignant B cells [14]. In contrast, ADCP mediated by fixed macrophages in the spleen and liver (Kupffer cells) has high cytotoxic capacity and plays a major role in rituximab-mediated clearance of circulating B cells [9–16]. ADCP activated by rituximab Fc binding to macrophage FcR is well described, but the role of activation of ADCP via the binding of complement C3b and its derivates to CR3 and CR expressed by macrophages is less well understood [14,16,22]. The relative role of CDC versus cADCP in the clinical activity of rituximab and other complement-activating anti-CD20 mAb is also not known.

The recognition that the major cytotoxic mechanism of anti-CD20 mAb is the innate immune system has profound consequences. Foremost among these is the likelihood that the finite cytotoxic capacity of the innate immune system limits the therapeutic effect of each dose of mAb and that subsequent "exhaustion" could have deleterious effects on therapy. We recently reported that hypophagia, the autoregulatory macrophage feedback mechanism that limits phagocytic capacity [16], could in part explain the observed rapid but finite clearance of CLL cells from the circulation by rituximab and ofatumumab [48–51]. Recovery of phagocytic activity in vitro as measured by quantitative ADCP assays takes approximately 24 h [13,16], a time scale similar to that observed in clinical trials using high-frequency low-dose rituximab therapy [48,51]. The cytotoxic capacity of activated complement via CDC and cADCP [23,24] during mAb therapy for B-cell malignancies is not well defined. A better understanding of the cytotoxic capacity of cADCP and the mechanistic overlap with Fc-FcR-mediated ADCP will be critical to developing therapeutic regimens that optimize mAb therapy. The goal of this optimization would be to develop therapeutic regimens that optimize patient outcome by maintaining a continuous rate of innate immune cytotoxicity without inducing "exhaustion".

4. Complement Activation and CDC

The therapeutic effect of mAb activation of complement is determined by mAb pharmacokinetics and pharmacodynamics, availability of complement, target cell antigen expression and intrinsic target lymphocyte susceptibility to complement-mediated cytotoxicity.

4.1. Pharmacokinetics

Human Fc wild-type IgG mAbs are cleared from the circulation by the liver and spleen in a manner similar to the mechanism of clearance of endogenous IgG and in addition by ligation to target cells [52]. In patients with circulating malignant B lymphocytes, the rate of clearance of the first dose of anti-CD20 mAb is proportional to the amount of circulating CD20 available for ligation [50]. Although there is a correlation between low post-treatment serum mAb concentration and poor clinical response [53], there are no mechanistic data showing that these low serum mAb levels are responsible for treatment failure. In patients treated with current standard doses of anti-CD20 mAb, serum levels are consistently higher than required to saturate target binding in the circulation [14,44,50]. This suggests that the lower serum concentrations seen in patients with poorer prognosis are indicative of higher tumor burden rather than an inadequate therapeutic dose and that increasing the dose of mAb is unlikely to have any beneficial therapeutic effect. In contrast, there are limited published data on mAb concentrations achieved in lymphoid tissue and the ability of mAb to achieve complement-activating concentrations in malignant lymphoid tissue has not been reported. The possibility that lymphoid tissue mAb levels are not sufficient to activate complement requires further evaluation.

4.2. Pharmacodynamics

mAb currently used to treat B-cell malignancies vary widely in their ability to activate complement. mAb that bind ligand epitopes closer to the cell membrane (e.g., ofatumumab) are more likely to mediate membrane capture of activated complement components. Although ofatumumab has similar binding affinity for CD20 compared to rituximab, it has a slower off rate, resulting in more durable binding and binding stoichiometry that causes closer association of multiple mAb Fc regions which further increases its ability to activate complement [29,54–57].

mAb ability to activate complement is determined by target cell membrane ligand density and the ability to generate the hexameric Fc configuration that efficiently activates C1q [55,58]. For example, complement activation by rituximab in CLL, a disease characterized by low cell membrane CD20 density, is considerably less than in other B-cell lymphomas with higher CD20 density such as follicular cell lymphoma. The type I (complement-activating) [59] anti-CD20 mAbs rituximab and ofatumumab bind cell membrane CD20 dimers at a ratio of 2:1 to form mAb superstructures, which then concentrate on the cell membrane (forming lipid rafts) to efficiently activate complement as shown in Figure 2 [55,57]. In contrast, the type II (non-complement-activating) [59] anti-CD20 mAb obinutuzumab binds CD20 at lower ratios of 1:2, does not induce lipid rafts or formation of mAb superstructures and is not able to efficiently activate complement [56,57,60].

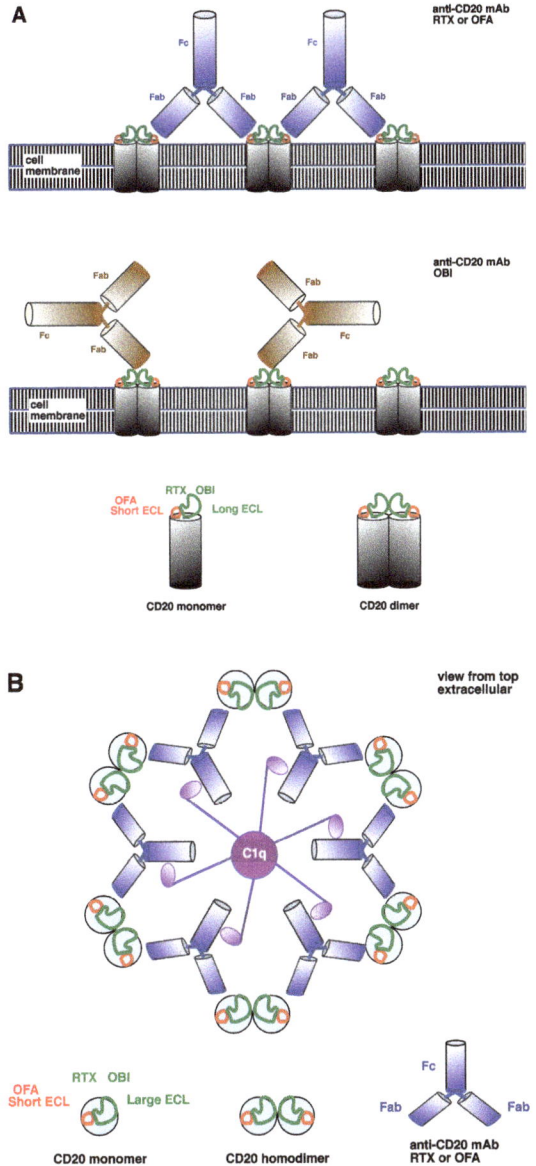

Figure 2. Anti-CD20 monoclonal antibody (mAb) ligation and activation of complement. (**A**) CD20 molecules form homodimers in the B-cell membrane. Rituximab (RTX) and obinutuzumab (OBI) ligate the long extracellular loop (ECL). RTX binds the long ECL in an area near the short ECL. OBI binds the long ECL in an area away from the short ECL. Ofatumumab (OFA) ligates the short ECL of the CD20 molecule. Type I complement-activating anti-CD20 mAb (RTX and OFA) Fabs can bind to two adjacent CD20 dimers. In contrast, the non-complement-activating anti-CD20 OBI binds only one CD20 dimer, resulting in a different Fc orientation to type I mAbs. (**B**) Model of the extracellular view from the top showing that type I anti-CD20 mAb RTX and OFA ligate adjacent CD20 dimers to form a hexamer that efficiently activates C1q.

In summary, characteristics of mAb that contribute to efficient activation of complement are high antigen affinity and low off rate, binding to antigen epitopes close to the cell membrane, antigen binding stoichiometry that facilitates Fc association, and lipid rafts.

4.3. Complement Levels

Patients with some B-cell malignancies (e.g., CLL) can have defective complement function which could decrease mAb-induced cytotoxicity [61]. Serum complement levels have been shown to decrease significantly after administration of mAbs that are efficient complement activators and this could limit treatment efficacy with repeat dosing [20,50,62]. However, in most of these studies, the complement levels did not decrease below levels known to be sufficient for activation of maximum complement levels in vitro, and rebound of complement levels to baseline did not result in additional clearance of circulating CLL cells despite adequate mAb levels. These data suggest that complement deficiency was not a major limiting mAb effect.

Therapy with fresh frozen plasma (FFP) has been reported to increase activity of rituximab in CLL patients but this was not formally demonstrated to be mediated by increased complement availability [63]. FFP contains a large number of proteins and it could be useful to determine what component (e.g., immunoglobulin) could have modified the mAb therapeutic effect.

4.4. Complement Regulatory Proteins (CRP)

CLL cells have low expression of the CRP CD46 and high expression of CD55 and CD59 [64]. Inhibition of CD55 or CD59 increases in vitro CDC of malignant B cells [64] and there is in vitro data suggesting that for B cells with high levels of CD20, increased expression of CRP could decrease CDC [44]. Use of a targeted CD59 inhibitor in a mouse lymphoma model decreased lymphoma growth [65] but this approach has not yet evolved into an established clinical modality. Of note, in vitro daratumumab-induced CDC of primary multiple myeloma cells did not correlate with expression of CRP [39]. In conclusion, current data suggest that CRP expressed by target B cells is unlikely to determine the therapeutic efficacy of mAb in B-cell malignancies.

4.5. mAb Antigen

CDC requires higher levels of mAb ligation of cell membrane antigens than ADCP [14,50,64]. Consequently, malignant B lymphocytes that generally express lower levels of a specific mAb antigen, such as CD20 in CLL cells, are less sensitive to CDC [64]. In addition, rapid (within hours) loss of B-cell membrane CD20 after initiation of anti-CD20 mAb therapy has been well documented in vivo and can cause acquired resistance to in vitro CDC [50]. The primary mechanism of antigen loss is trogocytosis, the transfer of cell surface molecules (ligand-mAb immune complex) from a donor cell (opsonized B cell) to effector cells (e.g., macrophage, monocyte, and granulocyte) [66–68]. We have recently shown that ADCP of opsonized B cells by macrophages occurs as a rapid burst of engulfment (<1 h) followed by a period of exhaustion (hypophagia) with minimal further phagocytosis for the subsequent 24 h [16]. However, data from in vitro experiments show that trogocytosis is a slower and ongoing process [69] and clinical trials suggest that decreased in CD20 levels of circulating B cells continues for at least 24 h after the first infusion of ofatumumab to reach levels of ~3% of baseline [50]. These data suggest that trogocytosis of immune complexes (CD20-mAb) from circulating B cells could be an ongoing process that occurs independently from ADCP. Loss of mAb ligand following initiation of therapy can also occur because of endocytosis of mAb-ligand by target cells [70] but this process is likely to be slower and of lesser magnitude than trogocytosis [69]. Apparent loss of antigen could also occur because of selective mAb-mediated cytotoxicity of target B cells with higher antigen levels. However, careful evaluation of target circulating cell population numbers and distribution of membrane CD20 before and after initiation of ofatumumab therapy did not show selected survival of a pre-existing subpopulation of CLL cells with low levels of CD20 [50].

4.6. Intrinsic Cellular Resistance

The terminal event of activation of the classical complement pathway by mAb is generation of MACs that insert in the cell membrane and cause cell necrosis or lysis. In vitro mAbs that are highly efficient at activating complement such as alemtuzumab are cytotoxic to over 90% of CLL cells [71]. Cytotoxicity could be significantly increased by addition of ofatumumab to alemtuzumab but over 1% of CLL cells still remained viable, demonstrating that these treatments are unlikely to be curative. CDC of nucleated cells is known to require generation of multiple MACs per cells and cells can recover by shedding MACs [43] but most of the viable cells in this study had high levels of MAC equivalent to those seen in cells undergoing apoptosis [71]. To further investigate this finding, we assessed complement activation in viable cells by measurement of iC3b and C9 and showed that the majority of these cells had evidence of complement activation and MAC generation that would be expected to be lethal [50,71]. The Taylor laboratory subsequently showed that in these resistant cells, MAC generation induced the expected calcium flux but that this was not lethal [72]. The mechanism of resistance remains undetermined but these data suggest that a subpopulation of circulating B cells from patients with CLL could be intrinsically resistant to CDC.

5. Complement Activation and cADCP

As already noted, mAb ligation on the target cell surface can also lead to deposition of complement fragments that trigger ADCP upon binding to CRs on phagocytes. While cADCP can mediate rapid clearance of mAb-ligated tumor cells in vitro, the relative contribution of cADCP to tumor cell clearance in vivo is likely a very important but still poorly understood killing mechanism of mAbs.

5.1. cADCP Signaling

Activation of complement by mAb on target cells leads to the covalent binding of C3 activation fragments (C3b, which can decay to cell-bound iC3b, C3d) that effectively opsonize the target cell surface. These opsonins can be recognized by CR1, CR3, and CR4 on phagocytes to trigger a form of engulfment that is biochemically distinct from FcγR-mediated ADCP [73]. CR3 and CR4 recognition of iC3b is the principal means by which macrophages mediate cADCP [74]. To date, CR3, also known as $\alpha_M\beta_2$ or CD11b, is the best-studied cADCP receptor. The signaling events that trigger phagocytosis downstream of CR3 are distinct from those of FcγR signaling. Activation of Rho family small GTPases (e.g., Rac, RhoA, and CDC42) is critical for driving the cytoskeletal reorganization that leads to target cell internalization [73]. Unlike FcγR ligation, the activation of CR3 during cADCP results in robust activation of RhoA but not Rac1 or Rac2 [75]. Active RhoA stimulates the nucleation and polymerization of actin at the phagocytic cup via activation of Rho kinase and mDia [76,77]. With regards to the role of Syk in cADCP, Kiefer et al. used macrophages from Syk-/- mice to establish definitively that Syk, a tyrosine kinase essential for FcγR ADCP, is dispensable for cADCP [78]. To date, the mechanisms and consequences of target degradation post-engulfment in FcγR ADCP and cADCP have not been investigated in-depth.

5.2. Crosstalk between FcγR- and cADCP

Part of understanding the relative contributions of both FcγR- and CR-activated ADCP pathways in therapeutic mAb-mediated cell clearance involves understanding the extent of crosstalk between these two pathways [79]. Early investigations into the connectedness of FcγR- and cADCP suggested the presence of C3 reduced the bound IgG levels that were needed to activate FcγR-ADCP; and found FcγR-mediated engulfment was lower when CR3 was blocked [80–82]. Jongstra-Bilen et al. showed that the engagement of IgG to FcγR resulted in increased CR3 lateral movement and enhanced iC3b binding to CR3 [83]. Additionally, Shushakova et al. showed that C5a-receptor signaling upregulated transcription of the activating FcγRI and FcγRIII was a pivotal component of FcγR-mediated signaling [84]. On the other hand, Huang et al. showed that the crosstalk between

FcγR- and cADCP was more complex, and that their synergistic relationship was dependent upon the FcγR subtype that was co-stimulated with CRs [85]. Even the involvement of Syk in cADCP remains under debate based on evidence that cADCP can result in Syk phosphorylation and expression of dominant-negative Syk can disrupt cADCP [86]. These findings suggest that a complex synergy exists between FcγR- and cADCP and that co-stimulation of certain components within each pathway may be integral for full activation. The extent of their crosstalk and signaling connectivity, however, remain to be fully elucidated.

5.3. Importance of cADCP in mAb Therapy

While in vitro studies have been useful in establishing the ability of different mAbs to activate complement and trigger cADCP by macrophages, our understanding of the role of cADCP in vivo is much less developed. Using C1q-deficient mice, Di Gaetano et al. showed that activation of complement was essential for anti-CD20 mAbs to control tumor burden in a lymphoma model [87]. Intriguingly, this phenotype is similar to that seen in FcγR-deficient mice treated with CD20 and HER2 mAbs [12,42]. Additionally, van Spriel et al. revealed that knocking out CR3 substantially reduced the efficacy of the mAb TA99 in a syngeneic melanoma model compared to wild-type mice [88]. While these studies support the idea of cADCP as a major cytotoxic mechanism of mAbs in vivo, future studies that measure cADCP in vivo are needed to establish the role of complement in mAb-mediated cell clearance. Finally, there is a paucity of data on cADCP in humans, although there is evidence that anti-CD20 mAb therapies are less effective in CLL patients with complement deficiencies [62].

6. Conclusions

The development of mAbs targeting B lymphocytes has significantly improved therapy for patients with B-cell malignancies. Despite the impressive empiric clinical data supporting the use of these mAbs both as monotherapy and in combination regimens, there is limited data about how mAbs cause malignant lymphocyte cytotoxicity and how a subpopulation of these cells resist this cytotoxicity. Available data support complement activation as an important innate immune cytotoxic mechanism for rituximab, ofatumumab, daratumumab, and alemtuzumab. We propose that additional studies of the roles of CDC and cADCP in the clinical efficacy of these mAbs are required to provide the data needed to optimize the use of these drugs; these studies should allow for the design of new drugs to enhance activity and overcome resistance. These investigations could focus on defining the cytotoxic capacity of the innate immune system in order to develop clinical regimens that prevent immune "exhaustion". It will be important to examine how nucleated cells can survive MAC-mediated calcium fluxes, and to determine the role of cADCP which has only limited overlap (and thus cross resistance) with CDC and ADCP. Current mAb-based therapeutic developments include engineered Fc with enhanced ability to form hexameric complement-activating structures [89], and bispecific mAb that decrease complement inhibitory proteins [90]. An improved understanding of the role of complement activation in the treatment of B-cell malignancies will both guide the development of these classes of drugs and provide the data required to develop novel drugs to improve complement-mediated cytotoxicity.

Author Contributions: C.S.Z., J.J.P., C.C.C. and M.R.E. wrote and edited this manuscript. All authors have read and agreed to the published version of the manuscript.

Funding: C.S.Z and C.C.C. have funding from the Hairy Cell Leukemia Foundation. M.R.E. was supported by grants from the National Institutes of Health (AI114554, DK119285). J.J.P. was supported in part by the University of Rochester Immunology Training T32 Grant from NIH (AI007285). This research was also funded through the University of Rochester from Acerta/AstraZeneca and TG Therapeutics.

Conflicts of Interest: C.S.Z. and C.C.C.: research funding from Acerta/AstraZeneca and TG Therapeutics.

References

1. Coiffier, B.; Lepage, E.; Brière, J.; Herbrecht, R.; Tilly, H.; Bouabdallah, R.; Morel, P.; Neste, E.V.D.; Salles, G.; Gaulard, P.; et al. CHOP Chemotherapy plus Rituximab Compared with CHOP Alone in Elderly Patients with Diffuse Large-B-Cell Lymphoma. *N. Engl. J. Med.* **2002**, *346*, 235–242. [CrossRef] [PubMed]
2. Habermann, T.M.; Weller, E.A.; Morrison, V.A.; Gascoyne, R.D.; Cassileth, P.A.; Cohn, J.B.; Dakhil, S.R.; Woda, B.; Fisher, R.I.; Peterson, B.A.; et al. Rituximab-CHOP Versus CHOP Alone or with Maintenance Rituximab in Older Patients with Diffuse Large B-Cell Lymphoma. *J. Clin. Oncol.* **2006**, *24*, 3121–3127. [CrossRef] [PubMed]
3. Marcus, R.; Imrie, K.; Belch, A.; Cunningham, D.; Flores, E.; Catalano, J.; Solal-Celigny, P.; Offner, F.; Walewski, J.; Raposo, J.; et al. CVP chemotherapy plus rituximab compared with CVP as first-line treatment for advanced follicular lymphoma. *Blood* **2005**, *105*, 1417–1423. [CrossRef] [PubMed]
4. Schulz, H.; Bohlius, J.F.; Trelle, S.; Skoetz, N.; Reiser, M.; Kober, T.; Schwarzer, G.; Herold, M.; Dreyling, M.; Hallek, M.; et al. Immunochemotherapy with Rituximab and Overall Survival in Patients with Indolent or Mantle Cell Lymphoma: A Systematic Review and Meta-analysis. *J. Natl. Cancer Inst.* **2007**, *99*, 706–714. [CrossRef] [PubMed]
5. Hallek, M.; Fischer, K.; Fingerle-Rowson, G.; Fink, A.M.; Busch, R.; Mayer, J.; Hensel, M.; Hopfinger, G.; Hess, G.; Von Grünhagen, U.; et al. Addition of rituximab to fludarabine and cyclophosphamide in patients with chronic lymphocytic leukaemia: A randomised, open-label, phase 3 trial. *Lancet* **2010**, *376*, 1164–1174. [CrossRef]
6. Uchida, J.; Hamaguchi, Y.; Oliver, J.A.; Ravetch, J.V.; Poe, J.C.; Haas, K.M.; Tedder, T.F. The Innate Mononuclear Phagocyte Network Depletes B Lymphocytes through Fc Receptor–dependent Mechanisms during Anti-CD20 Antibody Immunotherapy. *J. Exp. Med.* **2004**, *199*, 1659–1669. [CrossRef]
7. Bowles, J.A.; Wang, S.-Y.; Link, B.K.; Allan, B.; Beuerlein, G.; Campbell, M.-A.; Marquis, D.; Ondek, B.; Wooldridge, J.E.; Smith, B.J.; et al. Anti-CD20 monoclonal antibody with enhanced affinity for CD16 activates NK cells at lower concentrations and more effectively than rituximab. *Blood* **2006**, *108*, 2648–2654. [CrossRef]
8. Beum, P.V.; Lindorfer, M.A.; Taylor, R.P. Within Peripheral Blood Mononuclear Cells, Antibody-Dependent Cellular Cytotoxicity of Rituximab-Opsonized Daudi cells Is Promoted by NK Cells and Inhibited by Monocytes due to Shaving. *J. Immunol.* **2008**, *181*, 2916–2924. [CrossRef]
9. Montalvao, F.; Garcia, Z.; Celli, S.; Breart, B.; Deguine, J.; Van Rooijen, N.; Bousso, P. The mechanism of anti-CD20–mediated B cell depletion revealed by intravital imaging. *J. Clin. Investig.* **2013**, *123*, 5098–5103. [CrossRef]
10. Gül, N.; Babes, L.; Siegmund, K.; Korthouwer, R.; Bögels, M.; Braster, R.; Vidarsson, G.; Hagen, T.L.T.; Kubes, P.; Van Egmond, M. Macrophages eliminate circulating tumor cells after monoclonal antibody therapy. *J. Clin. Investig.* **2014**, *124*, 812–823. [CrossRef]
11. Gül, N.; Van Egmond, M. Antibody-Dependent Phagocytosis of Tumor Cells by Macrophages: A Potent Effector Mechanism of Monoclonal Antibody Therapy of Cancer. *Cancer Res.* **2015**, *75*, 5008–5013. [CrossRef] [PubMed]
12. Grandjean, C.L.; Montalvao, F.; Celli, S.; Michonneau, D.; Breart, B.; Garcia, Z.; Perro, M.; Freytag, O.; Gerdes, C.A.; Bousso, P. Intravital imaging reveals improved Kupffer cell-mediated phagocytosis as a mode of action of glycoengineered anti-CD20 antibodies. *Sci. Rep.* **2016**, *6*, srep34382. [CrossRef] [PubMed]
13. Church, A.K.; VanDerMeid, K.R.; Baig, N.A.; Baran, A.M.; Witzig, T.E.; Nowakowski, G.S.; Zent, C.S. Anti-CD20 monoclonal antibody-dependent phagocytosis of chronic lymphocytic leukaemia cells by autologous macrophages. *Clin. Exp. Immunol.* **2015**, *183*, 90–101. [CrossRef]
14. VanDerMeid, K.R.; Elliott, M.R.; Baran, A.M.; Barr, P.M.; Chu, C.C.; Zent, C.S. Cellular Cytotoxicity of Next-Generation CD20 Monoclonal Antibodies. *Cancer Immunol. Res.* **2018**, *6*, 1150–1160. [CrossRef] [PubMed]
15. Chu, C.C.; Pinney, J.J.; Whitehead, H.E.; Rivera-Escalera, F.; VanDerMeid, K.R.; Zent, C.S.; Elliott, M.R. High-resolution quantification of discrete phagocytic events by live cell time-lapse high-content microscopy imaging. *J. Cell Sci.* **2020**, *133*, jcs237883. [CrossRef]
16. Pinney, J.J.; Rivera-Escalera, F.; Chu, C.C.; Whitehead, H.E.; VanDerMeid, K.R.; Nelson, A.M.; Barbeau, M.C.; Zent, C.S.; Elliott, M.R. Macrophage hypophagia as a mechanism of innate immune exhaustion in mAb-induced cell clearance. *Blood* **2020**, *136*, 2065–2079. [CrossRef]

17. Pavlasova, G.; Mraz, M. The regulation and function of CD20: An "enigma" of B-cell biology and targeted therapy. *Haematologica* **2020**, *105*, 1494–1506. [CrossRef]
18. Reis, E.S.; Mastellos, D.C.; Ricklin, D.; Mantovani, A.; Lambris, J.D. Complement in cancer: Untangling an intricate relationship. *Nat. Rev. Immunol.* **2018**, *18*, 5–18. [CrossRef]
19. Bordron, A.; Bagacean, C.; Tempescul, A.; Berthou, C.; Bettacchioli, E.; Hillion, S.; Renaudineau, Y. Complement System: A Neglected Pathway in Immunotherapy. *Clin. Rev. Allergy Immunol.* **2020**, *58*, 155–171. [CrossRef]
20. Kennedy, A.D.; Beum, P.V.; Solga, M.D.; DiLillo, D.J.; Lindorfer, M.A.; Hess, C.E.; Densmore, J.J.; Williams, M.E.; Taylor, R.P. Rituximab Infusion Promotes Rapid Complement Depletion and Acute CD20 Loss in Chronic Lymphocytic Leukemia. *J. Immunol.* **2004**, *172*, 3280–3288. [CrossRef]
21. Zent, C.S.; Secreto, C.R.; LaPlant, B.R.; Bone, N.D.; Call, T.G.; Shanafelt, T.D.; Jelinek, D.F.; Tschumper, R.C.; Kay, N.E. Direct and complement dependent cytotoxicity in CLL cells from patients with high-risk early–intermediate stage chronic lymphocytic leukemia (CLL) treated with alemtuzumab and rituximab. *Leuk. Res.* **2008**, *32*, 1849–1856. [CrossRef] [PubMed]
22. Zent, C.S.; Elliott, M.R. Maxed out macs: Physiologic cell clearance as a function of macrophage phagocytic capacity. *FEBS J.* **2017**, *284*, 1021–1039. [CrossRef] [PubMed]
23. Lee, C.H.; Romain, G.; Yan, W.; Watanabe, M.; Charab, W.; Todorova, B.; Lee, J.; Triplett, K.; Donkor, M.; Lungu, O.I.; et al. IgG Fc domains that bind C1q but not effector Fcgamma receptors delineate the importance of complement-mediated effector functions. *Nat. Immunol.* **2017**, *18*, 889–898. [CrossRef] [PubMed]
24. Lukácsi, S.; Nagy-Baló, Z.; Erdei, A.; Sándor, N.; Bajtay, Z. The role of CR3 (CD11b/CD18) and CR4 (CD11c/CD18) in complement-mediated phagocytosis and podosome formation by human phagocytes. *Immunol. Lett.* **2017**, *189*, 64–72. [CrossRef]
25. Hamblin, T.J.; Abdul-Ahad, A.K.; Gordon, J.; Stevenson, F.K.; Stevenson, G.T. Preliminary experience in treating lymphocytic leukaemia with antibody to immunoglobulin idiotypes on the cell surfaces. *Br. J. Cancer* **1980**, *42*, 495–502. [CrossRef] [PubMed]
26. Maloney, D.G.; Grillo-Lopez, A.J.; White, C.A.; Bodkin, D.; Schilder, R.J.; Neidhart, J.A.; Janakiraman, N.; Foon, K.A.; Liles, T.-M.; Dallaire, B.K.; et al. IDEC-C2B8 (Rituximab) anti-CD20 monoclonal antibody therapy in patients with relapsed low-grade non-Hodgkin's lymphoma. *Blood* **1997**, *90*, 2188–2195. [CrossRef]
27. Coiffier, B.; Haioun, C.; Ketterer, N.; Engert, A.; Tilly, H.; Ma, D.; Johnson, P.; Lister, A.; Feuring-Buske, M.; Radford, J.A.; et al. Rituximab (anti-CD20 monoclonal antibody) for the treatment of patients with relapsing or refractory aggressive lymphoma: A multicenter phase II study. *Blood* **1998**, *92*, 27.
28. Teeling, J.L.; French, R.R.; Cragg, M.S.; Brakel, J.V.D.; Pluyter, M.; Huang, H.; Chan, C.; Parren, P.W.H.I.; Hack, C.E.; DeChant, M.; et al. Characterization of new human CD20 monoclonal antibodies with potent cytolytic activity against non-Hodgkin lymphomas. *Blood* **2004**, *104*, 1793–1800. [CrossRef]
29. Teeling, J.L.; Mackus, W.J.M.; Wiegman, L.J.J.M.; Brakel, J.H.N.V.D.; Beers, S.A.; French, R.R.; Van Meerten, T.; Ebeling, S.; Vink, T.; Slootstra, J.W.; et al. The Biological Activity of Human CD20 Monoclonal Antibodies Is Linked to Unique Epitopes on CD20. *J. Immunol.* **2006**, *177*, 362–371. [CrossRef]
30. Mössner, E.; Brünker, P.; Moser, S.; Püntener, U.; Schmidt, C.; Herter, S.; Grau, R.; Gerdes, C.; Nopora, A.; Van Puijenbroek, E.; et al. Increasing the efficacy of CD20 antibody therapy through the engineering of a new type II anti-CD20 antibody with enhanced direct and immune effector cell–mediated B-cell cytotoxicity. *Blood* **2010**, *115*, 4393–4402. [CrossRef]
31. Hale, G.; Clark, M.R.; Marcus, R.; Winter, G.; Dyer, M.J.; Phillips, J.; Riechmann, L.; Waldmann, H. Remission induction in non-hodgkin lymphoma with reshaped human monoclonal antibody campath-1h. *Lancet* **1988**, *332*, 1394–1399. [CrossRef]
32. Xia, M.Q.; Hale, G.; Waldmann, H.; Meng-Qi, X. Efficient complement-mediated lysis of cells containing the CAMPATH-1 (CDw52) antigen. *Mol. Immunol.* **1993**, *30*, 1089–1096. [CrossRef] [PubMed]
33. Österborg, A.; Fassas, A.S.; Anagnostopoulos, A.; Dyer, M.J.S.; Catovsky, D.; Mellstedt, H. Humanized CD52 monoclonal antibody campath-1H as first-line treatment in chronic lymphocytic leukaemia. *Br. J. Haematol.* **1996**, *93*, 151–153. [CrossRef] [PubMed]
34. Keating, M.J.; Flinn, I.; Jain, V.; Binet, J.-L.; Hillmen, P.; Byrd, J.; Albitar, M.; Brettman, L.; Santabarbara, P.; Wacker, B.; et al. Therapeutic role of alemtuzumab (Campath-1H) in patients who have failed fludarabine: Results of a large international study. *Blood* **2002**, *99*, 3554–3561. [CrossRef] [PubMed]

35. Bowen, A.L.; Zomas, A.; Emmett, E.; Matutes, E.; Dyer, M.J.; Catovsky, D. Subcutaneous CAMPATH-1H in fludarabine-resistant/relapsed chronic lymphocytic and B-prolymphocytic leukaemia. *Br. J. Haematol.* **1997**, *96*, 617–619. [CrossRef] [PubMed]
36. Hillmen, P.; Skotnicki, A.B.; Robak, T.; Jaksic, B.; Dmoszynska, A.; Wu, J.; Sirard, C.; Mayer, J. Alemtuzumab Compared with Chlorambucil As First-Line Therapy for Chronic Lymphocytic Leukemia. *J. Clin. Oncol.* **2007**, *25*, 5616–5623. [CrossRef] [PubMed]
37. Cross, M.; Dearden, C.E. B and T cell prolymphocytic leukaemia. *Best Pr. Res. Clin. Haematol.* **2019**, *32*, 217–228. [CrossRef]
38. Van De Donk, N.W.; Usmani, S.Z. CD38 Antibodies in Multiple Myeloma: Mechanisms of Action and Modes of Resistance. *Front. Immunol.* **2018**, *9*, 2134. [CrossRef] [PubMed]
39. De Weers, M.; Tai, Y.-T.; Van Der Veer, M.S.; Bakker, J.M.; Vink, T.; Jacobs, D.C.H.; Oomen, L.A.; Peipp, M.; Valerius, T.; Slootstra, J.W.; et al. Daratumumab, a Novel Therapeutic Human CD38 Monoclonal Antibody, Induces Killing of Multiple Myeloma and Other Hematological Tumors. *J. Immunol.* **2011**, *186*, 1840–1848. [CrossRef]
40. Moreno, L.; Perez, C.; Zabaleta, A.; Manrique, I.; Alignani, D.; Ajona, D.; Blanco, L.; Lasa, M.; Maiso, P.; Rodriguez, I.; et al. The Mechanism of Action of the Anti-CD38 Monoclonal Antibody Isatuximab in Multiple Myeloma. *Clin. Cancer Res.* **2019**, *25*, 3176–3187. [CrossRef]
41. Golay, J.; Zaffaroni, L.; Vaccari, T.; Lazzari, M.; Borleri, G.M.; Bernasconi, S.; Tedesco, F.; Rambaldi, A.; Introna, M. Biologic response of B lymphoma cells to anti-CD20 monoclonal antibody rituximab in vitro: CD55 and CD59 regulate complement-mediated cell lysis. *Blood* **2000**, *95*, 3900–3908. [CrossRef] [PubMed]
42. Clynes, R.A.; Towers, T.L.; Presta, L.G.; Ravetch, J.V. Inhibitory Fc receptors modulate in vivo cytoxicity against tumor targets. *Nat. Med.* **2000**, *6*, 443–446. [CrossRef] [PubMed]
43. Kennedy, A.D.; Solga, M.D.; Schuman, T.A.; Chi, A.W.; Lindorfer, M.A.; Sutherland, W.M.; Foley, P.L.; Taylor, R.P. An anti-C3b(i) mAb enhances complement activation, C3b(i) deposition, and killing of CD20+ cells by rituximab. *Blood* **2003**, *101*, 1071–1079. [CrossRef] [PubMed]
44. Manches, O.; Lui, G.; Chaperot, L.; Gressin, R.; Molens, J.-P.; Jacob, M.-C.; Sotto, J.-J.; Leroux, D.; Bensa, J.-C.; Plumas, J. In vitro mechanisms of action of rituximab on primary non-Hodgkin lymphomas. *Blood* **2003**, *101*, 949–954. [CrossRef] [PubMed]
45. Zent, C.S.; Chen, J.B.; Kurten, R.C.; Kaushal, G.P.; Lacy, H.M.; Schichman, S.A. Alemtuzumab (CAMPATH 1H) does not kill chronic lymphocytic leukemia cells in serum free medium. *Leuk. Res.* **2004**, *28*, 495–507. [CrossRef] [PubMed]
46. Golay, J.; Manganini, M.; Rambaldi, A.; Introna, M. Effect of alemtuzumab on neoplastic B cells. *Haematologica* **2004**, *89*, 1476–1483.
47. Reff, M.E.; Carner, K.; Chambers, K.S.; Chinn, P.C.; Leonard, J.E.; Raab, R.; Newman, R.A.; Hanna, N.; Anderson, D.R. Depletion of B cells in vivo by a chimeric mouse human monoclonal antibody to CD20. *Blood* **1994**, *83*, 435–445. [CrossRef]
48. Williams, M.E.; Densmore, J.J.; Pawluczkowycz, A.W.; Beum, P.V.; Kennedy, A.D.; Lindorfer, M.A.; Hamil, S.H.; Eggleton, J.C.; Taylor, R.P. Thrice-Weekly Low-Dose Rituximab Decreases CD20 Loss via Shaving and Promotes Enhanced Targeting in Chronic Lymphocytic Leukemia. *J. Immunol.* **2006**, *177*, 7435–7443. [CrossRef]
49. Aue, G.; Lindorfer, M.A.; Beum, P.V.; Pawluczkowycz, A.W.; Vire, B.; Hughes, T.; Taylor, R.P.; Wiestner, A. Fractionated subcutaneous rituximab is well-tolerated and preserves CD20 expression on tumor cells in patients with chronic lymphocytic leukemia. *Haematologica* **2009**, *95*, 329–332. [CrossRef]
50. Baig, N.A.; Taylor, R.P.; Lindorfer, M.A.; Church, A.K.; LaPlant, B.R.; Pettinger, A.M.; Shanafelt, T.D.; Nowakowski, G.S.; Zent, C.S. Induced Resistance to Ofatumumab-Mediated Cell Clearance Mechanisms, Including Complement-Dependent Cytotoxicity, in Chronic Lymphocytic Leukemia. *J. Immunol.* **2014**, *192*, 1620–1629. [CrossRef]
51. Zent, C.S.; Taylor, R.P.; Lindorfer, M.A.; Beum, P.V.; LaPlant, B.; Wu, W.; Call, T.G.; Bowen, D.A.; Conte, M.J.; Frederick, L.A.; et al. Chemoimmunotherapy for relapsed/refractory and progressive 17p13-deleted chronic lymphocytic leukemia (CLL) combining pentostatin, alemtuzumab, and low-dose rituximab is effective and tolerable and limits loss of CD20 expression by circulating CLL cells. *Am. J. Hematol.* **2014**, *89*, 757–765. [CrossRef] [PubMed]

52. Cartron, G.; Blasco, H.; Paintaud, G.; Watier, H.; Le Guellec, C. Pharmacokinetics of rituximab and its clinical use: Thought for the best use? *Crit. Rev. Oncol.* **2007**, *62*, 43–52. [CrossRef]
53. Berinstein, N.L.; Grillo-Lopez, A.J.; White, C.A.; Bence-Bruckler, I.; Maloney, D.; Czuczman, M.; Green, D.; Rosenberg, J.; McLaughlin, P.; Shen, D. Association of serum Rituximab (IDEC–C2B8) concentration and anti-tumor response in the treatment of recurrent low-grade or follicular non-Hodgkin's lymphoma. *Ann. Oncol.* **1998**, *9*, 995–1001. [CrossRef]
54. Pawluczkowycz, A.W.; Beurskens, F.J.; Beum, P.V.; Lindorfer, M.A.; Van De Winkel, J.G.J.; Parren, P.W.H.I.; Taylor, R.P. Binding of Submaximal C1q Promotes Complement-Dependent Cytotoxicity (CDC) of B Cells Opsonized with Anti-CD20 mAbs Ofatumumab (OFA) or Rituximab (RTX): Considerably Higher Levels of CDC Are Induced by OFA than by RTX. *J. Immunol.* **2009**, *183*, 749–758. [CrossRef]
55. Bondza, S.; Broeke, T.T.; Nestor, M.; Leusen, J.H.; Buijs, J. Bivalent binding on cells varies between anti-CD20 antibodies and is dose-dependent. *mAbs* **2020**, *12*, 1792673. [CrossRef] [PubMed]
56. Kumar, A.; Planchais, C.; Fronzes, R.; Mouquet, H.; Reyes, N. Binding mechanisms of therapeutic antibodies to human CD20. *Science* **2020**, *369*, 793–799. [CrossRef] [PubMed]
57. Rougé, L.; Chiang, N.; Steffek, M.; Kugel, C.; Croll, T.I.; Tam, C.; Estevez, A.; Arthur, C.P.; Koth, C.M.; Ciferri, C.; et al. Structure of CD20 in complex with the therapeutic monoclonal antibody rituximab. *Science* **2020**, *367*, 1224–1230. [CrossRef]
58. Diebolder, C.A.; Beurskens, F.J.; De Jong, R.N.; Koning, R.I.; Strumane, K.; Lindorfer, M.A.; Voorhorst, M.; Ugurlar, D.; Rosati, S.; Heck, A.J.R.; et al. Complement Is Activated by IgG Hexamers Assembled at the Cell Surface. *Science* **2014**, *343*, 1260–1263. [CrossRef]
59. Cragg, M.S.; Glennie, M.J. Antibody specificity controls in vivo effector mechanisms of anti-CD20 reagents. *Blood* **2004**, *103*, 2738–2743. [CrossRef]
60. Herter, S.; Herting, F.; Mundigl, O.; Waldhauer, I.; Weinzierl, T.; Fauti, T.; Muth, G.; Ziegler-Landesberger, D.; Van Puijenbroek, E.; Lang, S.; et al. Preclinical Activity of the Type II CD20 Antibody GA101 (Obinutuzumab) Compared with Rituximab and Ofatumumab In Vitro and in Xenograft Models. *Mol. Cancer Ther.* **2013**, *12*, 2031–2042. [CrossRef]
61. Schlesinger, M.; Broman, I.; Lugassy, G. The complement system is defective in chronic lymphatic leukemia patients and in their healthy relatives. *Leukemia* **1996**, *10*, 1509–1513. [PubMed]
62. Middleton, O.; Cosimo, E.; Dobbin, E.; McCaig, A.M.; Clarke, C.L.; Brant, A.M.; Leach, M.; Michie, A.M.; Wheadon, H. Complement deficiencies limit CD20 monoclonal antibody treatment efficacy in CLL. *Leukemia* **2015**, *29*, 107–114. [CrossRef] [PubMed]
63. Klepfish, A.; Rachmilewitz, E.; Kotsianidis, I.; Patchenko, P.; Schattner, A. Adding fresh frozen plasma to rituximab for the treatment of patients with refractory advanced CLL. *QJM Int. J. Med.* **2008**, *101*, 737–740. [CrossRef] [PubMed]
64. Golay, J.; Lazzari, M.; Facchinetti, V.; Bernasconi, S.; Borleri, G.; Barbui, T.; Rambaldi, A.; Introna, M. CD20 levels determine the in vitro susceptibility to rituximab and complement of B-cell chronic lymphocytic leukemia: Further regulation by CD55 and CD59. *Blood* **2001**, *98*, 3383–3389. [CrossRef]
65. Hu, W.; Ge, X.; You, T.; Xu, T.; Zhang, J.; Wu, G.; Peng, Z.; Chorev, M.; Aktas, B.H.; Halperin, J.A.; et al. Human CD59 Inhibitor Sensitizes Rituximab-Resistant Lymphoma Cells to Complement-Mediated Cytolysis. *Cancer Res.* **2011**, *71*, 2298–2307. [CrossRef]
66. Beum, P.V.; Kennedy, A.D.; Williams, M.E.; Lindorfer, M.A.; Taylor, R.P. The Shaving Reaction: Rituximab/CD20 Complexes Are Removed from Mantle Cell Lymphoma and Chronic Lymphocytic Leukemia Cells by THP-1 Monocytes. *J. Immunol.* **2006**, *176*, 2600–2609. [CrossRef]
67. Taylor, R.P.; Lindorfer, M.A. Fcgamma-receptor-mediated trogocytosis impacts mAb-based therapies: Historical precedence and recent developments. *Blood* **2015**, *125*, 762–766. [CrossRef]
68. Valgardsdottir, R.; Cattaneo, I.; Klein, C.; Introna, M.; Figliuzzi, M.; Golay, J. Human neutrophils mediate trogocytosis rather than phagocytosis of CLL B cells opsonized with anti-CD20 antibodies. *Blood* **2017**, *129*, 2636–2644. [CrossRef]
69. Beum, P.V.; Peek, E.M.; Lindorfer, M.A.; Beurskens, F.J.; Engelberts, P.J.; Parren, P.W.H.I.; Van De Winkel, J.G.J.; Taylor, R.P.; Labrijn, A.F.; Meesters, J.; et al. Loss of CD20 and Bound CD20 Antibody from Opsonized B Cells Occurs More Rapidly Because of Trogocytosis Mediated by Fc Receptor-Expressing Effector Cells Than Direct Internalization by the B Cells. *J. Immunol.* **2011**, *187*, 3438–3447. [CrossRef]

70. Beers, S.A.; French, R.R.; Chan, H.T.C.; Lim, S.H.; Jarrett, T.C.; Vidal, R.M.; Wijayaweera, S.S.; Dixon, S.V.; Kim, H.; Cox, K.L.; et al. Antigenic modulation limits the efficacy of anti-CD20 antibodies: Implications for antibody selection. *Blood* **2010**, *115*, 5191–5201. [CrossRef]
71. Baig, N.A.; Taylor, R.P.; Lindorfer, M.A.; Church, A.K.; Laplant, B.R.; Pavey, E.S.; Nowakowski, G.S.; Zent, C.S. Complement dependent cytotoxicity (CDC) in chronic lymphocytic leukemia (CLL): Ofatumumab enhances alemtuzumab CDC and reveals cells resistant to activated complement. *Leuk. Lymphoma* **2012**, *53*, 2218–2227. [CrossRef] [PubMed]
72. Lindorfer, M.A.; Cook, E.M.; Tupitza, J.C.; Zent, C.S.; Burack, R.; De Jong, R.N.; Beurskens, F.J.; Schuurman, J.; Parren, P.W.; Taylor, R.P. Real-time analysis of the detailed sequence of cellular events in mAb-mediated complement-dependent cytotoxicity of B-cell lines and of chronic lymphocytic leukemia B-cells. *Mol. Immunol.* **2016**, *70*, 13–23. [CrossRef] [PubMed]
73. Flannagan, R.S.; Jaumouillé, V.; Grinstein, S. The Cell Biology of Phagocytosis. *Annu. Rev. Pathol. Mech. Dis.* **2012**, *7*, 61–98. [CrossRef] [PubMed]
74. Ross, G.D.; Reed, W.; Dalzell, J.G.; Becker, S.E.; Hogg, N. Macrophage cytoskeleton association with CR3 and CR4 regulates receptor mobility and phagocytosis of iC3b-opsonized erythrocytes. *J. Leukoc. Biol.* **1992**, *51*, 109–117. [CrossRef]
75. Wiedemann, A.; Patel, J.C.; Lim, J.; Tsun, A.; van Kooyk, Y.; Caron, E. Two distinct cytoplasmic regions of the beta2 integrin chain regulate RhoA function during phagocytosis. *J Cell Biol.* **2006**, *172*, 1069–1079. [CrossRef] [PubMed]
76. Olazabal, I.M.; Caron, E.; May, R.C.; Schilling, K.; Knecht, D.A.; Machesky, L.M. Rho-Kinase and Myosin-II Control Phagocytic Cup Formation during CR, but Not FcγR, Phagocytosis. *Curr. Biol.* **2002**, *12*, 1413–1418. [CrossRef]
77. Colucci-Guyon, E.; Niedergang, F.; Wallar, B.J.; Peng, J.; Alberts, A.S.; Chavrier, P. A Role for Mammalian Diaphanous-Related Formins in Complement Receptor (CR3)-Mediated Phagocytosis in Macrophages. *Curr. Biol.* **2005**, *15*, 2007–2012. [CrossRef] [PubMed]
78. Kiefer, F.; Brumell, J.; Al-Alawi, N.; Latour, S.; Cheng, A.; Veillette, A.; Grinstein, S.; Pawson, T. The Syk protein tyrosine kinase is essential for Fcgamma receptor signaling in macrophages and neutrophils. *Mol. Cell Biol.* **1998**, *18*, 4209–4220. [CrossRef] [PubMed]
79. Lindorfer, M.A.; Kohl, J.; Taylor, R.P. Interactions between the complement system and Fcg receptors. In *Antibody Fc: Linking Adaptive and Innate Immunity*; Ackerman, M.E., Nimmerhahn, F., Eds.; Elsevier Press: Philadelphia, PA, USA, 2014; pp. 49–74.
80. Schreiber, A.D.; Frank, M.M. Role of antibody and complement in the immune clearance and destruction of erythrocytes. I. In vivo effects of IgG and IgM complement-fixing sites. *J. Clin. Investig.* **1972**, *51*, 575–582. [CrossRef]
81. Schreiber, A.D.; Frank, M.M. Role of Antibody and Complement in the Immune Clearance and Destruction of Erythrocytes II. Molecular nature of igg and igm complement-fixing sites and effects of their interaction with serum. *J. Clin. Investig.* **1972**, *51*, 583–589. [CrossRef]
82. Brown, E.J.; Bohnsack, J.F.; Gresham, H.D. Mechanism of inhibition of immunoglobulin G-mediated phagocytosis by monoclonal antibodies that recognize the Mac-1 antigen. *J. Clin. Investig.* **1988**, *81*, 365–375. [CrossRef] [PubMed]
83. Jongstra-Bilen, J.; Harrison, R.; Grinstein, S. Fcgamma-receptors induce Mac-1 (CD11b/CD18) mobilization and accumulation in the phagocytic cup for optimal phagocytosis. *J. Biol. Chem.* **2003**, *278*, 45720–45729. [CrossRef] [PubMed]
84. Shushakova, N.; Skokowa, J.; Schulman, J.; Baumann, U.; Zwirner, J.; Schmidt, R.E.; Gessner, J.E. C5a anaphylatoxin is a major regulator of activating versus inhibitory FcgammaRs in immune complex-induced lung disease. *J. Clin. Investig.* **2002**, *110*, 1823–1830. [CrossRef] [PubMed]
85. Huang, Z.-Y.; Hunter, S.; Chien, P.; Kim, M.-K.; Han-Kim, T.-H.; Indik, Z.K.; Schreiber, A.D. Interaction of Two Phagocytic Host Defense Systems. *J. Biol. Chem.* **2011**, *286*, 160–168. [CrossRef] [PubMed]
86. Shi, Y.; Tohyama, Y.; Kadono, T.; He, J.; Miah, S.M.S.; Hazama, R.; Tanaka, C.; Tohyama, K.; Yamamura, H. Protein-tyrosine kinase Syk is required for pathogen engulfment in complement-mediated phagocytosis. *Blood* **2006**, *107*, 4554–4562. [CrossRef] [PubMed]

87. Di Gaetano, N.; Cittera, E.; Nota, R.; Vecchi, A.; Grieco, V.; Scanziani, E.; Botto, M.; Introna, M.; Golay, J. Complement Activation Determines the Therapeutic Activity of Rituximab In Vivo. *J. Immunol.* **2003**, *171*, 1581–1587. [CrossRef] [PubMed]
88. Van Spriel, A.B.; Van Ojik, H.H.; Bakker, A.; Jansen, M.J.H.; Van De Winkel, J.G.J. Mac-1 (CD11b/CD18) is crucial for effective Fc receptor–mediated immunity to melanoma. *Blood* **2003**, *101*, 253–258. [CrossRef]
89. Taylor, R.P.; Lindorfer, M.A.; Cook, E.M.; Beurskens, F.J.; Schuurman, J.; Parren, P.W.; Zent, C.S.; VanDerMeid, K.R.; Burack, R.; Mizuno, M.; et al. Hexamerization-enhanced CD20 antibody mediates complement-dependent cytotoxicity in serum genetically deficient in C9. *Clin. Immunol.* **2017**, *181*, 24–28. [CrossRef]
90. Macor, P.; Secco, E.; Mezzaroba, N.; Zorzet, S.; Durigutto, P.; Gaiotto, T.; De Maso, L.; Biffi, S.; Garrovo, C.; Capolla, S.; et al. Bispecific antibodies targeting tumor-associated antigens and neutralizing complement regulators increase the efficacy of antibody-based immunotherapy in mice. *Leukemia* **2015**, *29*, 406–414. [CrossRef]

Publisher's Note: MDPI stays neutral with regard to jurisdictional claims in published maps and institutional affiliations.

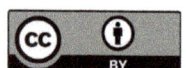 © 2020 by the authors. Licensee MDPI, Basel, Switzerland. This article is an open access article distributed under the terms and conditions of the Creative Commons Attribution (CC BY) license (http://creativecommons.org/licenses/by/4.0/).

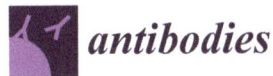

Review

The Role of Complement in the Mechanism of Action of Therapeutic Anti-Cancer mAbs

Josée Golay [1,2,*] and Ronald P. Taylor [3,*]

[1] Center of Cellular Therapy "G. Lanzani", Division of Hematology, Azienda Socio Sanitaria Territoriale Papa Giovanni XXIII, 24127 Bergamo, Italy
[2] Fondazione per la Ricerca Ospedale Maggiore, 24127 Bergamo, Italy
[3] Department of Biochemistry and Molecular Genetics, University of Virginia School of Medicine, Charlottesville, VA 22908, USA
* Correspondence: jgolay@fondazionefrom.it (J.G.); rpt@virginia.edu (R.P.T.)

Received: 14 August 2020; Accepted: 21 September 2020; Published: 28 October 2020

Abstract: Unconjugated anti-cancer IgG1 monoclonal antibodies (mAbs) activate antibody-dependent cellular cytotoxicity (ADCC) by natural killer (NK) cells and antibody-dependent cellular phagocytosis (ADCP) by macrophages, and these activities are thought to be important mechanisms of action for many of these mAbs in vivo. Several mAbs also activate the classical complement pathway and promote complement-dependent cytotoxicity (CDC), although with very different levels of efficacy, depending on the mAb, the target antigen, and the tumor type. Recent studies have unraveled the various structural factors that define why some IgG1 mAbs are strong mediators of CDC, whereas others are not. The role of complement activation and membrane inhibitors expressed by tumor cells, most notably CD55 and CD59, has also been quite extensively studied, but how much these affect the resistance of tumors in vivo to IgG1 therapeutic mAbs still remains incompletely understood. Recent studies have demonstrated that complement activation has multiple effects beyond target cell lysis, affecting both innate and adaptive immunity mediated by soluble complement fragments, such as C3a and C5a, and by stimulating complement receptors expressed by immune cells, including NK cells, neutrophils, macrophages, T cells, and dendritic cells. Complement activation can enhance ADCC and ADCP and may contribute to the vaccine effect of mAbs. These different aspects of complement are also briefly reviewed in the specific context of FDA-approved therapeutic anti-cancer IgG1 mAbs.

Keywords: therapeutic monoclonal antibodies (mAbs); complement; antibody dependent cellular cytotoxicity; phagocytosis; complement receptors

1. Introduction

Human IgG1 monoclonal antibodies (mAbs), after antigen binding, have the ability to activate the classical pathway of the complement cascade and mediate complement-dependent cytotoxicity (CDC) [1,2]. They can also cross-link Fcγ receptors expressed by immune cells, including natural killer (NK) cells, monocytes/macrophages, and neutrophils, and thereby activate cell-mediated innate immunity [2–4]. IgG1 mAbs therefore have the ability to activate both the humoral and cellular immune system for the immunological control of tumor growth and metastasis. These two pathways may also interact with each other, with potential synergy [5]. This is why most therapeutic mAbs that target a tumor antigen have been designed to bear a functional or even enhanced human IgG1 Fc portion. The tumor-specific unconjugated mAbs approved by the Food and Drug Administration (FDA) and European Medicines Agency (EMA) are listed in Table 1. The first part of the table lists mAbs approved for hematological malignancies, and the second part lists mAbs approved to target solid tumors. The gold standard for these mAbs is the anti-CD20 rituximab, which was the first approved anti-cancer mAb (in 1997) and has shown considerable therapeutic activity in several B cell tumor subtypes, initially as monotherapy, and subsequently in combination with chemotherapy. Indeed multiple phase III clinical studies have demonstrated the clinical efficacy of rituximab in combination with chemotherapy or as maintenance therapy in B-cell non-Hodgkin's lymphoma (B-NHL) (in particular follicular lymphoma and diffuse large B cell lymphoma) and, to a lesser extent, chronic lymphocytic leukemia (CLL), Burkitt's lymphoma, and mantle cell lymphomas (reviewed in Past, Present, and Future of Rituximab-The World's First Oncology Monoclonal Antibody Therapy [6]). Rituximab efficiently activates CDC, antibody-dependent cellular cytotoxicity (ADCC), and antibody-dependent cellular phagocytosis (ADCP) in vitro, and these different mechanisms must all contribute to its efficacy [4,7]. CD20 is well expressed in most mature B-cell leukemias and lymphomas and is nearly exclusively restricted to the B cell lineage, a factor likely contributing to the success of rituximab and other anti-CD20 antibodies.

Beyond their activation of innate immune mechanisms mentioned above, mAbs targeting tumor antigens may also act by blocking (neutralizing) the antigen receptor or enzymatic function through their Fab portion, either by interference with ligand binding or through internalization and degradation of the receptor or both, leading to inhibition of cell growth or of metastasis [8–10]. Some mAbs also induce direct cell death after antigen binding [11–13]. Table 1 reports the principal mechanisms of action that are thought to be at the base of the efficacy of the unconjugated IgG1 anti-tumor antigen mAbs approved for anti-tumor therapy. Some have antigen neutralizing functions, as expected, since they target important growth factor receptors such as human epidermal growth factor receptor 2 (HER2), epidermal growth factor receptor (EGFR), chemokine receptor 4 (CCR4), or enzymes (CD38) expressed on the plasma membranes of the cancer cells [4,8]. As noted above, mAbs can activate innate immune cells through their Fc regions and promote ADCC by NK cells and ADCP by macrophages [14–19]. Anti-SLAMF7 antibody elotuzumab also directly activates NK cells expressing this receptor in addition to inducing FcγR mediated ADCC and ADCP [20]. Some mAbs—most notably rituximab, ofatumumab, alemtuzumab, and daratumumab—also activate the complement cascade and induce CDC [2,4,8,21–23] (Table 1). Given the complexity of the immune activation induced by all of these mAbs, understanding which of these different mechanisms is most important for their efficacy in vivo is an important and complex question that has yet to be resolved. In particular, the role of complement in the mechanisms of action of rituximab and certain other therapeutic mAbs remains an active area of research [2]. In the next paragraphs, we will describe what is known about the role of complement in the mechanism of action of unconjugated IgG1 antibodies targeting tumor antigens, including the indirect effects that complement activation may have beyond target cell lysis.

Table 1. Approved unconjugated IgG1 monoclonal antibodies (mAbs) targeting tumor antigen.

Name	Target Antigen	Antibody Type	1st Indication	Year of 1st Approval [1]	Major Mechanism of Action
Rituximab	CD20	Chimeric IgG1	B-NHL	1997	CDC, ADCC, ADCP
Ofatumumab	CD20	Human IgG1	CLL	2009	CDC, ADCC, ADCP
Obinutuzumab	CD20	Humaniz. IgG1, Glycoengin.	CLL	2013	ADCC, ADCP, PCD
Daratumumab	CD38	Human IgG1	MM	2015	CDC, ADCC, ADCP, neutral.
Isatuximab	CD38	Chimeric IgG1k	MM	2020	Neutral. ADCC, ADCP
Alemtuzumab	CD52	Humanized IgG1	CLL	2001	CDC, ADCC, ADCP
Elotuzumab	SLAMF7	Humanized IgG1	MM	2015	ADCC. NK agonist, ADCP
Mogamulizumab	CCR4	Humanized IgG1, low fucose	T leuk/lymph	2012 Japan 2018 EU	ADCC, ADCP, Treg elimin.
Trastuzumab	HER2	Humanized IgG1	Breast cancer	1998	ADCC, neutral.
Pertuzumab	HER2	Humanized IgG1	Breast cancer	2012	Neutral. (HER2/HER3 dimerization)
Cetuximab	EGFR	Chimeric IgG1	CRC	2004	Neutral, ADCC, CDC
Panitumumab	EGFR	Human IgG2	CRC	2006	Neutral., PMN mediated ADCC
Necitumumab	EGFR	Human IgG1	NSCLC	2015	ADCC, neutral.
Dinutuximab	GD2	Chimeric IgG1	Neuroblastoma	2015	CDC, ADCC, ADCP

[1] Food and Drug Administration (FDA) and/or European Medicines Agency (EMA) approval. B-NHL: B- Non Hodgkin's lymphoma; CLL: Chronic lymphocytic leukemia; MM: Multiple myeloma; CRC: Colorectal carcinoma; NSCLC: Non small cell lung carcinoma; CDC: Complement dependent cytotoxicity; ADCC: Antibody dependent cellular cytotoxicity; ADCP: Antibody dependent cellular phagocytosis.

2. Complement Activation by Human IgG1 mAbs

The main steps of the classical complement cascade on mAb-opsonized tumor cells are illustrated in Figure 1 (top). The initial binding of the IgG1 antibody to the multiple target antigens expressed on the plasma membrane is rapidly followed by aggregation and, in optimal circumstances, hexamerization of the antibody on the surface [24,25], allowing the efficient binding of the C1q (hexameric)/(C1r)$_2$/(C1s)$_2$ complex, which in a series of proteolytic steps sequentially leads to activation of C1r, C1s, and subsequent activation of soluble C4 and C2 to yield C4b and C2a. C4b fragments attach covalently (opsonization) to the membrane in the vicinity of the antibody or to the antibody itself, and this is followed by non-covalent binding of C2a to generate the C3 convertase enzyme (C4bC2a). The C3 convertase binds and cleaves soluble C3 into C3a, a potent anaphylatoxin, and into C3b, which binds to the C4b/C2a complex and forms the C5 convertase (C4bC2aC3b). C3b also binds covalently (opsonizes) to target acceptor sites (amino and hydroxyl groups) on the cell membrane as well as to the cell-bound IgG mAb. Cleavage of C5 by the C5 convertase produces C5a, another important anaphylatoxin, as well as C5b. Production of C5b catalyzes formation of the C5b/C6/C7/C8 complex and initiation of C9 polymerization, inducing formation of the pore-forming membrane attack complex (MAC). Insertion of a sufficient number of MACs in the membrane above a threshold level leads to the rapid lysis of the target cells [26–31].

As also described in other chapters of this series, C3 is central to the complement cascade. It is also part of the alternative pathway of complement, a pathway that relies on Factor B, Factor D, Properdin (FP), and aqueous phase hydrolyzed C3 (C3H$_2$O) instead of C2 and C4, to form the C3 and C5 convertases (C3bBb and C3bBbC3b, respectively, both stabilized by Properdin) (Figure 1, bottom). C3(H$_2$O) is constantly generated at low levels in a tick-over mechanism (i.e., a weak but constant hydrolytic activation of C3), but the alternative pathway can amplify complement activation (via nascent C3b) first generated by the classical pathway (Figure 1) [26,27].

In view of the cytotoxic and inflammatory nature of complement, it is not surprising that multiple independent controls serve to provide protection of normal cells and tissues from the ravages of complement. For example, C3 deposition, whether produced by the classical or alternative pathway, is tightly regulated by membrane and soluble inhibitors: C3b is rapidly inactivated (proteolyzed) to iC3b (inactive C3b) and then to C3d and C3dg and soluble C3c by Factor I (FI), a soluble protease that inhibits the complement cascade [26]. The transmembrane ubiquitous protein CD46 (membrane cofactor protein or MCP) and Factor H (FH) both act as a cofactors for Factor I and therefore enhance C3 convertase downmodulation. CD55 (decay-activating factor, or DAF) is a glycosylphosphatidylinositol (GPI)-linked membrane protein that accelerates the dissociation of C3b from the C3 convertase, thus inhibiting the cascade. Other inhibitors, in particular membrane-bound GPI-linked protein CD59, inhibit the final steps of the cascade, i.e., the polymerization of C9 for MAC formation. C3b deposition and convertase formation are central regulated steps and do not necessarily lead to MAC formation, depending on the balance between the strength of initial activation and the level of inhibition by the regulators. This is why both C3b deposition (the first phase of complement activation) and the generation of soluble C5b-9 along with MAC binding to the cells (corresponding to the last phase: MAC formation on the cell membrane) are the parameters most commonly measured to identify the first and second phase of the cascade. On this basis, it should be clear that C9 polymerization generally correlates with effective cell lysis [30,32,33].

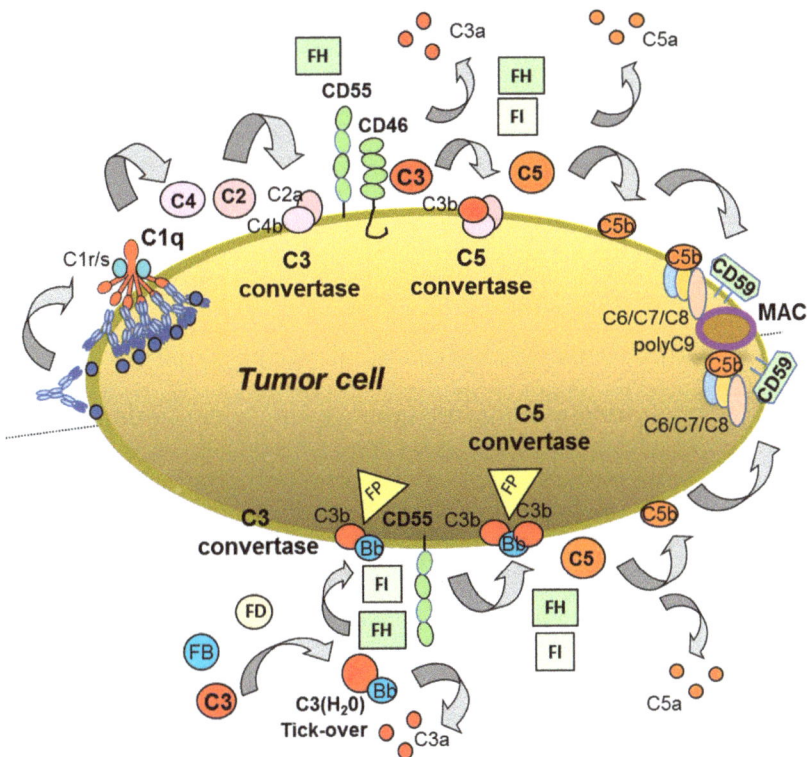

Figure 1. The classical and alternative complement pathways. The classical pathway (**top**): Human IgG1 antibodies bind antigen, form hexamers that allow C1q binding and the activation of the classical complement cascade. This is followed by C2 and C4 cleavage to produce the membrane bound C3 convertase (C4bC2a complex). Further cleavage of C3 to C3a and C3b forms the C5 convertase (C4bC2aC3b). C5 is cleaved to C5a and C5b allows further recruitment and activation of the C6, C7 and C8 components which catalyze C9 polymerization forming the membrane attack complex (MAC). The alternative pathway (**bottom**): it is initiated by tick-over activation of C3 in the fluid phase (C3(H$_2$O)). It is further activated by Factors B and D to form the alternative C3 convertase (C3bBb) which is stabilized by Properdin (FP, yellow triangle). Further C3 cleavage forms the C5 convertase (C3bBbC3b) (also stabilized by Properdin). The alternative pathway amplifies the classical pathway. Both pathways are inhibited by the soluble inhibitors Factor H (FH) and Factor I (FI) and by membrane bound inhibitors: CD46 and CD55 at the level of the C3 convertase and CD59, which inhibits C9 polymerization. Complement pathway inhibitors are shown in green.

3. The Interaction of Complement Components with Immune Cells

The complement cascade induced by an IgG1 mAb like rituximab may lead to the formation of the MAC and target cell lysis. However, complement is also at the center stage of a crosstalk with immune cells, and this crosstalk can be equally important to achieve immune-mediated elimination of tumor cells in vivo. For example, C3a and C5a are released following complement activation and are strong anaphylatoxins, thereby interacting with C3aR and C5aR1 (CD88) expressed on a variety of effector cells, including mast cells, macrophages, polymorphonuclear neutrophils (PMN), and dendritic cells (DCs). They can induce chemotaxis of the cells to the tumors and the generation of a profound pro-inflammatory state [26,34]. C3a and C5a also increase the permeability of small blood vessels through this inflammatory reaction and facilitate immune cell recruitment to sites of complement activation [35]. Immune cells express several different receptors for the cell-bound complement fragments—in particular, C3b and its degradation products iC3b and C3d(g)—as well as C4b and C1q. Several of these receptors, such as cC1qR (collagen C1q receptor), CR1 (complement receptor 1, CD35), CR3 (complement receptor 3, CD11b/CD18), and CRIg (complement receptor of the immunoglobulin superfamily), are implicated in the activation of macrophages and neutrophils and also function as mediators of phagocytosis and ADCC of opsonized target cells. These complex interactions are nicely reviewed by Lukacsi et al. [36]. Thus, macrophages can mediate phagocytosis of targets through both FcγRs and CRs, and the potential synergy in this process was recognized long ago [5,37–41]. DCs also express receptors for complement fragments such as C3a and C5a, and signaling through these receptors increase major histocompatibility complex (MHC) expression, antigen internalization, and antigen presentation. Complement factors also modulate T cell responses directly through CR1, CR2 (complement receptor 2, CD21), C1q, C3aR, and C5aRs receptors [42,43]. The multiple role of complement and complement receptors expressed by immune cells are summarized in Figure 2.

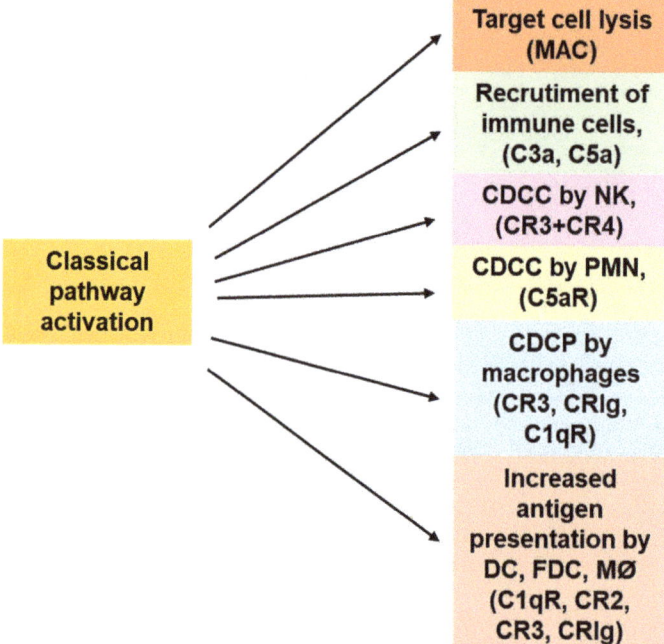

Figure 2. Multiple possible roles of complement for tumor control by IgG1 MAbs. Complement activation leads to complement mediated cell lysis but also to recruitment and activation of immune cells through complement fragments and their receptors which amplify the Fc-mediated ADCC and ADCP of IgG1 antibodies. CDCC: Complement dependent cellular cytotoxicity; CDCP: Complement dependent cellular phagocytosis; DC: dendritic cell; FDC: Follicular dendritic cells, MAC: membrane attack complex. MØ: macrophages; PMN: polymorphonuclear neutrophil; C1qR: C1q receptor, CR2, CR3, CR4, and CRIg: Receptors for complement fragments.

4. Main Factors Affecting Complement Activation by IgG1 Anti-Tumor Antibodies

4.1. Antigen Density and Hexamerization

The need for IgG1 hexamerization to allow for most effective chelation of hexavalent C1q and robust activation of the classical complement pathway explains why some mAbs activate complement efficiently and others do not, since the capacity to form hexamers depends on the density of the antigen on the surface, the capacity of the antibody to cluster multiple copies of the antigen, the specific orientation of the bound antibody molecules with each other, the closeness of the epitope to the cell membrane, and the specific epitope recognized [24,44–47]. For example, different anti-CD20 antibodies vary in their capacity to activate complement, with ofatumumab being the most effective, followed by rituximab [48,49] (both so-called type I anti-CD20 antibodies). Ofatumumab binds to CD20 at a site closer to the cell membrane, thus allowing for more efficient C1q binding and deposition of nascently activated C4b and C3b on the cell, and it is well-established that, for a variety of substrate cells, substantially more CDC is mediated by ofatumumab than by rituximab [48–50]. In contrast, obinutuzumab is only a weak complement activator [11,50] (a type II antibody). Rituximab and ofatumumab, but not obinutuzumab, are capable of relocating CD20 into lipid rafts, concentrating the antigen to small regions of the membrane, which will favor hexamerization of the antibody. In fact, the capacity of different anti-CD20 mAbs to translocate CD20 to lipid rafts correlates with their efficiency at inducing CDC [47,51]. CDC also correlates with the capacity of anti-CD20 or other antibodies to form hexamers.

Recently cryogenic electron microscopy and crystal structure studies of different anti-CD20 mAbs bound to purified CD20 or CD20 peptides have allowed for the precise analysis of the structure of type I and II anti-CD20 mAbs and their orientation with respect to CD20 itself and to adjacent antibody molecules [52–54]. CD20 forms a dimer rather than a tetramer as previously suggested and the studies show that each CD20 dimer binds 2 rituximab or ofatumumab Fabs (2:2 stoichiometry) but only one obinutuzumab Fab (2:1 stoichiometry), fully confirming the known binding behavior of these antibodies identified by flow cytometry. These studies altogether suggest that the epitope recognized by rituximab is more extended than previously thought and in part overlaps with that of ofatumumab. Furthermore the orientation of binding of the different mAbs to CD20 are distinct so that that rituximab and ofatumumab binding rapidly leads to CD20 concatenation and hexamerization of the mAbs on the cell surface, appropriate for C1q binding [52,53]. In contrast, obinutuzumab Fabs bind CD20 with a 2:1 stoichiometry (CD20:Fab) due to the steric hindrance between the 2 Fabs. This different orientation and steric hindrance explain its decreased ability to form hexamers and therefore to activate complement [52]. These studies nicely show how the specific epitope recognition of different mAbs can lead to different binding orientations, inter-molecular interactions, and structural constrictions that, in turn, lead to quite different capacities to activate complement, even if the mAbs are directed against the same antigen (CD20) and bind partially overlapping epitopes [47,51,54]. Thus, even though distance of the epitopes from the membrane, as well as antibody affinity, may affect CDC as well as ADCC/ADCP [55], recent data suggest that major role intermolecular interactions and the capacity of the mAbs to form hexamers are major determinants for CDC.

Similarly, among a panel of anti-CD38 antibodies, only daratumumab was found to be a potent complement activator, although the epitope recognized by daratumumab overlaps with that of other antibodies that are poor activators, suggesting that, in this case, the specific orientation of daratumumab may allow for more efficient hexamerization [21,56]. Fc mutations that favor hexamerization of antibodies targeting EGFR, CD38, or CD37 can render them strong effectors through CDC [24,25,44,45,57,58] and are being developed for clinical use [59,60].

The need for antibody clustering and hexamerization explains why the level of expression of antigen on the target cell membrane at least in part determines whether specific mAbs will be able to efficiently activate complement and lead to CDC. There is indeed a threshold level of CD20 required to allow for robust complement activation, sufficient to lead to high levels of activation of C3 followed by adequate activation of C5, thus leading to efficient downstream MAC deposition and cell lysis [4,29,61–63]. Indeed, CLL cells are less sensitive to CDC mediated by rituximab than most B-NHL cells that may express 10-fold higher levels of CD20 on their surfaces [63]. This rather low level of complement-mediated lysis of CLL cells in vitro by rituximab is increased considerably when using ofatumumab, in agreement with the higher capacity of the latter antibody to activate complement. Nonetheless, ofatumumab-mediated CDC is still antigen density dependent [62,64].

4.2. Membrane and Soluble Complement Inhibitors

CDC induced by IgG1 mAbs is also regulated by both membrane and soluble complement inhibitors that protect normal cells and tissues from complement. Cancer cells are known to express, and sometimes overexpress, the membrane complement inhibitor proteins CD46, CD55, and CD59 [33]. CD55 and CD59 have been shown to substantially inhibit the complement cascade in vitro, induced by rituximab and ofatumumab, reducing MAC binding and subsequent CDC [63–72]. Targeting the third short consensus repeat (SCR3) of CD55 with antibodies or small molecules appears to be required for CDC enhancement [73]. CD55 and CD59 activities are species-specific, explaining why the complement of some species like guinea pig are hyperactive against human cells [74]. CD55 and CD59 act synergistically to protect cells so that blocking both molecules simultaneously generally leads to the best enhancement of CDC [63,65,75]. The cooperation between CD55 and CD59 is explained by the different steps in the complement cascade that these two molecules inhibit (Figure 1).

Overexpression of CD55/CD59 also downmodulates complement-mediated lysis induced by other therapeutic IgG mAbs, such as trastuzumab in HER2-overexpressing carcinoma cell lines [76–78]. Blocking CD55 and in particular CD59 increased in vitro CDC of acute lymphoblastic leukemia, MM, and sarcoma cells induced by alemtuzumab, daratumumab, rituximab, and anti-CD24, respectively [79–81].

Whether CD55 and/or CD59 play a role in protecting cancer cells from mAb-mediated CDC in vivo is not completely clear. Increased CD55/CD59 expression was observed on cell lines selected in vitro for resistance to rituximab and complement [82]. Inhibiting CD55 and CD59 has also been shown to enhance the activity of rituximab in mouse xenograft models [83,84]. However, Williams et al. reported that CLL cells that persisted in the circulation after infusion of large amounts of rituximab had reduced levels of CD55 and CD59 due to "innocent bystander" loss of these membrane-associated proteins induced by trogocytosis of nearby CD20 [85]. As a result of the loss of CD20, these cells are resistant to rituximab-mediated complement activation, but this is clearly not due to CD55 and or CD59 up-regulation.

In contrast to CD55/CD59, there is little evidence, using antibodies, that blocking CD46 alone has any effect on IgG1 triggered CDC [86]. However, the lack of effect of anti-CD46 mAbs may be due to incomplete functional block of the protein, since an adenovirus-derived recombinant ligand of CD46, called Ad35K++, which induces cross-linking and internalization of the molecule, also significantly increased rituximab efficacy in vitro and in vivo in mouse and monkey studies [87]. These data indeed provide considerable evidence that CD46, like CD55 and CD59, modulates the efficacy of at least some IgG1 therapeutic antibodies [88].

As already mentioned above, soluble FI and FH function as inhibitors of the classical complement cascade and of the alternative pathway amplification loop by accelerating the dissociation of the C3 convertases as well as proteolytically inactivating C3b and C4b (Figure 1). FH has been shown to diminish the efficacy of ofatumumab-mediated CDC of CLL cells in vitro [89,90]. FH inhibition also enhances CDC of a subset of CLL samples and cooperates with anti-CD59 [91]. Membrane protein sialylation also inhibits complement at least in part by promoting binding of FH [92] and this has been suggested as an additional mechanism of resistance of CLL cells to anti-CD20 mediated lysis. That is, due to substantial α2-6 sialyl transferase activity, high levels of surface sialic acid are expressed on the cells, leading to binding of the complement inhibitor FH and subsequent downmodulation of complement activation [93]. FH also binds to cell surfaces and to apoptotic cells by recognition of other molecules, such as extracellular matrix proteins, DNA, soluble pattern recognition molecules, etc., thereby protecting them from complement attack [94]. With respect to FI, Lindorfer et al. reported that blocking its action increases CDC of CLL cells mediated by rituximab or ofatumumab [95]. The possible use of FI inhibition to enhance anti-tumor antibody activity is vivo is still unknown but of obvious interest.

It is clear that manipulation of the complement cascade, through the design of anti-tumor mAbs with increased ability to activate complement [44,59,96], or with mAbs that hyperactivate the complement cascade [97] or block soluble or membrane bound inhibitors [63,84,91], may all be feasible strategies to enhance the CDC activity of mAbs for cancer immunotherapy. However, there is still the need for the demonstration that each of these strategies has efficacy in vivo.

5. The Role of Complement in the Therapeutic Activity of Anti-Tumor mAbs

5.1. Studies In Vitro and in Animal Models

The importance of complement activation by unconjugated IgG1 mAbs in contributing to the anti-tumor response in vivo has been the subject of a considerable series of investigations, even for rituximab, which has been the most studied therapeutic mAb [2,4,98]. The fact that most approved IgG1 mAbs are able to activate complement upon binding to target cells suggested a positive role for complement in tumor control. Indeed rituximab [63,65], ofatumumab [48,62,70], alemtuzumab [22], daratumumab [21], trastuzumab [77], and cetuximab [99] have all been reported to activate complement in vitro, albeit with highly variable efficacy. However, other mAbs, such as isatuzumab and obinutuzumab as well as others, are effective in vivo even though they are poor complement activators [100–102].

Most anti-tumor IgG1 mAbs have also been demonstrated to promote ADCC and ADCP (Table 1). FcγR and cell-dependent mechanisms, ADCP in particular, have been clearly and consistently shown to be crucial for efficacy in most animal tumor models [11,103–105]. Murine models are, in contrast, rather discordant with regard to the role of complement in vivo for complement activating mAbs like rituximab. Some models suggest a role of complement in vivo in murine syngeneic models in which C3 knock down or complement depletion by cobra venom factor diminished or abolished the therapeutic efficacy of rituximab [2,106,107] or cetuximab [99]. However, other studies did not confirm this finding in different models [108]. Rather, most murine models suggest that FcγRs and myeloid cells are required and suggest a strong role of ADCP in the mechanism of action of many unconjugated mAbs, including rituximab, ofatumumab, obinutuzumab, cetuximab, trastuzumab, and daratumumab [11,103,108–113], as reviewed by Stevenson [114]. Some data that may reconcile some of the above-mentioned contrasting results indicate that the complement requirement for anti-CD20 activity in vivo may differ according to CD20 expression levels and tumor burden [109,115–118]. Furthermore, immune cells, including macrophages, PMN, T cells, NK cells, and dendritic cells express complement receptors, and some of these molecules participate in complement dependent cellular cytotoxicity (CDCC) or complement dependent phagocytosis (CDCP) (Figure 2) [119]. In other words, NK cells and macrophages recognize tumor-cell-associated complement fragments—in particular C3b, iC3b, and C3d and mediate cytotoxicity or phagocytosis [36]. Thus, complement may control tumor growth directly through CDC or indirectly through CDCC and CDCP as well as through the chemotaxis and activation of immune cells by C3a and C5a. These reactions may eliminate the tumor cells through either FcγRs or complement receptors or both. In support of this concept are studies of mutant anti-CD20 antibodies able to activate complement but unable to bind to FcγRs, which indicate that CDCC by NK cells and CDCP by macrophages does play a role in vitro and in vivo in a murine immunocompetent model [120]. Similarly, an immunodeficient NOD scid gamma (NSG) mouse model with active complement suggests a contribution of both complement and immune cells for tumor control by rituximab [121]. Such interactions between complement and immune cells may also explain the need for both in some in vivo models, such as the BJAB xenograft model treated with rituximab [122] and in the syngeneic EL4-CD20 model [123]. Similar cross-talk has been shown for other antibodies such as cetuximab [9] and a complement optimized anti-EGFR mAb was found to induce enhanced ADCC by PMNs [124].

Deposition of C3 fragments on B cells mediated by rituximab may have unexpected negative consequences. In a series of provocative papers, Weiner et al. reported that NK-cell-mediated killing (ADCC) of rituximab-opsonized B cells is substantially reduced if complement is activated; their results suggest that the deposited C3 fragments sterically hinder interaction of NK cell FcγRIII (CD16) with the Fc region of cell-bound rituximab. Moreover, this "problem" does not occur when obinutuzumab is examined, most likely because it poorly activates complement and C3b deposition is low and/or because it has higher affinity for FcγRIII [125,126]. Thus, complement activation may in some circumstances antagonize ADCC.

Several groups have shown that antibodies can induce a vaccinal effect; in particular, anti-CD20 mAbs induce presentation of tumor antigens (e.g., mutant proteins or aberrantly expressed differentitation antigens) to T cells by DCs [127,128]. Whereas DC antigen uptake for a vaccine effect has been shown to be mediated by FcγRs [129], complement components could also play a role, since DCs express several complement receptors [36]. However, the physiological significance of these observations is unclear; in particular, there is virtually no evidence that ofatumumab or rituximab treatment in humans promotes an immune response to either malignant or normal B cells. Furthermore the expression of complement receptors on different immune cell types including DCs is not identical between mice and men, making the study of the relevance of a possible vaccine effect via these molecules even more difficult [130].

Anti-CD38 daratumumab is an example of another mAb that eliminates tumor cells based on multiple mechanisms of action, including complement, which may synergize with each other for maximal antibody efficacy in vivo. Daratumumab, similar to rituximab, induces CDC, ADCC, and ADCP in vitro. Moreover CDC, as well as ADCC in vitro, correlates with CD38 expression levels on MM cells and is enhanced by antibodies blocking CD55 and CD59 [21,110,131]. Daratumumab and isatuximab have also been reported to deplete CD38$^+$ immune regulatory cells, such as Treg, Breg, and myeloid derived suppressor cells (MDSCs) in vitro and in vivo [132,133]. We suggest that these activities may reflect, in part, daratumumab mediated "trogocytosis" of CD38 (i.e., the transfer of the target molecule, CD38, together with bound antibody from the tumor cell to phagocytes mediated by FcγRs on the acceptor cells), and so the issue may be more complex [132,134]. Finally anti-CD38 mAbs inhibit the CD38 ectoenzyme activity [135], thus diminishing immunosuppressive adenosine production. Thus the multiple effects of anti-CD38 antibodies, including daratumumab, probably all contribute to their efficacy in vivo and CDC may be dispensable in some cases [100].

5.2. Ex Vivo and In Vivo Human Studies

The major caveat of studies in mice is that both complement and FcγRs differ considerably between mice and humans, and some complement inhibitory proteins are species specific, so that the relative roles of CDC, ADCC, and ADCP in mice may not fully recapitulate the human situation [74,136]. For this reason, some groups have attempted to measure the role of complement and immune cells in human whole blood assays, which may at least better reflect what takes place in the circulation immediately after mAb infusion in patients [50,64,137]. The best compounds to block coagulation in these assays are hirudin and its derivatives, since these molecules block thrombin activation but do not affect the complement cascade, unlike most other anticoagulants [50,64,119]. With such assays, it was possible to show that the most effective short-term depletion of neoplastic B cells in whole blood by rituximab and ofatumumab, but not obinutuzumab, requires complement and can be blocked by anti-C5 eculizumab [50,64]. These data suggest that, at least in the circulation in humans, the first mechanism of rituximab and ofatumumab for B depletion is via CDC. These in vitro assays have limitations, since they do not fully model the flowing circulation along blood vessels and the effects of mAbs beyond 24 h of treatment.

Analyses of blood samples have been performed in patients treated with therapeutic IgG1 mAbs. Rapid complement activation with deposition of C3b and iC3b on the CLL cell membrane has been demonstrated very soon after rituximab and ofatumumab infusion [138,139]. The opsonized cells can then be effectively removed from the circulation by fixed tissue macrophages that have receptors for cell-bound IgG and C3 fragments, as first demonstrated for other substrates almost 50 years ago [37,40,41]. C5a production, as well as consumption of complement components with exhaustion of rate limiting factors, in particular C2 and C4, has been observed following rituximab or ofatumumab infusion in patients with CLL [138–143]. These data clearly show that complement is rapidly activated, and the results are consistent with the whole blood assays. Some investigators have also observed a correlation between CDC in vitro and response of CLL patients to rituximab in vivo, in support of a role of complement in vivo in humans, either directly or indirectly, by enhancing cell-mediated mechanisms [93]. Similarly, Manches et al. found a correlation between differential sensitivities of B cell lymphoma subtypes to rituximab-mediated CDC in vitro and clinical responses to rituximab. They found that lymphomas in which the patients' primary B cells were highly sensitive to CDC (e.g., follicular lymphoma cells) showed overall a better clinical response to rituximab therapy than in neoplasias in which the B cells (CLL cells) were only weakly killed by rituximab-mediated CDC [144].

Baig et al. first reported that alemtuzumab and ofatumumab could synergize in promoting CDC of CLL B cells, reaching close to quantitative killing of the cells. CDC was not at all correlated with levels of CD55 or CD59. They then isolated B cells from the bloodstream of CLL patients soon after they were treated with ofatumumab. These cells could not be killed in vitro by CDC upon addition of more ofatumumab because CD20 had been removed from the cells due to trogocytosis. However, the sensitivity of the cells to alemtuzumab-mediated CDC remained quite high, indicating that the CD52 epitope on the cells recognized by alemtuzumab was clearly still expressed at high levels, and that complement control proteins on the cells were not upregulated to provide protection against the alemtuzumab [141,145].

The demonstrated exhaustion of complement activity and of specific complement components after antibody infusion led to the suggestion that fresh frozen plasma could be used to replenish missing factors and overcome resistance due to complement exhaustion [138]. Fresh frozen plasma has been used in CLL patients treated with rituximab with some positive results [138,146–149]. Nonetheless the efficacy of such an approach may be limited by the downmodulation of CD20 expression that follows mAb infusion and take place mostly through trogocytosis of CD20, together with bound antibody from the tumor cell to phagocytes expressing FcγRs [134,150–154]. Trogocytosis has been shown to occur both in vitro and in vivo in CLL patients and is likely to be another mechanism of resistance to complement and cell-mediated cytotoxicity [85]. Thus, in vivo, exhaustion of effector mechanisms, including complement and effector cells such as NK and macrophages, as well as loss of target antigen by trogocytosis or internalization, can limit the efficacy of anti-tumor mAbs [18,134,139,152,155,156].

Several analyses of polymorphic elements associated with complement related genes in relation to the clinical response of follicular lymphoma and diffuse large B cell lymphoma patients treated with rituximab have been conducted, but the results have not offered clear-cut answers about the role of complement in the efficacy of this antibody [157–159].

With regard to complement inhibitors, in particular CD55 and CD59, several studies have attempted to determine whether high expression levels of these proteins correlated with resistance or with relapse after mAb treatment. Although some correlations have been found in cases of lymphoma patients treated with rituximab and chemotherapy [160,161], this has not been confirmed in other studies [162], even with rituximab used as monotherapy [163]. A correlation between CD55 and CD59 expression and response of breast cancer patients to trastuzumab has been suggested [164]. Interestingly, in MM patients who progressed after daratumumab treatment, their malignant plasma cells had elevated levels of CD55 and CD59, but not of CD46, suggesting that resistance to daratumumab in vivo may be related at least in part to resistance to CDC [80]. In conclusion, the data derived from clinical correlation studies suggest that in some patients, complement may play a role in antibody therapy, but clearly, due to the multiple mechanisms of therapeutic antibodies, there are no clear-cut answers about the role of complement in vivo.

Another clue about the role of complement may come from the results of the clinical investigations with anti-CD20 mAbs and patient CLL cells, which show very different capacities to activate complement in vitro. For example, as noted above, ofatumumab is much more effective than rituximab in mediating CDC of CLL cells, and it is noteworthy that ofatumumab (but not rituximab) was approved as a single agent for the treatment of CLL [165]. On the other hand, obinuzutumab is ineffective as measured by CDC, but it is much more effective in killing CLL cells by other mechanisms and was also approved as a single agent for CLL [47].

It should thus be clear that comparison of these three mAbs is made difficult by the fact they have mechanisms of action independent of complement, and most investigations have not been performed as head-to-head comparisons. In some cases, the studies that have compared obinutuzumab with rituximab have shown a significant advantage of the former, particularly in CLL in combination with chlorambucil [166,167]. In other B-NHL types, the advantage of obinutuzumab has not been consistently demonstrated (reviewed by Pierpont [6]). In addition, the phase III clinical trials comparing obinutuzumab with rituximab have used higher doses and a different schedule of obinutuzumab, making rigorous comparison more difficult. There have also been few direct comparisons between ofatumumab and rituximab in the clinic [168]. Overall, ofatumumab seems to induce similar response rates as rituximab in B-NHL [6]. Therefore, one can conclude that the three anti-CD20 antibodies used for B-NHL and CLL treatment along with chemotherapy do not show greatly different efficacies in vivo, at least not such differences as were hoped for when they were selected and developed on the basis of their higher efficacy or different mechanisms of action in vitro [169,170]. These conclusions support the idea that the ultimate mechanisms are multifaceted, that combinations of mechanisms probably work, and some may predominate more than others in different patients, also depending upon the sites in which the tumors are targeted. Furthermore, exhaustion of most of the involved mechanisms has been shown in vivo, including complement and cell-mediated cytotoxic mechanisms [138,171], as well as down modulation of target antigen through trogocytosis [134]. This means that an antibody with a greater CDC or ADCC potential in vitro may in any case be limited in vivo by these mechanisms [2,141,172].

6. Conclusions and Future Perspective

Unconjugated IgG1 anti-tumor mAbs often show a variety of mechanisms of action that may operate simultaneously and interact with each other: neutralization of the target antigen/receptor, activation of cell-mediated cytotoxicity, and complement activation. More recent evidence suggests that these mechanisms probably interact with each other, either positively or negatively. In particular, evidence suggests that complement factors and receptors synergize to enhance ADCC and ADCP. Complement fragments may also affect T-cell-mediated immunity by interaction with DCs and T cells, perhaps explaining the delayed or long-term effects of antibody treatment that has been suggested in some cases [173]. Also, the direct effects of the mAbs can, in some cases, synergize with immune-mediated mechanisms, as is the case for NK activation by anti-SLAMF7 mAb elotuzumab [174] or the T-cell-activating effect of anti-CD38 mAbs [100]. Given this plethora of activities and interactions, understanding the relative contribution of each of the potential mechanisms of action of IgG1 therapeutic mAbs is difficult to clearly establish and remains unsolved even for the best-known mAbs. In particular, a substantial literature of in vitro studies and in vivo correlations cited in this review strongly support (but do not prove) the importance of complement in the action of several anti-tumor mAbs. These observations and the finding that exhaustion mechanisms may limit efficacy should, in our view, lead to development of optimized schedules/combination treatments in the clinic, including combination with cell therapy approaches, as well as optimized mAbs capable of multiple effector functions. The latter is becoming possible thanks to a better understanding of mutations or modifications that may enhance different mechanisms (CDC, ADCC, ADCP) and perhaps abolish the negative interference that is sometimes observed between these effects or through the use of mAb combinations that may be specifically favorable for these mechanisms [175]. The effects of chemotherapy on the different mechanisms of unconjugated therapeutic IgG1 antibodies is another area of particular interest, and it will be important to identify the best drug combinations and schedules required to achieve synergy between small drug and mAb therapy. Indeed, chemotherapy may negatively affect the cell-mediated mechanisms of therapeutic mAbs, but could also potentially affect complement mediated mechanisms, if modulation of target antigen or of complement factors is induced by drug treatment [176,177]. A precise understanding of these interactions will therefore be needed for optimized treatments.

Funding: This work was funded by the "Associazione Italiana Ricerca contro il Cancro" (AIRC, Individual Grant to JG, n° IG19036, AIRC 5 × 1000 Grant "ISM"), the Fondazione Regionale per la Ricerca Biomedica (Regione Lombardia), project nr. 2015-0042 FRBB and the "Associazione Italiana control le Leucemie-linfomi e mieloma (AIL-sezione Paolo Belli, Bergamo).

Conflicts of Interest: The authors declare no conflict of interest.

References

1. Melis, J.P.; Strumane, K.; Ruuls, S.R.; Beurskens, F.J.; Schuurman, J.; Parren, P.W. Complement in therapy and disease: Regulating the complement system with antibody-based therapeutics. *Mol. Immunol.* **2015**, *67*, 117–130. [CrossRef] [PubMed]
2. Taylor, R.P.; Lindorfer, M.A. Cytotoxic mechanisms of immunotherapy: Harnessing complement in the action of anti-tumor monoclonal antibodies. *Semin. Immunol.* **2016**, *28*, 309–316. [CrossRef] [PubMed]
3. Weiner, G.J. Building better monoclonal antibody-based therapeutics. *Nat. Rev. Cancer* **2015**, *15*, 361–370. [CrossRef] [PubMed]
4. Golay, J. Direct targeting of cancer cells with antibodies: What can we learn from the successes and failure of unconjugated antibodies for lymphoid neoplasias? *J. Autoimmun.* **2017**, *85*, 6–19. [CrossRef] [PubMed]
5. Lindorfer, M.A.; Koehl, J.; Taylor, R.P. Interactions between the complement system and Fcgamma receptors. In *IgG Fc: Linking Adaptive and Innate Immunity*; Nimmerhahn, F., Ackerman, M.E., Eds.; Elsevier Press: Amsterdam, The Netherlands, 2013; pp. 49–74.
6. Pierpont, T.M.; Limper, C.B.; Richards, K.L. Past, Present, and Future of Rituximab-The World's First Oncology Monoclonal Antibody Therapy. *Front. Oncol.* **2018**, *8*, 163. [CrossRef] [PubMed]
7. Taylor, R.P.; Lindorfer, M.A. Immunotherapeutic mechanisms of anti-CD20 monoclonal antibodies. *Curr. Opin. Immunol.* **2008**, *20*, 444–449. [CrossRef] [PubMed]
8. Carter, P.J.; Lazar, G.A. Next generation antibody drugs: Pursuit of the 'high-hanging fruit'. *Nat. Rev. Drug Discov.* **2018**, *17*, 197–223. [CrossRef]
9. Garcia-Foncillas, J.; Sunakawa, Y.; Aderka, D.; Wainberg, Z.; Ronga, P.; Witzler, P.; Stintzing, S. Distinguishing Features of Cetuximab and Panitumumab in Colorectal Cancer and Other Solid Tumors. *Front. Oncol.* **2019**, *9*, 849. [CrossRef]
10. Hudis, C.A. Trastuzumab—Mechanism of action and use in clinical practice. *NEJM* **2007**, *357*, 39–51. [CrossRef]
11. Moessner, E.; Bruenker, P.; Moser, S.; Puentener, U.; Schmidt, C.; Herter, S.; Grau, R.; Gerdes, C.; Nopora, A.; van Puijenbroek, E.; et al. Increasing the efficacy of CD20 antibody therapy through the engineering of a new type II anti-CD20 with enhanced direct and immune effector cell-mediated B-cell cytotoxicity. *Blood* **2010**, *115*, 4393–4402. [CrossRef]
12. Jiang, H.; Acharya, C.; An, G.; Zhong, M.; Feng, X.; Wang, L.; Dasilva, N.; Song, Z.; Yang, G.; Adrian, F.; et al. SAR650984 directly induces multiple myeloma cell death via lysosomal-associated and apoptotic pathways, which is further enhanced by pomalidomide. *Leukemia* **2016**, *30*, 399–408. [CrossRef] [PubMed]
13. Lapalombella, R.; Yeh, Y.Y.; Wang, L.; Ramanunni, A.; Rafiq, S.; Jha, S.; Staubli, J.; Lucas, D.M.; Mani, R.; Herman, S.E.; et al. Tetraspanin CD37 directly mediates transduction of survival and apoptotic signals. *Cancer Cell* **2012**, *21*, 694–708. [CrossRef]
14. Plesner, T.; Krejcik, J. Daratumumab for the Treatment of Multiple Myeloma. *Front. Immunol.* **2018**, *9*, 1228. [CrossRef]

15. Musolino, A.; Boggiani, D.; Pellegrino, B.; Zanoni, D.; Sikokis, A.; Missale, G.; Silini, E.M.; Maglietta, G.; Frassoldati, A.; Michiara, M. Role of innate and adaptive immunity in the efficacy of anti-HER2 monoclonal antibodies for HER2-positive breast cancer. *Crit. Rev. Oncol./Hematol.* **2020**, *149*, 102927. [CrossRef]
16. Costa, D.; Vene, R.; Benelli, R.; Romairone, E.; Scabini, S.; Catellani, S.; Rebesco, B.; Mastracci, L.; Grillo, F.; Minghelli, S.; et al. Targeting the Epidermal Growth Factor Receptor Can Counteract the Inhibition of Natural Killer Cell Function Exerted by Colorectal Tumor-Associated Fibroblasts. *Front. Immunol.* **2018**, *9*, 1150. [CrossRef]
17. Ferris, R.L.; Jaffee, E.M.; Ferrone, S. Tumor antigen-targeted, monoclonal antibody-based immunotherapy: Clinical response, cellular immunity, and immunoescape. *J. Clin. Oncol.* **2010**, *28*, 4390–4399. [CrossRef] [PubMed]
18. Zent, C.S.; Elliott, M.R. Maxed out macs: Physiologic cell clearance as a function of macrophage phagocytic capacity. *FEBS J.* **2017**, *284*, 1021–1039. [CrossRef] [PubMed]
19. VanDerMeid, K.R.; Elliott, M.R.; Baran, A.M.; Barr, P.M.; Chu, C.C.; Zent, C.S. Cellular Cytotoxicity of Next-Generation CD20 Monoclonal Antibodies. *Cancer Immunol. Res.* **2018**, *6*, 1150–1160. [CrossRef]
20. Campbell, K.S.; Cohen, A.D.; Pazina, T. Mechanisms of NK Cell Activation and Clinical Activity of the Therapeutic SLAMF7 Antibody, Elotuzumab in Multiple Myeloma. *Front. Immunol.* **2018**, *9*, 2551. [CrossRef]
21. de Weers, M.; Tai, Y.T.; van der Veer, M.S.; Bakker, J.M.; Vink, T.; Jacobs, D.C.; Oomen, L.A.; Peipp, M.; Valerius, T.; Slootstra, J.W.; et al. Daratumumab, a novel therapeutic human CD38 monoclonal antibody, induces killing of multiple myeloma and other hematological tumors. *J. Immunol.* **2011**, *186*, 1840–1848. [CrossRef]
22. Zent, C.S.; Chen, J.B.; Kurten, R.C.; Kaushal, G.P.; Marie Lacy, H.; Schichman, S.A. Alemtuzumab (CAMPATH 1H) does not kill chronic lymphocytic leukemia cells in serum free medium. *Leuk. Res.* **2004**, *28*, 495–507. [CrossRef] [PubMed]
23. Golay, J.; Manganini, M.; Rambaldi, A.; Introna, M. Effect of alemtuzumab on neoplastic B cells. *Haematologica* **2004**, *89*, 1476–1483. [PubMed]
24. Diebolder, C.A.; Beurskens, F.J.; de Jong, R.N.; Koning, R.I.; Strumane, K.; Lindorfer, M.A.; Voorhorst, M.; Ugurlar, D.; Rosati, S.; Heck, A.J.; et al. Complement is activated by IgG hexamers assembled at the cell surface. *Science* **2014**, *343*, 1260–1263. [CrossRef]
25. Wang, G.; de Jong, R.N.; van den Bremer, E.T.; Beurskens, F.J.; Labrijn, A.F.; Ugurlar, D.; Gros, P.; Schuurman, J.; Parren, P.W.; Heck, A.J. Molecular Basis of Assembly and Activation of Complement Component C1 in Complex with Immunoglobulin G1 and Antigen. *Mol. Cell* **2016**, *63*, 135–145. [CrossRef] [PubMed]
26. Merle, N.S.; Church, S.E.; Fremeaux-Bacchi, V.; Roumenina, L.T. Complement System Part I—Molecular Mechanisms of Activation and Regulation. *Front. Immunol.* **2015**, *6*, 262. [CrossRef]
27. Goldberg, B.S.; Ackerman, M.E. Antibody-mediated complement activation in pathology and protection. *Immunol. Cell Biol.* **2020**, *98*, 305–317. [CrossRef] [PubMed]
28. Bordron, A.; Bagacean, C.; Tempescul, A.; Berthou, C.; Bettacchioli, E.; Hillion, S.; Renaudineau, Y. Complement System: A Neglected Pathway in Immunotherapy. *Clin. Rev. Allergy Immunol.* **2020**, *58*, 155–171. [CrossRef] [PubMed]
29. Lindorfer, M.A.; Cook, E.M.; Tupitza, J.C.; Zent, C.S.; Burack, R.; de Jong, R.N.; Beurskens, F.J.; Schuurman, J.; Parren, P.W.; Taylor, R.P. Real-time analysis of the detailed sequence of cellular events in mAb-mediated complement-dependent cytotoxicity of B-cell lines and of chronic lymphocytic leukemia B-cells. *Mol. Immunol.* **2016**, *70*, 13–23. [CrossRef]
30. Morgan, B.P.; Walters, D.; Serna, M.; Bubeck, D. Terminal complexes of the complement system: New structural insights and their relevance to function. *Immunol. Rev.* **2016**, *274*, 141–151. [CrossRef]
31. Reis, E.S.; Mastellos, D.C.; Ricklin, D.; Mantovani, A.; Lambris, J.D. Complement in cancer: Untangling an intricate relationship. *Nat. Rev. Immunol.* **2018**, *18*, 5–18. [CrossRef]
32. Merle, N.S.; Noe, R.; Halbwachs-Mecarelli, L.; Fremeaux-Bacchi, V.; Roumenina, L.T. Complement System Part II: Role in Immunity. *Front. Immunol.* **2015**, *6*, 257. [CrossRef] [PubMed]
33. Geller, A.; Yan, J. The Role of Membrane Bound Complement Regulatory Proteins in Tumor Development and Cancer Immunotherapy. *Front. Immunol.* **2019**, *10*, 1074. [CrossRef]
34. Laumonnier, Y.; Karsten, C.M.; Kohl, J. Novel insights into the expression pattern of anaphylatoxin receptors in mice and men. *Mol. Immunol.* **2017**, *89*, 44–58. [CrossRef] [PubMed]

35. Karsten, C.M.; Pandey, M.K.; Figge, J.; Kilchenstein, R.; Taylor, P.R.; Rosas, M.; McDonald, J.U.; Orr, S.J.; Berger, M.; Petzold, D.; et al. Anti-inflammatory activity of IgG1 mediated by Fc galactosylation and association of FcgammaRIIB and dectin-1. *Nat. Med.* **2012**, *18*, 1401–1406. [CrossRef]
36. Lukacsi, S.; Macsik-Valent, B.; Nagy-Balo, Z.; Kovacs, K.G.; Kliment, K.; Bajtay, Z.; Erdei, A. Utilization of complement receptors in immune cell-microbe interaction. *FEBS Lett.* **2020**, *594*, 2695–2713. [CrossRef]
37. Fries, L.F.; Siwik, S.A.; Malbran, A.; Frank, M.M. Phagocytosis of target particles bearing C3b-IgG covalent complexes by human monocytes and polymorphonuclear leucocytes. *Immunology* **1987**, *62*, 45–51. [PubMed]
38. Brown, E.J.; Joiner, K.A.; Cole, R.M.; Berger, M. Localization of complement component 3 on Streptococcus pneumoniae: Anti-capsular antibody causes complement deposition on the pneumococcal capsule. *Infect. Immun.* **1983**, *39*, 403–409. [CrossRef]
39. Ehlenberger, A.G.; Nussenzweig, V. The role of membrane receptors for C3b and C3d in phagocytosis. *J. Exp. Med.* **1977**, *145*, 357–371. [CrossRef]
40. Schreiber, A.D.; Frank, M.M. Role of antibody and complement in the immune clearance and destruction of erythrocytes. I. In vivo effects of IgG and IgM complement-fixing sites. *J. Clin. Investig.* **1972**, *51*, 575–582. [CrossRef]
41. Atkinson, J.P.; Frank, M.M. Studies on the in vivo effects of antibody. Interaction of IgM antibody and complement in the immune clearance and destruction of erythrocytes in man. *J. Clin. Investig.* **1974**, *54*, 339–348. [CrossRef]
42. Zaal, A.; van Ham, S.M.; Ten Brinke, A. Differential effects of anaphylatoxin C5a on antigen presenting cells, roles for C5aR1 and C5aR2. *Immunol. Lett.* **2019**, *209*, 45–52. [CrossRef] [PubMed]
43. Wang, Y.; Zhang, H.; He, Y.W. The Complement Receptors C3aR and C5aR Are a New Class of Immune Checkpoint Receptor in Cancer Immunotherapy. *Front. Immunol.* **2019**, *10*, 1574. [CrossRef]
44. Tammen, A.; Derer, S.; Schwanbeck, R.; Rosner, T.; Kretschmer, A.; Beurskens, F.J.; Schuurman, J.; Parren, P.W.; Valerius, T. Monoclonal Antibodies against Epidermal Growth Factor Receptor Acquire an Ability To Kill Tumor Cells through Complement Activation by Mutations That Selectively Facilitate the Hexamerization of IgG on Opsonized Cells. *J. Immunol.* **2017**, *198*, 1585–1594. [CrossRef] [PubMed]
45. Cook, E.M.; Lindorfer, M.A.; van der Horst, H.; Oostindie, S.; Beurskens, F.J.; Schuurman, J.; Zent, C.S.; Burack, R.; Parren, P.W.; Taylor, R.P. Antibodies That Efficiently Form Hexamers upon Antigen Binding Can Induce Complement-Dependent Cytotoxicity under Complement-Limiting Conditions. *J. Immunol.* **2016**, *197*, 1762–1775. [CrossRef] [PubMed]
46. Taylor, R.P.; Lindorfer, M.A.; Cook, E.M.; Beurskens, F.J.; Schuurman, J.; Parren, P.; Zent, C.S.; VanDerMeid, K.R.; Burack, R.; Mizuno, M.; et al. Hexamerization-enhanced CD20 antibody mediates complement-dependent cytotoxicity in serum genetically deficient in C9. *Clin. Immunol.* **2017**, *181*, 24–28. [CrossRef]
47. Marshall, M.J.E.; Stopforth, R.J.; Cragg, M.S. Therapeutic Antibodies: What Have We Learnt from Targeting CD20 and Where Are We Going? *Front. Immunol.* **2017**, *8*, 1245. [CrossRef] [PubMed]
48. Teeling, J.L.; French, R.R.; Cragg, M.S.; van den Brakel, J.; Pluyter, M.; Huang, H.; Chan, C.; Parren, P.W.; Hack, C.E.; Dechant, M.; et al. Characterization of new human CD20 monoclonal antibodies with potent cytolytic activity against non-Hodgkin lymphomas. *Blood* **2004**, *104*, 1793–1800. [CrossRef]
49. Pawluczkowycz, A.W.; Beurskens, F.J.; Beum, P.V.; Lindorfer, M.A.; van de Winkel, J.G.; Parren, P.W.; Taylor, R.P. Binding of submaximal C1q promotes complement-dependent cytotoxicity (CDC) of B cells opsonized with anti-CD20 mAbs ofatumumab (OFA) or rituximab (RTX): Considerably higher levels of CDC are induced by OFA than by RTX. *J. Immunol.* **2009**, *183*, 749–758. [CrossRef]
50. Bologna, L.; Gotti, E.; Manganini, M.; Rambaldi, A.; Intermesoli, T.; Introna, M.; Golay, J. Mechanism of action of type II, glycoengineered, anti-CD20 monoclonal antibody GA101 in B-chronic lymphocytic leukemia whole blood assays in comparison with rituximab and alemtuzumab. *J. Immunol.* **2011**, *186*, 3762–3769. [CrossRef]
51. Cragg, M.S.; Morgan, S.M.; Chan, H.T.; Morgan, B.P.; Filatov, A.V.; Johnson, P.W.; French, R.R.; Glennie, M.J. Complement-mediated lysis by anti-CD20 mAb correlates with segregation into lipid rafts. *Blood* **2003**, *101*, 1045–1052. [CrossRef]
52. Rouge, L.; Chiang, N.; Steffek, M.; Kugel, C.; Croll, T.I.; Tam, C.; Estevez, A.; Arthur, C.P.; Koth, C.M.; Ciferri, C.; et al. Structure of CD20 in complex with the therapeutic monoclonal antibody rituximab. *Science* **2020**, *367*, 1224–1230. [CrossRef] [PubMed]

53. Kumar, A.; Planchais, C.; Fronzes, R.; Mouquet, H.; Reyes, N. Binding mechanisms of therapeutic antibodies to human CD20. *Science* **2020**, *369*, 793–799. [CrossRef]
54. Niederfellner, G.; Lammens, A.; Mundigl, O.; Georges, G.J.; Schaefer, W.; Schwaiger, M.; Franke, A.; Wiechmann, K.; Jenewein, S.; Slootstra, J.W.; et al. Epitope characterization and crystal structure of GA101 provide insights into the molecular basis for type I/II distinction of CD20 antibodies. *Blood* **2010**, *118*, 358–367. [CrossRef] [PubMed]
55. Cleary, K.L.S.; Chan, H.T.C.; James, S.; Glennie, M.J.; Cragg, M.S. Antibody Distance from the Cell Membrane Regulates Antibody Effector Mechanisms. *J. Immunol.* **2017**, *198*, 3999–4011. [CrossRef] [PubMed]
56. Beum, P.V.; Lindorfer, M.A.; Peek, E.M.; Stukenberg, P.T.; de Weers, M.; Beurskens, F.J.; Parren, P.W.; van de Winkel, J.G.; Taylor, R.P. Penetration of antibody-opsonized cells by the membrane attack complex of complement promotes Ca(2+) influx and induces streamers. *Eur. J. Immunol.* **2011**, *41*, 2436–2446. [CrossRef]
57. de Jong, R.N.; Beurskens, F.J.; Verploegen, S.; Strumane, K.; van Kampen, M.D.; Voorhorst, M.; Horstman, W.; Engelberts, P.J.; Oostindie, S.C.; Wang, G.; et al. A Novel Platform for the Potentiation of Therapeutic Antibodies Based on Antigen-Dependent Formation of IgG Hexamers at the Cell Surface. *PLoS Biol.* **2016**, *14*, e1002344. [CrossRef]
58. Schutze, K.; Petry, K.; Hambach, J.; Schuster, N.; Fumey, W.; Schriewer, L.; Rockendorf, J.; Menzel, S.; Albrecht, B.; Haag, F.; et al. CD38-Specific Biparatopic Heavy Chain Antibodies Display Potent Complement-Dependent Cytotoxicity Against Multiple Myeloma Cells. *Front. Immunol.* **2018**, *9*, 2553. [CrossRef]
59. Oostindie, S.C.; van der Horst, H.J.; Kil, L.P.; Strumane, K.; Overdijk, M.B.; van den Brink, E.N.; van den Brakel, J.H.N.; Rademaker, H.J.; van Kessel, B.; van den Noort, J.; et al. DuoHexaBody-CD37((R)), a novel biparatopic CD37 antibody with enhanced Fc-mediated hexamerization as a potential therapy for B-cell malignancies. *Blood Cancer J.* **2020**, *10*, 30. [CrossRef]
60. Gulati, S.; Beurskens, F.J.; de Kreuk, B.J.; Roza, M.; Zheng, B.; DeOliveira, R.B.; Shaughnessy, J.; Nowak, N.A.; Taylor, R.P.; Botto, M.; et al. Complement alone drives efficacy of a chimeric antigonococcal monoclonal antibody. *PLoS Biol.* **2019**, *17*, e3000323. [CrossRef]
61. van Meerten, T.; van Rijn, R.S.; Hol, S.; Hagenbeek, A.; Ebeling, S.B. Complement-induced cell death by rituximab depends on CD20 expression level and acts complementary to antibody-dependent cellular cytotoxicity. *Clin. Cancer Res.* **2006**, *12*, 4027–4035. [CrossRef]
62. van Meerten, T.; Rozemuller, H.; Hol, S.; Moerer, P.; Zwart, M.; Hagenbeek, A.; Mackus, W.J.; Parren, P.W.; van de Winkel, J.G.; Ebeling, S.B.; et al. HuMab-7D8, a monoclonal antibody directed against the membrane-proximal small loop epitope of CD20 can effectively eliminate CD20 low expressing tumor cells that resist rituximab-mediated lysis. *Haematologica* **2010**, *95*, 2063–2071. [CrossRef]
63. Golay, J.; Lazzari, M.; Facchinetti, V.; Bernasconi, S.; Borleri, G.; Barbui, T.; Rambaldi, A.; Introna, M. CD20 levels determine the in vitro susceptibility to rituximab and complement of B-cell chronic lymphocytic leukemia: Further regulation by CD55 and CD59. *Blood* **2001**, *98*, 3383–3389. [CrossRef] [PubMed]
64. Bologna, L.; Gotti, E.; Da Roit, F.; Intermesoli, T.; Rambaldi, A.; Introna, M.; Golay, J. Ofatumumab is more efficient than rituximab in lysing B chronic lymphocytic leukemia cells in whole blood and in combination with chemotherapy. *J. Immunol.* **2013**, *190*, 231–239. [CrossRef] [PubMed]
65. Golay, J.; Zaffaroni, L.; Vaccari, T.; Lazzari, M.; Borleri, G.M.; Bernasconi, S.; Tedesco, F.; Rambaldi, A.; Introna, M. Biologic response of B lymphoma cells to anti-CD20 monoclonal antibody rituximab in vitro: CD55 and CD59 regulate complement-mediated cell lysis. *Blood* **2000**, *95*, 3900–3908. [CrossRef]
66. Sebejova, L.; Borsky, M.; Jaskova, Z.; Potesil, D.; Navrkalova, V.; Malcikova, J.; Sramek, M.; Doubek, M.; Loja, T.; Pospisilova, S.; et al. Distinct in vitro sensitivity of p53-mutated and ATM-mutated chronic lymphocytic leukemia cells to ofatumumab and rituximab. *Exp. Hematol.* **2014**, *42*, 867–874.e861. [CrossRef] [PubMed]
67. Terui, Y.; Sakurai, T.; Mishima, Y.; Mishima, Y.; Sugimura, N.; Sasaoka, C.; Kojima, K.; Yokoyama, M.; Mizunuma, N.; Takahashi, S.; et al. Blockade of bulky lymphoma-associated CD55 expression by RNA interference overcomes resistance to complement-dependent cytotoxicity with rituximab. *Cancer Sci.* **2006**, *97*, 72–79. [CrossRef] [PubMed]
68. Hu, W.; Ge, X.; You, T.; Xu, T.; Zhang, J.; Wu, G.; Peng, Z.; Chorev, M.; Aktas, B.H.; Halperin, J.A.; et al. Human CD59 inhibitor sensitizes rituximab-resistant lymphoma cells to complement-mediated cytolysis. *Cancer Res.* **2011**, *71*, 2298–2307. [CrossRef]

69. Ge, X.; Wu, L.; Hu, W.; Fernandes, S.; Wang, C.; Li, X.; Brown, J.R.; Qin, X. rILYd4, a human CD59 inhibitor, enhances complement-dependent cytotoxicity of ofatumumab against rituximab-resistant B-cell lymphoma cells and chronic lymphocytic leukemia. *Clin. Cancer Res.* **2011**, *17*, 6702–6711. [CrossRef]
70. Barth, M.J.; Hernandez-Ilizaliturri, F.J.; Mavis, C.; Tsai, P.C.; Gibbs, J.F.; Deeb, G.; Czuczman, M.S. Ofatumumab demonstrates activity against rituximab-sensitive and -resistant cell lines, lymphoma xenografts and primary tumour cells from patients with B-cell lymphoma. *Br. J. Haematol.* **2011**, *156*, 490–498. [CrossRef]
71. Barth, M.J.; Mavis, C.; Czuczman, M.S.; Hernandez-Ilizaliturri, F.J. Ofatumumab Exhibits Enhanced In Vitro and In Vivo Activity Compared to Rituximab in Preclinical Models of Mantle Cell Lymphoma. *Clin. Cancer Res.* **2015**, *21*, 4391–4397. [CrossRef]
72. Beum, P.V.; Mack, D.A.; Pawluczkowycz, A.W.; Lindorfer, M.A.; Taylor, R.P. Binding of rituximab, trastuzumab, cetuximab, or mAb T101 to cancer cells promotes trogocytosis mediated by THP-1 cells and monocytes. *J. Immunol.* **2008**, *181*, 8120–8132. [CrossRef] [PubMed]
73. Guo, B.; Ma, Z.W.; Li, H.; Xu, G.L.; Zheng, P.; Zhu, B.; Wu, Y.Z.; Zou, Q. Mapping of binding epitopes of a human decay-accelerating factor monoclonal antibody capable of enhancing rituximab-mediated complement-dependent cytotoxicity. *Clin. Immunol.* **2008**, *128*, 155–163. [CrossRef]
74. Morgan, B.P.; Berg, C.W.; Harris, C.L. "Homologous restriction" in complement lysis: Roles of membrane complement regulators. *Xenotransplantation* **2005**, *12*, 258–265. [CrossRef] [PubMed]
75. Harjunpaa, A.; Junnikkala, S.; Meri, S. Rituximab (anti-CD20) therapy of B-cell lymphomas: Direct complement killing is superior to cellular effector mechanisms. *Scand. J. Immunol.* **2000**, *51*, 634–641. [CrossRef]
76. Bellone, S.; Roque, D.; Cocco, E.; Gasparrini, S.; Bortolomai, I.; Buza, N.; Abu-Khalaf, M.; Silasi, D.A.; Ratner, E.; Azodi, M.; et al. Downregulation of membrane complement inhibitors CD55 and CD59 by siRNA sensitises uterine serous carcinoma overexpressing Her2/neu to complement and antibody-dependent cell cytotoxicity in vitro: Implications for trastuzumab-based immunotherapy. *Br. J. Cancer* **2012**, *106*, 1543–1550. [CrossRef]
77. Zhao, W.P.; Zhu, B.; Duan, Y.Z.; Chen, Z.T. Neutralization of complement regulatory proteins CD55 and CD59 augments therapeutic effect of herceptin against lung carcinoma cells. *Oncol. Rep.* **2009**, *21*, 1405–1411. [CrossRef] [PubMed]
78. Wang, Y.; Yang, Y.J.; Wang, Z.; Liao, J.; Liu, M.; Zhong, X.R.; Zheng, H.; Wang, Y.P. CD55 and CD59 expression protects HER2-overexpressing breast cancer cells from trastuzumab-induced complement-dependent cytotoxicity. *Oncol. Lett.* **2017**, *14*, 2961–2969. [CrossRef] [PubMed]
79. Loeff, F.C.; van Egmond, H.M.E.; Nijmeijer, B.A.; Falkenburg, J.H.F.; Halkes, C.J.; Jedema, I. Complement-dependent cytotoxicity induced by therapeutic antibodies in B-cell acute lymphoblastic leukemia is dictated by target antigen expression levels and augmented by loss of membrane-bound complement inhibitors. *Leuk. Lymphoma* **2017**, *58*, 1–14. [CrossRef] [PubMed]
80. Nijhof, I.S.; Casneuf, T.; van Velzen, J.; van Kessel, B.; Axel, A.E.; Syed, K.; Groen, R.W.; van Duin, M.; Sonneveld, P.; Minnema, M.C.; et al. CD38 expression and complement inhibitors affect response and resistance to daratumumab therapy in myeloma. *Blood* **2016**, *128*, 959–970. [CrossRef] [PubMed]
81. You, T.; Hu, W.; Ge, X.; Shen, J.; Qin, X. Application of a novel inhibitor of human CD59 for the enhancement of complement-dependent cytolysis on cancer cells. *Cell. Mol. Immunol.* **2011**, *8*, 157–163. [CrossRef]
82. Takei, K.; Yamazaki, T.; Sawada, U.; Ishizuka, H.; Aizawa, S. Analysis of changes in CD20, CD55, and CD59 expression on established rituximab-resistant B-lymphoma cell lines. *Leuk. Res.* **2006**, *30*, 625–631. [CrossRef]
83. Macor, P.; Tripodo, C.; Zorzet, S.; Piovan, E.; Bossi, F.; Marzari, R.; Amadori, A.; Tedesco, F. In vivo targeting of human neutralizing antibodies against CD55 and CD59 to lymphoma cells increases the antitumor activity of rituximab. *Cancer Res.* **2007**, *67*, 10556–10563. [CrossRef]
84. Macor, P.; Secco, E.; Mezzaroba, N.; Zorzet, S.; Durigutto, P.; Gaiotto, T.; De Maso, L.; Biffi, S.; Garrovo, C.; Capolla, S.; et al. Bispecific antibodies targeting tumor-associated antigens and neutralizing complement regulators increase the efficacy of antibody-based immunotherapy in mice. *Leukemia* **2015**, *29*, 406–414. [CrossRef] [PubMed]
85. Williams, M.E.; Densmore, J.J.; Pawluczkowycz, A.W.; Beum, P.V.; Kennedy, A.D.; Lindorfer, M.A.; Hamil, S.H.; Eggleton, J.C.; Taylor, R.P. Thrice-weekly low-dose rituximab decreases CD20 loss via shaving and promotes enhanced targeting in chronic lymphocytic leukemia. *J. Immunol.* **2006**, *177*, 7435–7443. [CrossRef] [PubMed]

86. Mamidi, S.; Hone, S.; Teufel, C.; Sellner, L.; Zenz, T.; Kirschfink, M. Neutralization of membrane complement regulators improves complement-dependent effector functions of therapeutic anticancer antibodies targeting leukemic cells. *Oncoimmunology* **2015**, *4*, e979688. [CrossRef]
87. Beyer, I.; Cao, H.; Persson, J.; Wang, H.; Liu, Y.; Yumul, R.; Li, Z.; Woodle, D.; Manger, R.; Gough, M.; et al. Transient removal of CD46 is safe and increases B-cell depletion by rituximab in CD46 transgenic mice and macaques. *Mol. Ther.* **2013**, *21*, 291–299. [CrossRef] [PubMed]
88. Carter, D.; Lieber, A. Protein engineering to target complement evasion in cancer. *FEBS Lett.* **2014**, *588*, 334–340. [CrossRef]
89. Horl, S.; Banki, Z.; Huber, G.; Ejaz, A.; Windisch, D.; Muellauer, B.; Willenbacher, E.; Steurer, M.; Stoiber, H. Reduction of complement factor H binding to CLL cells improves the induction of rituximab-mediated complement-dependent cytotoxicity. *Leukemia* **2013**, *27*, 2200–2208. [CrossRef]
90. Horl, S.; Banki, Z.; Huber, G.; Ejaz, A.; Mullauer, B.; Willenbacher, E.; Steurer, M.; Stoiber, H. Complement factor H-derived short consensus repeat 18–20 enhanced complement-dependent cytotoxicity of ofatumumab on chronic lymphocytic leukemia cells. *Haematologica* **2013**, *98*, 1939–1947. [CrossRef]
91. Winkler, M.T.; Bushey, R.T.; Gottlin, E.B.; Campa, M.J.; Guadalupe, E.S.; Volkheimer, A.D.; Weinberg, J.B.; Patz, E.F., Jr. Enhanced CDC of B cell chronic lymphocytic leukemia cells mediated by rituximab combined with a novel anti-complement factor H antibody. *PLoS ONE* **2017**, *12*, e0179841. [CrossRef]
92. Meri, S.; Pangburn, M.K. Discrimination between activators and nonactivators of the alternative pathway of complement: Regulation via a sialic acid/polyanion binding site on factor H. *Proc. Natl. Acad. Sci. USA* **1990**, *87*, 3982–3986. [CrossRef] [PubMed]
93. Bordron, A.; Bagacean, C.; Mohr, A.; Tempescul, A.; Bendaoud, B.; Deshayes, S.; Dalbies, F.; Buors, C.; Saad, H.; Berthou, C.; et al. Resistance to complement activation, cell membrane hypersialylation and relapses in chronic lymphocytic leukemia patients treated with rituximab and chemotherapy. *Oncotarget* **2018**, *9*, 31590–31605. [CrossRef] [PubMed]
94. Cserhalmi, M.; Papp, A.; Brandus, B.; Uzonyi, B.; Jozsi, M. Regulation of regulators: Role of the complement factor H-related proteins. *Semin. Immunol.* **2019**, *45*, 101341. [CrossRef]
95. Lindorfer, M.A.; Beum, P.V.; Taylor, R.P. CD20 mAb-Mediated Complement Dependent Cytotoxicity of Tumor Cells is Enhanced by Blocking the Action of Factor I. *Antibodies* **2013**, *2*, 598–616. [CrossRef]
96. Felberg, A.; Urban, A.; Borowska, A.; Stasilojc, G.; Taszner, M.; Hellmann, A.; Blom, A.M.; Okroj, M. Mutations resulting in the formation of hyperactive complement convertases support cytocidal effect of anti-CD20 immunotherapeutics. *Cancer Immunol. Immunother.* **2019**, *68*, 587–598. [CrossRef]
97. Kennedy, A.D.; Solga, M.D.; Schuman, T.A.; Chi, A.W.; Lindorfer, M.A.; Sutherland, W.M.; Foley, P.L.; Taylor, R.P. An anti-C3b(i) mAb enhances complement activation, C3b(i) deposition, and killing of CD20+ cells by rituximab. *Blood* **2003**, *101*, 1071–1079. [CrossRef] [PubMed]
98. Rogers, L.M.; Veeramani, S.; Weiner, G.J. Complement in monoclonal antibody therapy of cancer. *Immunol. Res.* **2014**, *59*, 203–210. [CrossRef]
99. Hsu, Y.F.; Ajona, D.; Corrales, L.; Lopez-Picazo, J.M.; Gurpide, A.; Montuenga, L.M.; Pio, R. Complement activation mediates cetuximab inhibition of non-small cell lung cancer tumor growth in vivo. *Mol. Cancer* **2010**, *9*, 139. [CrossRef]
100. Franssen, L.E.; Stege, C.A.M.; Zweegman, S.; van de Donk, N.; Nijhof, I.S. Resistance Mechanisms Towards CD38-Directed Antibody Therapy in Multiple Myeloma. *J. Clin. Med.* **2020**, *9*, 1195. [CrossRef]
101. Plesner, T.; van de Donk, N.; Richardson, P.G. Controversy in the Use of CD38 Antibody for Treatment of Myeloma: Is High CD38 Expression Good or Bad? *Cells* **2020**, *9*, 378. [CrossRef]
102. Mamidi, S.; Cinci, M.; Hasmann, M.; Fehring, V.; Kirschfink, M. Lipoplex mediated silencing of membrane regulators (CD46, CD55 and CD59) enhances complement-dependent anti-tumor activity of trastuzumab and pertuzumab. *Mol. Oncol.* **2013**, *7*, 580–594. [CrossRef] [PubMed]
103. Clynes, R.A.; Towers, T.L.; Presta, L.G.; Ravetch, J.V. Inhibitory Fc receptors modulate in vivo cytoxicity against tumor targets. *Nat. Med.* **2000**, *6*, 443–446. [CrossRef]
104. Beers, S.A.; Chan, C.H.; James, S.; French, R.R.; Attfield, K.E.; Brennan, C.M.; Ahuja, A.; Shlomchik, M.J.; Cragg, M.S.; Glennie, M.J. Type II (tositumomab) anti-CD20 monoclonal antibody out performs type I (rituximab-like) reagents in B-cell depletion regardless of complement activation. *Blood* **2008**, *112*, 4170–4177. [CrossRef] [PubMed]

105. Uchida, J.; Hamaguchi, Y.; Oliver, J.A.; Ravetch, J.V.; Poe, J.C.; Haas, K.M.; Tedder, T.F. The innate mononuclear phagocyte network depletes B lymphocytes through Fc receptor-dependent mechanisms during anti-CD20 antibody immunotherapy. *J. Exp. Med.* **2004**, *199*, 1659–1669. [CrossRef]
106. Di Gaetano, N.; Cittera, E.; Nota, R.; Vecchi, A.; Grieco, V.; Scanziani, E.; Botto, M.; Introna, M.; Golay, J. Complement activation determines the therapeutic activity of rituximab in vivo. *J. Immunol.* **2003**, *171*, 1581–1587. [CrossRef] [PubMed]
107. Golay, J.; Cittera, E.; Di Gaetano, N.; Manganini, M.; Mosca, M.; Nebuloni, M.; Van Rooijen, N.; Vago, L.; Introna, M. Complement is required for the therapeutic activity of rituximab in a murine B lymphoma model homing in lymph nodes. *Haematologica* **2006**, *91*, 176–183. [PubMed]
108. Minard-Colin, V.; Xiu, Y.; Poe, J.C.; Horikawa, M.; Magro, C.M.; Hamaguchi, Y.; Haas, K.M.; Tedder, T.F. Lymphoma depletion during CD20 immunotherapy in mice is mediated by macrophage FcγRI, FcγRIII, and FcγRIV. *Blood* **2008**, *112*, 1205–1213. [CrossRef] [PubMed]
109. Hamaguchi, Y.; Uchida, J.; Cain, D.W.; Venturi, G.M.; Poe, J.C.; Haas, K.M.; Tedder, T.F. The peritoneal cavity provides a protective niche for B1 and conventional B lymphocytes during anti-CD20 immunotherapy in mice. *J. Immunol.* **2005**, *174*, 4389–4399. [CrossRef]
110. Overdijk, M.B.; Verploegen, S.; Bogels, M.; van Egmond, M.; Lammerts van Bueren, J.J.; Mutis, T.; Groen, R.W.; Breij, E.; Martens, A.C.; Bleeker, W.K.; et al. Antibody-mediated phagocytosis contributes to the anti-tumor activity of the therapeutic antibody daratumumab in lymphoma and multiple myeloma. *mAbs* **2015**, *7*, 311–321. [CrossRef]
111. Grandjean, C.L.; Montalvao, F.; Celli, S.; Michonneau, D.; Breart, B.; Garcia, Z.; Perro, M.; Freytag, O.; Gerdes, C.A.; Bousso, P. Intravital imaging reveals improved Kupffer cell-mediated phagocytosis as a mode of action of glycoengineered anti-CD20 antibodies. *Sci. Rep.* **2016**, *6*, 34382. [CrossRef]
112. Montalvao, F.; Garcia, Z.; Celli, S.; Breart, B.; Deguine, J.; Van Rooijen, N.; Bousso, P. The mechanism of anti-CD20-mediated B cell depletion revealed by intravital imaging. *J. Clin. Investig.* **2013**, *123*, 5098–5103. [CrossRef]
113. Gul, N.; Babes, L.; Siegmund, K.; Korthouwer, R.; Bogels, M.; Braster, R.; Vidarsson, G.; ten Hagen, T.L.; Kubes, P.; van Egmond, M. Macrophages eliminate circulating tumor cells after monoclonal antibody therapy. *J. Clin. Investig.* **2014**, *124*, 812–823. [CrossRef] [PubMed]
114. Stevenson, G.T. Three major uncertainties in the antibody therapy of cancer. *Haematologica* **2014**, *99*, 1538–1546. [CrossRef] [PubMed]
115. Boross, P.; Jansen, J.H.; de Haij, S.; Beurskens, F.J.; van der Poel, C.E.; Bevaart, L.; Nederend, M.; Golay, J.; van de Winkel, J.G.; Parren, P.W.; et al. The in vivo mechanism of action of CD20 monoclonal antibodies depends on local tumor burden. *Haematologica* **2011**, *96*, 1822–1830. [CrossRef]
116. Gong, Q.; Ou, Q.; Ye, S.; Lee, W.P.; Cornelius, J.; Diehl, L.; Lin, W.Y.; Hu, Z.; Lu, Y.; Chen, Y.; et al. Importance of cellular microenvironment and circulatory dynamics in B cell immunotherapy. *J. Immunol.* **2005**, *174*, 817–826. [CrossRef] [PubMed]
117. Lux, A.; Seeling, M.; Baerenwaldt, A.; Lehmann, B.; Schwab, I.; Repp, R.; Meidenbauer, N.; Mackensen, A.; Hartmann, A.; Heidkamp, G.; et al. A humanized mouse identifies the bone marrow as a niche with low therapeutic IgG activity. *Cell Rep.* **2014**, *7*, 236–248. [CrossRef]
118. Gordan, S.; Albert, H.; Danzer, H.; Lux, A.; Biburger, M.; Nimmerjahn, F. The Immunological Organ Environment Dictates the Molecular and Cellular Pathways of Cytotoxic Antibody Activity. *Cell Rep.* **2019**, *29*, 3033–3046.e4. [CrossRef]
119. Mollnes, T.E.; Brekke, O.L.; Fung, M.; Fure, H.; Christiansen, D.; Bergseth, G.; Videm, V.; Lappegard, K.T.; Kohl, J.; Lambris, J.D. Essential role of the C5a receptor in E coli-induced oxidative burst and phagocytosis revealed by a novel lepirudin-based human whole blood model of inflammation. *Blood* **2002**, *100*, 1869–1877.
120. Lee, C.H.; Romain, G.; Yan, W.; Watanabe, M.; Charab, W.; Todorova, B.; Lee, J.; Triplett, K.; Donkor, M.; Lungu, O.I.; et al. IgG Fc domains that bind C1q but not effector Fcgamma receptors delineate the importance of complement-mediated effector functions. *Nat. Immunol.* **2017**, *18*, 889–898. [CrossRef]
121. Verma, M.K.; Clemens, J.; Burzenski, L.; Sampson, S.B.; Brehm, M.A.; Greiner, D.L.; Shultz, L.D. A novel hemolytic complement-sufficient NSG mouse model supports studies of complement-mediated antitumor activity in vivo. *J. Immunol. Methods* **2017**, *446*, 47–53. [CrossRef]

122. Cittera, E.; Leidi, M.; Buracchi, C.; Pasqualini, F.; Sozzani, S.; Vecchi, A.; Waterfield, J.D.; Introna, M.; Golay, J. The CCL3 family of chemokines and innate immunity cooperate in vivo in the eradication of an established lymphoma xenograft by rituximab. *J. Immunol.* **2007**, *178*, 6616–6623. [CrossRef]
123. Betting, D.J.; Yamada, R.E.; Kafi, K.; Said, J.; van Rooijen, N.; Timmerman, J.M. Intratumoral but not systemic delivery of CpG oligodeoxynucleotide augments the efficacy of anti-CD20 monoclonal antibody therapy against B cell lymphoma. *J. Immunother.* **2009**, *32*, 622–631. [CrossRef] [PubMed]
124. Derer, S.; Cossham, M.; Rosner, T.; Kellner, C.; Beurskens, F.J.; Schwanbeck, R.; Lohse, S.; Sina, C.; Peipp, M.; Valerius, T. A Complement-Optimized EGFR Antibody Improves Cytotoxic Functions of Polymorphonuclear Cells against Tumor Cells. *J. Immunol.* **2015**, *195*, 5077–5087. [CrossRef]
125. Wang, S.Y.; Veeramani, S.; Racila, E.; Cagley, J.; Fritzinger, D.; Vogel, C.W.; St John, W.; Weiner, G.J. Depletion of the C3 component of complement enhances the ability of rituximab-coated target cells to activate human NK cells and improves the efficacy of monoclonal antibody therapy in an in vivo model. *Blood* **2009**, *114*, 5322–5330. [CrossRef]
126. Kern, D.J.; James, B.R.; Blackwell, S.; Gassner, C.; Klein, C.; Weiner, G.J. GA101 induces NK-cell activation and antibody-dependent cellular cytotoxicity more effectively than rituximab when complement is present. *Leuk. Lymphoma* **2013**, *54*, 2500–2505. [CrossRef]
127. Abes, R.; Gelize, E.; Fridman, W.H.; Teillaud, J.L. Long-lasting antitumor protection by anti-CD20 antibody through cellular immune response. *Blood* **2010**, *116*, 926–934. [CrossRef]
128. Deligne, C.; Metidji, A.; Fridman, W.H.; Teillaud, J.L. Anti-CD20 therapy induces a memory Th1 response through the IFN-gamma/IL-12 axis and prevents protumor regulatory T-cell expansion in mice. *Leukemia* **2015**, *29*, 947–957. [CrossRef] [PubMed]
129. DiLillo, D.J.; Ravetch, J.V. Differential Fc-Receptor Engagement Drives an Anti-tumor Vaccinal Effect. *Cell* **2015**, *161*, 1035–1045. [CrossRef]
130. Erdei, A.; Lukacsi, S.; Macsik-Valent, B.; Nagy-Balo, Z.; Kurucz, I.; Bajtay, Z. Non-identical twins: Different faces of CR3 and CR4 in myeloid and lymphoid cells of mice and men. *Semin. Cell Dev. Biol.* **2019**, *85*, 110–121. [CrossRef]
131. Nijhof, I.S.; Lammerts van Bueren, J.J.; van Kessel, B.; Andre, P.; Morel, Y.; Lokhorst, H.M.; van de Donk, N.W.; Parren, P.W.; Mutis, T. Daratumumab-mediated lysis of primary multiple myeloma cells is enhanced in combination with the human anti-KIR antibody IPH2102 and lenalidomide. *Haematologica* **2015**, *100*, 263–268. [CrossRef] [PubMed]
132. Krejcik, J.; Casneuf, T.; Nijhof, I.S.; Verbist, B.; Bald, J.; Plesner, T.; Syed, K.; Liu, K.; van de Donk, N.W.; Weiss, B.M.; et al. Daratumumab depletes CD38+ immune regulatory cells, promotes T-cell expansion, and skews T-cell repertoire in multiple myeloma. *Blood* **2016**, *128*, 384–394. [CrossRef] [PubMed]
133. van de Donk, N.; Usmani, S.Z. CD38 Antibodies in Multiple Myeloma: Mechanisms of Action and Modes of Resistance. *Front. Immunol.* **2018**, *9*, 2134. [CrossRef] [PubMed]
134. Taylor, R.P.; Lindorfer, M.A. Fcgamma-receptor-mediated trogocytosis impacts mAb-based therapies: Historical precedence and recent developments. *Blood* **2015**, *125*, 762–766. [CrossRef]
135. Hogan, K.A.; Chini, C.C.S.; Chini, E.N. The Multi-faceted Ecto-enzyme CD38: Roles in Immunomodulation, Cancer, Aging, and Metabolic Diseases. *Front. Immunol.* **2019**, *10*, 1187. [CrossRef]
136. Bruhns, P. Properties of mouse and human IgG receptors and their contribution to disease models. *Blood* **2012**, *119*, 5640–5649. [CrossRef] [PubMed]
137. Natsume, A.; Shimizu-Yokoyama, Y.; Satoh, M.; Shitara, K.; Niwa, R. Engineered anti-CD20 antibodies with enhanced complement-activating capacity mediate potent anti-lymphoma activity. *Cancer Sci.* **2009**, *100*, 2411–2418. [CrossRef] [PubMed]
138. Kennedy, A.D.; Beum, P.V.; Solga, M.D.; DiLillo, D.J.; Lindorfer, M.A.; Hess, C.E.; Densmore, J.J.; Williams, M.E.; Taylor, R.P. Rituximab infusion promotes rapid complement depletion and acute CD20 loss in chronic lymphocytic leukemia. *J. Immunol.* **2004**, *172*, 3280–3288. [CrossRef] [PubMed]
139. Beurskens, F.J.; Lindorfer, M.A.; Farooqui, M.; Beum, P.V.; Engelberts, P.; Mackus, W.J.; Parren, P.W.; Wiestner, A.; Taylor, R.P. Exhaustion of cytotoxic effector systems may limit monoclonal antibody-based immunotherapy in cancer patients. *J. Immunol.* **2012**, *188*, 3532–3541. [CrossRef] [PubMed]
140. van der Kolk, L.E.; Grillo-Lopez, A.J.; Baars, J.W.; Hack, C.E.; van Oers, M.H. Complement activation plays a key role in the side-effects of rituximab treatment. *Br. J. Haematol.* **2001**, *115*, 807–811. [CrossRef]

141. Baig, N.A.; Taylor, R.P.; Lindorfer, M.A.; Church, A.K.; LaPlant, B.R.; Pettinger, A.M.; Shanafelt, T.D.; Nowakowski, G.S.; Zent, C.S. Induced resistance to ofatumumab-mediated cell clearance mechanisms, including complement-dependent cytotoxicity, in chronic lymphocytic leukemia. *J. Immunol.* **2014**, *192*, 1620–1629. [CrossRef]
142. Tempescul, A.; Bagacean, C.; Riou, C.; Bendaoud, B.; Hillion, S.; Debant, M.; Buors, C.; Berthou, C.; Renaudineau, Y. Ofatumumab capacity to deplete B cells from chronic lymphocytic leukaemia is affected by C4 complement exhaustion. *Eur. J. Haematol.* **2016**, *96*, 229–235. [CrossRef]
143. Middleton, O.; Cosimo, E.; Dobbin, E.; McCaig, A.M.; Clarke, C.; Brant, A.M.; Leach, M.T.; Michie, A.M.; Wheadon, H. Complement deficiencies limit CD20 monoclonal antibody treatment efficacy in CLL. *Leukemia* **2015**, *29*, 107–114. [CrossRef] [PubMed]
144. Manches, O.; Lui, G.; Chaperot, L.; Gressin, R.; Molens, J.P.; Jacob, M.C.; Sotto, J.J.; Leroux, D.; Bensa, J.C.; Plumas, J. In vitro mechanisms of action of rituximab on primary non-Hodgkin lymphomas. *Blood* **2003**, *101*, 949–954. [CrossRef]
145. Baig, N.A.; Taylor, R.P.; Lindorfer, M.A.; Church, A.K.; Laplant, B.R.; Pavey, E.S.; Nowakowski, G.S.; Zent, C.S. Complement dependent cytotoxicity in chronic lymphocytic leukemia: Ofatumumab enhances alemtuzumab complement dependent cytotoxicity and reveals cells resistant to activated complement. *Leuk. Lymphoma* **2012**, *53*, 2218–2227. [CrossRef] [PubMed]
146. Taylor, R. Fresh frozen plasma as a complement source. *Lancet Oncol.* **2007**, *8*, 370–371. [CrossRef]
147. Klepfish, A.; Schattner, A.; Ghoti, H.; Rachmilewitz, E.A. Addition of fresh frozen plasma as a source of complement to rituximab in advanced chronic lymphocytic leukaemia. *Lancet Oncol.* **2007**, *8*, 361–362. [CrossRef]
148. Xu, W.; Miao, K.R.; Zhu, D.X.; Fang, C.; Zhu, H.Y.; Dong, H.J.; Wang, D.M.; Wu, Y.J.; Qiao, C.; Li, J.Y. Enhancing the action of rituximab by adding fresh frozen plasma for the treatment of fludarabine refractory chronic lymphocytic leukemia. *Int. J. Cancer* **2011**, *128*, 2192–2201. [CrossRef]
149. Tuscano, J.; Poh, C.; Rosenberg, A.; Jonas, B.; Abedi, M.; Barisone, G.; Schwab, E.; Lundeberg, K.; Kaesberg, P. Ofatumumab and Complement Replacement in Relapsed/Refractory Chronic Lymphocytic Leukemia. *J. Hematol.* **2020**, *9*, 79–83. [CrossRef]
150. Beum, P.V.; Kennedy, A.D.; Williams, M.E.; Lindorfer, M.A.; Taylor, R.P. The shaving reaction: Rituximab/CD20 complexes are removed from mantle cell lymphoma and chronic lymphocytic leukemia cells by THP-1 monocytes. *J. Immunol.* **2006**, *176*, 2600–2609. [CrossRef]
151. Beum, P.V.; Lindorfer, M.A.; Taylor, R.P. Within peripheral blood mononuclear cells, antibody-dependent cellular cytotoxicity of rituximab-opsonized Daudi cells is promoted by NK cells and inhibited by monocytes due to shaving. *J. Immunol.* **2008**, *181*, 2916–2924. [CrossRef]
152. Beum, P.V.; Peek, E.M.; Lindorfer, M.A.; Beurskens, F.J.; Engelberts, P.J.; Parren, P.W.; van de Winkel, J.G.; Taylor, R.P. Loss of CD20 and bound CD20 antibody from opsonized B cells occurs more rapidly because of trogocytosis mediated by Fc receptor-expressing effector cells than direct internalization by the B cells. *J. Immunol.* **2011**, *187*, 3438–3447. [CrossRef]
153. Valgardsdottir, R.; Cattaneo, I.; Klein, C.; Introna, M.; Figliuzzi, M.; Golay, J. Human neutrophils mediate trogocytosis rather than phagocytosis of CLL B cells opsonized with anti-CD20 antibodies. *Blood* **2017**, *129*, 2636–2644. [CrossRef] [PubMed]
154. Boross, P.; Jansen, J.H.; Pastula, A.; van der Poel, C.E.; Leusen, J.H. Both activating and inhibitory Fc gamma receptors mediate rituximab-induced trogocytosis of CD20 in mice. *Immunol. Lett.* **2012**, *143*, 44–52. [CrossRef]
155. Beers, S.A.; French, R.R.; Chan, C.H.; Lim, S.H.; Jarrett, T.C.; Mora Vidal, R.; Wijayaweera, S.S.; Dixon, S.V.; Kim, H.J.; Cox, K.L.; et al. Antigenic modulation limits the efficacy of anti-CD20 antibodies: Implications for antibody selection. *Blood* **2010**, *115*, 5191–5201. [CrossRef] [PubMed]
156. Glennie, M.J.; French, R.R.; Cragg, M.S.; Taylor, R.P. Mechanisms of killing by anti-CD20 monoclonal antibodies. *Mol. Immunol.* **2007**, *44*, 3823–3837. [CrossRef]
157. Racila, E.; Link, B.K.; Weng, W.K.; Witzig, T.E.; Ansell, S.; Maurer, M.J.; Huang, J.; Dahle, C.; Halwani, A.; Levy, R.; et al. A polymorphism in the complement component C1qA correlates with prolonged response following rituximab therapy of follicular lymphoma. *Clin. Cancer Res.* **2008**, *14*, 6697–6703. [CrossRef] [PubMed]

158. Charbonneau, B.; Maurer, M.J.; Fredericksen, Z.S.; Zent, C.S.; Link, B.K.; Novak, A.J.; Ansell, S.M.; Weiner, G.J.; Wang, A.H.; Witzig, T.E.; et al. Germline variation in complement genes and event-free survival in follicular and diffuse large B-cell lymphoma. *Am. J. Hematol.* **2012**, *87*, 880–885. [CrossRef]
159. Rogers, L.M.; Mott, S.L.; Smith, B.J.; Link, B.K.; Sahin, D.; Weiner, G.J. Complement-Regulatory Proteins CFHR1 and CFHR3 and Patient Response to Anti-CD20 Monoclonal Antibody Therapy. *Clin. Cancer Res.* **2017**, *23*, 954–961. [CrossRef]
160. Song, G.; Song, G.; Ni, H.; Gu, L.; Liu, H.; Chen, B.; He, B.; Pan, Y.; Wang, S.; Cho, W.C. Deregulated expression of miR-224 and its target gene: CD59 predicts outcome of diffuse large B-cell lymphoma patients treated with R-CHOP. *Curr. Cancer Drug Targets* **2014**, *14*, 659–670. [CrossRef]
161. Song, G.; Cho, W.C.; Gu, L.; He, B.; Pan, Y.; Wang, S. Increased CD59 protein expression is associated with the outcome of patients with diffuse large B-cell lymphoma treated with R-CHOP. *Med. Oncol.* **2014**, *31*, 56. [CrossRef]
162. Dzietczenia, J.; Wrobel, T.; Mazur, G.; Poreba, R.; Jazwiec, B.; Kuliczkowski, K. Expression of complement regulatory proteins: CD46, CD55, and CD59 and response to rituximab in patients with CD20+ non-Hodgkin's lymphoma. *Med. Oncol.* **2010**, *27*, 743–746. [CrossRef]
163. Weng, W.K.; Levy, R. Expression of complement inhibitors CD46, CD55, and CD59 on tumor cells does not predict clinical outcome after rituximab treatment in follicular non-Hodgkin lymphoma. *Blood* **2001**, *98*, 1352–1357. [CrossRef] [PubMed]
164. Liu, M.; Yang, Y.J.; Zheng, H.; Zhong, X.R.; Wang, Y.; Wang, Z.; Wang, Y.G.; Wang, Y.P. Membrane-bound complement regulatory proteins are prognostic factors of operable breast cancer treated with adjuvant trastuzumab: A retrospective study. *Oncol. Rep.* **2014**, *32*, 2619–2627. [CrossRef]
165. Lindorfer, M.A.; Bakker, P.W.H.I.; Parren, P.W.; Taylor, R.P. Ofatumumab: A next-generation human therapeutic CD20 antibody with potent complement-dependent cytotoxicity. In *Handbook of Therapeutic Antibodies*; Duebel, S., Reichert, J.M., Eds.; Wiley-VCH: Weinberg, Germany, 2013; pp. 1733–1744.
166. Goede, V.; Fischer, K.; Busch, R.; Engelke, A.; Eichhorst, B.; Wendtner, C.M.; Chagorova, T.; de la Serna, J.; Dilhuydy, M.S.; Illmer, T.; et al. Obinutuzumab plus Chlorambucil in Patients with CLL and Coexisting Conditions. *NEJM* **2014**, *370*, 1101–1110. [CrossRef]
167. Goede, V.; Fischer, K.; Engelke, A.; Schlag, R.; Lepretre, S.; Montero, L.F.; Montillo, M.; Fegan, C.; Asikanius, E.; Humphrey, K.; et al. Obinutuzumab as frontline treatment of chronic lymphocytic leukemia: Updated results of the CLL11 study. *Leukemia* **2015**, *29*, 1602–1604. [CrossRef] [PubMed]
168. van Imhoff, G.W.; McMillan, A.; Matasar, M.J.; Radford, J.; Ardeshna, K.M.; Kuliczkowski, K.; Kim, W.; Hong, X.; Goerloev, J.S.; Davies, A.; et al. Ofatumumab Versus Rituximab Salvage Chemoimmunotherapy in Relapsed or Refractory Diffuse Large B-Cell Lymphoma: The ORCHARRD Study. *J. Clin. Oncol.* **2017**, *35*, 544–551. [CrossRef]
169. Freeman, C.L.; Sehn, L.H. A tale of two antibodies: Obinutuzumab versus rituximab. *Br. J. Haematol.* **2018**, *182*, 29–45. [CrossRef] [PubMed]
170. Offner, F.; Robak, T.; Janssens, A.; Govind Babu, K.; Kloczko, J.; Grosicki, S.; Mayer, J.; Panagiotidis, P.; Schuh, A.; Pettitt, A.; et al. A five-year follow-up of untreated patients with chronic lymphocytic leukaemia treated with ofatumumab and chlorambucil: Final analysis of the Complement 1 phase 3 trial. *Br. J. Haematol.* **2020**. [CrossRef] [PubMed]
171. Capuano, C.; Romanelli, M.; Pighi, C.; Cimino, G.; Rago, A.; Molfetta, R.; Paolini, R.; Santoni, A.; Galandrini, R. Anti-CD20 Therapy Acts via FcgammaRIIIA to Diminish Responsiveness of Human Natural Killer Cells. *Cancer Res.* **2015**, *75*, 4097–4108. [CrossRef] [PubMed]
172. Moreno, L.; Perez, C.; Zabaleta, A.; Manrique, I.; Alignani, D.; Ajona, D.; Blanco, L.; Lasa, M.; Maiso, P.; Rodriguez, I.; et al. The Mechanism of Action of the Anti-CD38 Monoclonal Antibody Isatuximab in Multiple Myeloma. *Clin. Cancer Res.* **2019**, *25*, 3176–3187. [CrossRef]
173. Cartron, G.; Watier, H.; Golay, J.; Solal-Celigny, P. From the bench to the bedside: Ways to improve rituximab efficacy. *Blood* **2004**, *104*, 2635–2642. [CrossRef] [PubMed]
174. Balasa, B.; Yun, R.; Belmar, N.A.; Fox, M.; Chao, D.T.; Robbins, M.D.; Starling, G.C.; Rice, A.G. Elotuzumab enhances natural killer cell activation and myeloma cell killing through interleukin-2 and TNF-alpha pathways. *Cancer Immunol. Immunother.* **2015**, *64*, 61–73. [CrossRef] [PubMed]

175. Oostindie, S.C.; van der Horst, H.J.; Lindorfer, M.A.; Cook, E.M.; Tupitza, J.C.; Zent, C.S.; Burack, R.; VanDerMeid, K.R.; Strumane, K.; Chamuleau, M.E.D.; et al. CD20 and CD37 antibodies synergize to activate complement by Fc-mediated clustering. *Haematologica* **2019**, *104*, 1841–1852. [CrossRef] [PubMed]
176. Da Roit, F.; Engelberts, P.J.; Taylor, R.P.; Breij, E.C.; Gritti, G.; Rambaldi, A.; Introna, M.; Parren, P.W.; Beurskens, F.J.; Golay, J. Ibrutinib interferes with the cell-mediated anti-tumor activities of therapeutic CD20 antibodies: Implications for combination therapy. *Haematologica* **2015**, *100*, 77–86. [CrossRef]
177. Evers, M.; Jak, M.; Leusen, J.H.W. The latest developments with anti-CD20 monoclonal antibodies in chronic lymphocytic leukemia. *Expert Opin. Biol. Ther.* **2018**, *18*, 973–982. [CrossRef]

Publisher's Note: MDPI stays neutral with regard to jurisdictional claims in published maps and institutional affiliations.

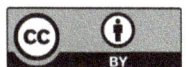 © 2020 by the authors. Licensee MDPI, Basel, Switzerland. This article is an open access article distributed under the terms and conditions of the Creative Commons Attribution (CC BY) license (http://creativecommons.org/licenses/by/4.0/).

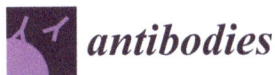

Review

How Do mAbs Make Use of Complement to Kill Cancer Cells? The Role of Ca^{2+}

Ronald P. Taylor * and Margaret A. Lindorfer

Department of Biochemistry and Molecular Genetics, University of Virginia School of Medicine, Charlottesville, VA 22908, USA; mal9e@virginia.edu
* Correspondence: rpt@virginia.edu; Tel.: +1-434-987-1964

Received: 28 July 2020; Accepted: 26 August 2020; Published: 4 September 2020

Abstract: We examined the kinetics and mechanisms by which monoclonal antibodies (mAbs) utilize complement to rapidly kill targeted cancer cells. Based on results from flow cytometry, confocal microscopy and high-resolution digital imaging experiments, The general patterns which have emerged reveal cytotoxic activities mediated by substantial and lethal Ca^{2+} fluxes. The Ca^{2+} fluxes are common to the reported pathways that have been utilized by other toxins in killing nucleated cells. These reactions terminate in very high levels of cell killing, and based on these considerations, we suggest additional strategies to further enhance mAb-based targeting of cancer with complement.

Keywords: complement; therapeutic monoclonal antibodies (mAbs); Ca^{2+}; fluorescence microscopy

1. Introduction

Complement was first described and characterized by Bordet more than 100 years ago [1]; he demonstrated it to be a heat-labile factor in serum that promoted destruction (lysis) of bacteria and/or hemolysis of erythrocytes, each opsonized with the antibodies in immune sera. Complement is an important "first responder" that orchestrates the rapid clearance and destruction of a variety of microbial invaders as well as damaged and dying cells. It is therefore quite reasonable to anticipate that it should also be capable of destroying antibody-opsonized tumor cells. The importance of complement (C) in health and disease is now very well recognized and several outstanding reviews that describe its pathways and biological actions are available [2–4].

The first figure in the review in this volume by Golay and Taylor succinctly summarizes the important steps and controls in C-mediated killing of malignant cells opsonized with specific mAbs [5]. The traditional view of the mechanism by which C mediates the killing of antibody-opsonized cells was based on classic experiments that focused on C-mediated lysis of non-nucleated sheep erythrocytes that were first opsonized with polyclonal rabbit antibodies before they were brought into contact with a source of C and then incubated for a considerable period of time at 37 °C to promote hemolysis [6–8]. The results of these studies led to the concept that insertion of the membrane attack complex (MAC) pore(s) into the erythrocyte cell membrane allowed for influx of water and ions into the cell, ultimately leading to swelling of the cells followed by osmotic lysis and killing of the cells [6–10]. This model system has of course proven to be invaluable for dissecting out and identifying virtually all of the key components of C, including pathways, activating factors and inhibitors.

2. Nucleated Cells Are More Complicated: Important Questions

However, a considerable body of evidence, based on a series of studies by Shin's group on the lysis of nucleated Ehrlich ascites cells (EACs) opsonized with rabbit polyclonal antibodies, suggested that the osmotic lysis concept could not explain how these nucleated cells were killed. Instead, The influx of Ca^{2+} mediated by MAC pores appeared to be the predominant lethal event [10–15].

The focus of these studies, completed more than 20 years ago, was on the terminal steps in the complement-dependent cytotoxicity (CDC) reaction. In the present review, in order to concentrate on mechanisms, we have examined multiple individual steps in the CDC reaction that start with mAb binding and end with cell death in a continuously monitored reaction mediated by Food and Drug Administration (FDA)-approved mAbs reacted with both cell lines and with primary malignant cells from patients with chronic lymphocytic leukemia (CLL) (Table 1).

Table 1. Observed consecutive steps in monoclonal antibody (mAb)-mediated complement-dependent cytotoxicity (CDC).

Step	Time Frame *	Method	Figure	References
mAb binding	30 s	Flow cytometry	8	[16]
C1q binding and colocalization with mAb	60 s	Flow cytometry	2, 8	[16,17]
C3b deposition and mAb colocalization	90 s	Flow cytometry, high-resolution digital imaging (HRDI)	3, 4, 10	[16,18,19]
C9 binding and colocalization of C9/C3b/mAb	60–120 s	HRDI, confocal	11, 12	[20]
Ca^{2+} influx, transition-state intermediate	40–135 s	Confocal, flow cytometry	9, 10, 15, 16	[16,21]
tunneling nanotube (TNT) generation	120 s	Spinning disk	4, 7	[19,22]
mitochondrial poisoning	180 s 60–180 s	HRDI, confocal	9–11	[16,20]
decay of transition-state intermediate	225 s	Confocal	9, 10, 15, 16	[16,21]
MAC formation and cell death	60–240 s	Confocal	8–10, 15	[16,20,21]

* Time estimates are based on a range of experiments and techniques.

In order to elucidate these mechanisms, we will address important questions with respect to the development of C-fixing mAbs to be used in cancer immunotherapy: How effective are these mAbs when they "attack" nucleated malignant cells in the presence of C (usually normal human serum (NHS))? What is the primary mechanism of cell killing? It would seem important to identify and optimize the primary killing mechanism to allow for efficient use of key resources, which comprise C and mAbs. Moreover, although the targeted malignant cells will employ a variety of defenses to ward off mAb-mediated attack [23–30], it is reasonable to ask that if the cells can be killed by CDC, then is there a common and general killing pathway? We developed several "complementary" (excuse the pun!) approaches to address these questions, based on quantitation and direct visualization and identification of many of the key separate steps in the CDC reaction. Many of our measurements of CDC made use of CD20 and CD37 mAbs in the killing of B cell lines and of CLL cells [16–22,31–33]. The similar patterns we have observed in these and other systems provide considerable evidence that there is indeed a common mechanism in the CDC reaction mediated by anti-tumor mAbs. In conducting these experiments, we followed the "ask-the-question" paradigm described by Nobel Prize investigator George Wald [34]:

"When it (scientific research) is going well, it is like a quiet conversation with Nature. One asks a question and gets an answer, then one asks the next question and gets the next answer. An experiment is a device to make Nature speak intelligibly. After that, one only has to listen."

3. Experimental Strategies

Our approaches make use of fluorescently-labeled probes and fluorescent indicators, which include anti-tumor mAbs (lightly labeled with Alexa (Al) dyes, so as not to interfere with their activities, but adequate to monitor their binding to cells); C1q; mAbs 7C12 and 3E7 (specific for C3b/iC3b deposited on the cell) [35,36]; mAb HB43, specific for the Fc region of human IgG and able to recognize cell-bound mAbs [37]; Fluo-4, a Ca^{2+} indicator which is very sensitive to increases in the Ca^{2+} concentration in the cytoplasm and mitochondria of the cell [16]; tetramethylrhodamine methyl ester (TMRME), which is highly fluorescent only in viable mitochondria [16]; mAb aE11, specific for membrane attack complex (MAC)-associated C9 deposited on cells [38]; and vital fluorescent dyes such as propidium iodide (PI), 7-aminoactinomycin D (7AAD) and TO-PRO-3 which enter dead permeabilized cells and, upon staining nuclear DNA, become highly fluorescent, thus providing reliable markers for cell death and successful CDC [16,19,22]. We have been able to use this array of reagents to interrogate the quantitative and kinetic details of mAb-mediated killing of cancer cells in parallel experiments based on flow cytometry, high-resolution digital imaging in a flow cytometry environment (HRDI, Amnis technology [18]), and real-time multicolor confocal fluorescent microscopy movies.

4. Quantitation and Visualization of Early Steps in mAb-Mediated CDC: In Vitro and In Vivo Studies

Table 1 summarizes the discrete events in mAb-mediated CDC that we have investigated. Initially, we were able to demonstrate rapid binding of the mAbs ofatumumab (OFA) and rituximab (RTX), specific for CD20, to B cell lines and to primary B cells from patients with chronic lymphocytic leukemia (CLL) [17]. We found that both RTX and OFA bound to the cells at the same levels (Figure 1, panels I–H). However, considerably more C1q was bound to the cells reacted with OFA (Figure 1, panels A–C) [17].

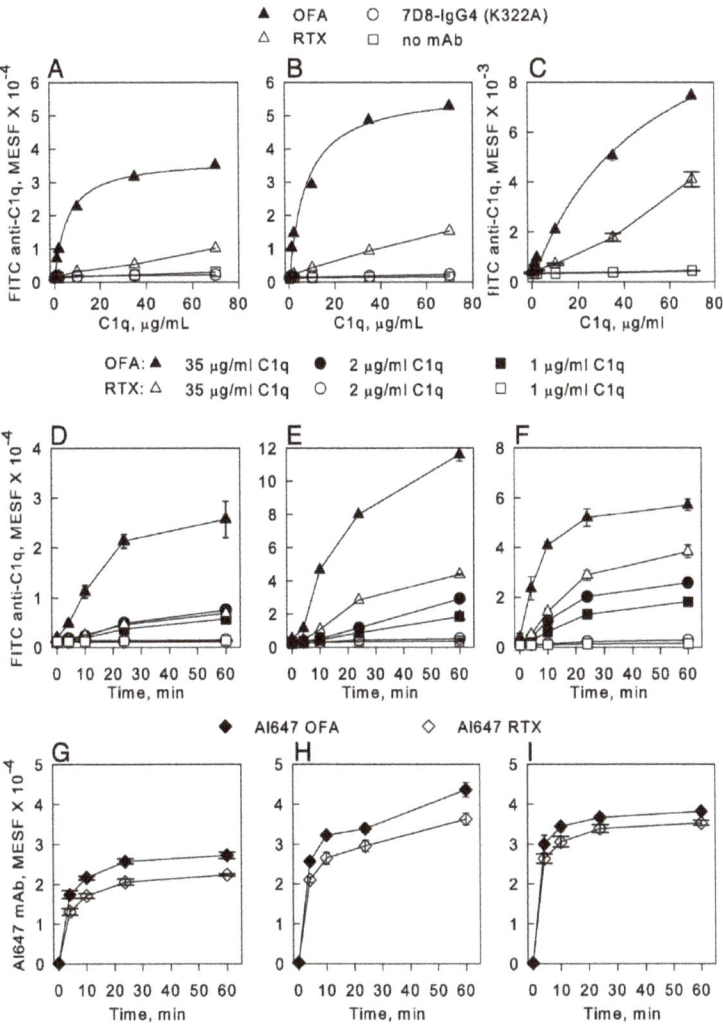

Figure 1. OFA-opsonized B cells bind more C1q than RTX-opsonized B cells. (**A,B**) Varying amounts of C1q were added to B cells suspended in complete RPMI 1640 medium and then reacted with either

Al647 OFA, Al647 RTX, or Al647 7D8-IgG4 (K322A, does not bind C1q), all at 10 µg/mL; alternatively, no mAb was added. After incubation for 60 min at 37 °C, cells were washed and C1q binding determined by probing with FITC rabbit anti-C1q, followed by flow cytometry. (**A**), Raji cells. (**B**), Daudi cells. The results for binding of C1q to OFA-opsonized Raji and Daudi cells were fit to a binding isotherm, giving a K_D of 12 and 16 nM, respectively. All Al647 mAbs bound at high levels to the cells and mAb binding was the same in the presence and absence of C1q (not shown). (**C**), Binding of C1q to CLL cells opsonized with either OFA or with RTX, similar conditions and analyses (K_D for OFA-opsonized cells = 106 nM). (**D–I**), Cells were combined in cold medium with Al647 mAb and varying amounts of C1q and then incubated at 37 °C. Aliquots were removed at the indicated times, quenched with ice-cold BSA-PBS, washed, probed with FITC anti-C1q, and then analyzed by flow cytometry for C1q binding (**D–F**) and mAb binding by secondary probing with mAb HB43, specific for the Fc region of human IgG (**G–I**). (**D,G**), Raji cells. (**E,H**), Daudi cells. (**F,I**), Z138 cells. Results in all panels are representative of at least two similar experiments [17].

It is well established that during C activation, innocent bystander opsonization or lysis of nearby non-targeted cells is negligible [4,39–41]. Therefore, implicit in the specificity of the lytic C cascade is the presumption that there is both concentration and localization of activated C components at the nexus of C activation, which, for the classical pathway, would be the cell-bound mAbs at the plasma membrane target site (e.g., CD20). We have demonstrated this phenomenon of colocalization of reactive proteins at multiple steps in the pathway, starting with C1q binding [17]. First, we observed a high level of colocalization of Al647 OFA with Al488 C1q on Daudi cells quantitated by HRDI measurements (Figure 2 and Table 2). However, when we performed the experiment under identical conditions with Al647 RTX-opsonized Daudi cells, we found that although the amount of cell-bound RTX was comparable to the amount of cell-bound OFA, there was a very modest level of C1q binding (Table 2) and considerably less colocalization of cell-bound C1q with RTX. Based on analyses of their CD20 epitope specificities, it is now well established that OFA binds much closer to the cell membrane and with a slower off rate than RTX [19,31,42–44], and this has also been reflected "downstream" in that OFA is able to mediate CDC of B cells much more effectively than does RTX. This is particularly apparent in the case of ARH77 cells and CLL B cells. These cells are more resistant to mAb-induced CDC than most B cell lines because they express low levels of CD20 but high levels of C control proteins CD55 and/or CD59, and therefore the differences in the CDC efficacy of OFA versus RTX are readily demonstrated [19,31,43,44].

Table 2. Binding of Al488-labeled C1q to mAb-opsonized Daudi cells and colocalization of C1q with mAb.

	Expt. 1			Expt. 2			Expt. 3 [a]		
	Al647 mAb (GMF) [b]	Al488 C1q (GMF)	BDSS [c]	Al647 mAb (GMF)	Al488 C1q (GMF)	BDSS	Al647 mAb (GMF)	Al488 C1q (GMF)	BDSS
Al647 OFA	181,000	162,000	3.0	116,000	113,000	3.4	206,000	30,000	2.5
Al647 RTX	186,000	7500	0.9	61,000	6600	2.1	155,000	2200	1.0
Al647 7D8 [d]	133,000	2300	0.6	104,000	1000	0.9	210,000	1300	0.7

[a] Different Al488 C1q preparation. [b] GMF, geometric mean fluorescence. [c] BDSS, bright detail similarity score. [d] IgG4 (K322A).

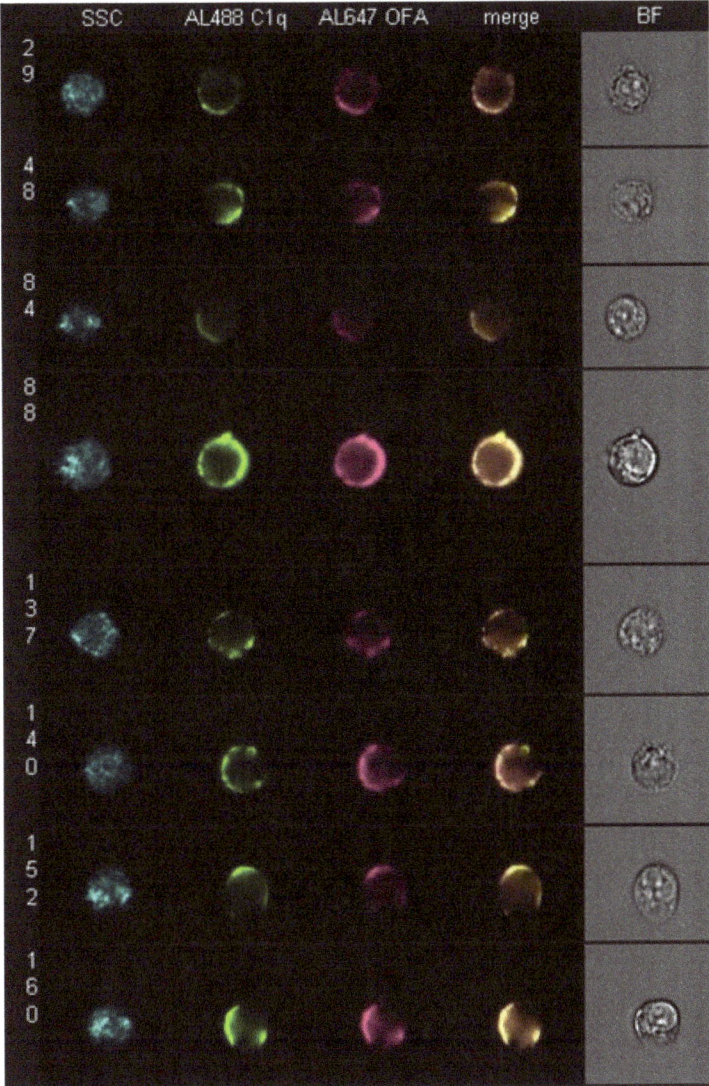

Figure 2. C1q colocalizes with bound OFA on daudi cells. Daudi cells were incubated with 10 μg/mL Al647 mAb and 1.6 μg/mL Al488 C1q in medium for 60 min at 37 °C. Samples were washed, fixed, concentrated, and then analyzed by multispectral high-resolution digital imaging (HRDI). Fluorescence signals for Al647 OFA-opsonized samples were analyzed for colocalization with bound Al488 C1q. Light scatter, fluorescence and bright field images of representative doubly positive cells. Results are representative of three similar experiments. Figures 1 and 2 were originally published in *The Journal of Immunology*. Pawluczkowycz, A.W. et al. 2009 Binding of submaximal C1q promotes CDC of B cells opsonized with anti-CD20 mAbs OFA or RTX: considerably higher levels of CDC are induced by OFA than by RTX. *J. Immunol.* 183: 749–758. Copyright © (2009) The American Association of Immunologists, Inc. [17].

Table 2 was originally published in *The Journal of Immunology*. Pawluczkowycz, A.W. et al. 2009 Binding of submaximal C1q promotes CDC of B cells opsonized with anti-CD20 mAbs OFA or RTX:

considerably higher levels of CDC are induced by OFA than by RTX. *J. Immunol.* 183: 749–758. Copyright © (2009) The American Association of Immunologists, Inc. [17].

These findings also speak to the issue of thresholds for C activation [9,45,46] and cell killing by the MAC. Binding of RTX to B cells does indeed allow for some C1q binding, C activation, and subsequent C3b deposition and colocalization of the deposited cell-bound C3b with cell-bound RTX (Figure 3) [18,19]. However, we found that on reaction in NHS, The amount of C3b deposited on OFA-reacted CLL cells was 5–10-fold greater than the amount of C3b deposited on RTX-opsonized CLL cells, quantitated with flow cytometry measurements [31]. Thus, although there is comparable binding of these CD20 mAbs to the CLL cells and there is enough C1q bound to RTX-opsonized cells to activate C, less C3b is deposited on the cells compared to the amount of C3b deposition mediated by OFA [17,31]. In other words, The C3b deposition threshold needed to achieve *adequate* generation of the MAC to enable cell killing is not reached for most RTX-opsonized CLL cells. It is therefore understandable why OFA is considerably more effective than RTX in promoting CDC of CLL cells.

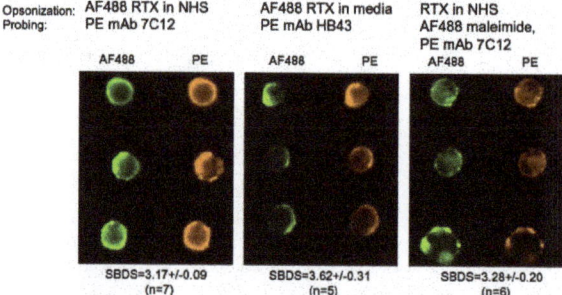

Figure 3. Deposited C3b colocalizes with bound RTX. Representative images from samples opsonized as indicated and then analyzed by HRDI. Similarity bright detail score (SBDS) values given below the images are the mean ± SD (*n*) for values obtained on '*n*' different replicate samples (at least 10,000 cells/sample) prepared and analyzed over a period of 18 months. The AF488 maleimide binds to the free SH group on C3b. Note how it is colocalized with mAb 7C12, specific for C3b. Reprinted from Journal of Immunological Methods, Vol. 317, 2006, Beum, P.V. et al., Quantitative analysis of protein colocalization on B cells opsonized with rituximab and complement using the ImageStream multispectral imaging flow cytometer, pp. 90–99, with permission from Elsevier, Amsterdam, The Netherlands [18].

However, RTX can promote very rapid C3b deposition on B cells in the circulation of non-human primates. We found that when RTX is infused intravenously into cynomolgus monkeys, it rapidly binds to circulating B cells and this is followed, within 2 min, by deposition of C3 fragments in close juxtaposition with B cell-bound RTX [36]. Moreover, we also obtained blood samples from CLL patients treated with either RTX or OFA, and we observed C3 fragments deposited on their B cells in close juxtaposition with cell-bound RTX/OFA on samples taken within an hour of the start of the mAb infusions [31,47,48]. We note that multiple lines of evidence indicate that mechanisms mediated by receptors for the Fc region of human IgG (FcγR) expressed on macrophages are principally responsible for the in vivo efficacy of RTX [49–51].

5. C3b Deposition Kinetics, a Key Intermediate Step in CDC; the "Discovery" of Streamers

We next asked whether the kinetics of C3b deposition and killing of B cell lines or of CLL cells opsonized with these CD20 mAbs would also reflect differences between OFA and RTX. We conducted real-time spinning disk confocal fluorescence microscopy experiments in which Alexa-labeled mAbs specific for CD20 were reacted with B cells and then incubated in NHS as a C source supplemented with Alexa-labeled mAb 3E7 as a marker to reveal C3b/iC3b deposition. Importantly, mAb 3E7 does not cross-react with C3 and therefore can report C3b deposition in situ. [19]. We confirmed that under these conditions, both RTX and OFA promoted rapid C activation (~2 min), and that substantial colocalization of deposited C3b with cell-bound RTX was easily demonstrable on Daudi cells (Figure 4, panels A–C). However, an unexpected and initially very puzzling observation set the stage for more detailed investigations that have ultimately allowed us to carefully decipher the intricacies of the CDC killing mechanism for nucleated cells. We found that *very soon after* the C3b deposition reaction could be detected, long very thin fragments of cell membrane extended from the Daudi cells *before* they were killed, and it was possible to detect both membrane-bound mAb (RTX or OFA) along with colocalized C3b on these fragments. Control experiments in the absence of mAb 3E7 clearly demonstrated that these structures were not an experimental artifact (Figure 4, panel D). We initially called these membrane fragments "streamers", but additional experiments revealed that we were studying the formation of tunneling nanotubules (TNTs), in a reaction that is mediated by rapid entry of large amounts of Ca^{2+} into a cell [22,52,53].

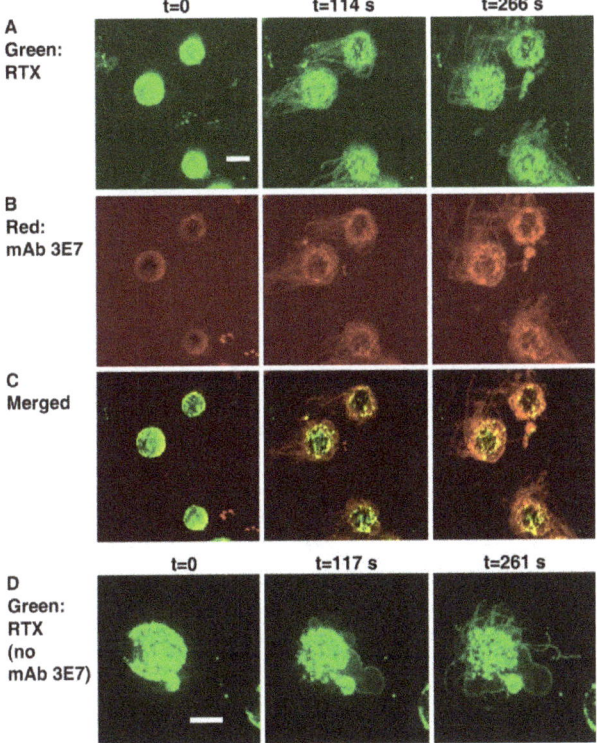

Figure 4. Binding of RTX to Daudi cells in NHS induces blebbing and streaming. (A–C), Images obtained at three different times for Daudi cells reacted with Al488 RTX, Al647 mAb 3E7, and NHS. (A), The 488 nm images show green RTX. (B), The 647 nm images show red mAb 3E7. (C), Merged images. Note that overlap of red and green produces orange or yellow. (D), Blebbing and streamers are generated in the absence of mAb 3E7. Daudi cells were opsonized with Al488 RTX and then reacted with NHS. Images for 488 nm are displayed at three time points. Green streamers can be seen to the left of the cells in panel A. The calibration bar in this and the following figures denotes 5 microns. The magnification in (A–C) was 40×, but, in panel (D) and all other figures derived from spinning disc confocal microscopy experiments, magnification at 63× was used [19].

We performed a similar experiment substituting ARH77 cells for Daudi cells. As noted previously, OFA, but not *RTX*, can mediate CDC of ARH77 cells. We observed colocalization of OFA or of RTX with C3b on ARH77 cells when the cells activated C in the presence of NHS. However, TNTs/streamers were released only by OFA-reacted ARH77 cells, but not by ARH77 cells reacted with RTX (Figure 5, panels A–D) [19]. This finding strongly suggests that C activation on ARH77 cells induced by RTX was not adequate to promote entry of Ca^{2+} into these cells. That is, in view of the large differentials in C3b deposition and cell killing for OFA versus RTX-opsonized CLL cells, these findings again support the idea that the threshold for C3b deposition required for generation downstream of sufficient amounts of the MAC to effectively permeabilize ARH77 cells and promote Ca^{2+} entry is not reached for RTX-reacted ARH77 cells. The patterns we have described (colocalization of mAb and C3b, formation of TNTs) are not unique to CD20 mAbs. Certain mAbs activate C very effectively on binding to target cells because they bind at very high levels (>80,000 mAbs per cell). These include HB28 (anti-β2 microglobulin, mouse (IgG2b), alemtuzumab (anti-CD52), and W6/32 (anti-HLA), and all of these mAbs have also been demonstrated to produce streamers/TNTs on binding to target cells in the presence of C [19,22,33,54].

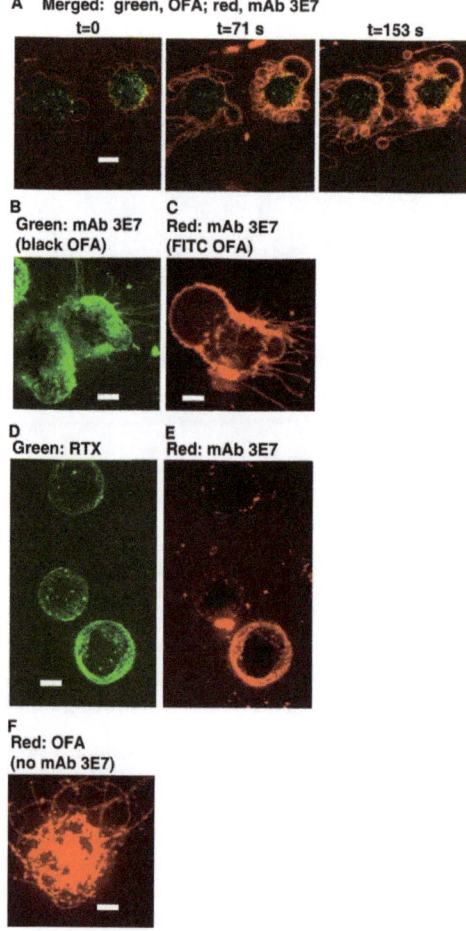

Figure 5. Binding of OFA to Daudi cells and ARH77 cells in NHS produces blebbing and streamers. (**A**), Daudi cells were opsonized with Al488 OFA, and then reacted with NHS and Al647 mAb 3E7; merged 488 nm/647 nm images at the indicated times. (**B**), ARH77 cells were opsonized with OFA,

and then reacted with NHS and Al488 mAb 3E7; the 488 nm image shows mAb 3E7. (**C**), ARH77 cells were opsonized with FITC OFA, and then reacted with NHS and Al647 mAb 3E7; the 647 nm image shows mAb 3E7. (**D,E**), ARH77 cells were opsonized with Al488 RTX, and then reacted with NHS and Al647 mAb 3E7; the 488 nm image (**D**) shows RTX and the 647 nm image (**E**) shows mAb 3E7. There is neither blebbing nor streamers in panels (**D,E**). (**F**), Blebbing and streamers are generated in the absence of mAb 3E7. Daudi cells were opsonized with Al647 OFA and then reacted with NHS. The 647 nm image is displayed. Figures 4 and 5 were originally published in *The Journal of Immunology*. Beum, P.V. et al., 2008, Complement activation on B lymphocytes opsonized with rituximab or ofatumumab produces substantial changes in membrane structure preceding cell lysis, *J. Immunol.* 181:822–832. Copyright © (2008) The American Association of Immunologists, Inc. [19].

6. On the Importance of Ca^{2+}

Based on these observations, we next focused on investigating the possible role of Ca^{2+} in the cell-killing phase of the CDC reaction [22]. Upstream deposition of C3b occurs in a process which requires Ca^{2+}, but the downstream terminal steps in the C cascade, in particular, generation of the MAC, do *not* directly require Ca^{2+}. Therefore, we briefly reacted Daudi cells with OFA in C5-depleted serum to deposit active C3b but not permit subsequent MAC formation. The cells were then washed and incubated in NHS-EDTA (to chelate Ca^{2+}) or in NHS. Under both conditions, The MAC is then generated and the cells are killed (Figure 6); however, TNTs are not produced when the cells are killed in NHS-EDTA, providing strong evidence that in NHS it is entry of Ca^{2+} into the cells that promotes TNT formation (Figure 7) [22]. The degree of killing for C3b-opsonized cells reacted in NHS-EDTA was somewhat lower and slower than in in NHS. We suggest that under these conditions, where Ca^{2+} entry into cells is precluded, we are instead studying "death by drowning" of the cells due to influx of large amounts of water and loss of cellular constituents upon permeabilization of the cell membrane. However, it is our working hypothesis that when the cells are killed under normal physiological conditions for CDC, it is the influx of lethal amounts of Ca^{2+} that provides the most immediate fatal blow. A similar finding of slower cell killing was reported by Papadimitriou et al., who examined MAC killing of EACs in the presence of EGTA in which Ca^{2+} was chelated, thus precluding its rapid entry into the cells [14,15].

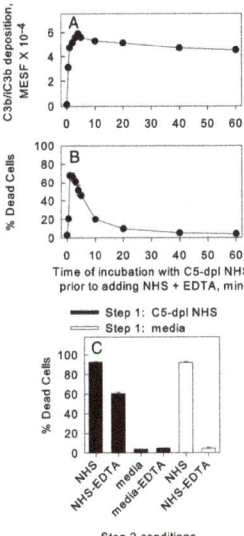

Figure 6. Two-step CDC. Reaction of OFA-opsonized Daudi cells in C5-depleted (C5-dpl) NHS in step

1 promotes C3b/iC3b deposition and these cells are killed when they are incubated in either NHS or NHS + EDTA in step 2. (**A**) C3b/iC3b deposition was assayed with PE mAb 7C12 and is expressed as molecules of equivalent soluble fluorochrome (MESF). In a control to block C3b deposition, cells were opsonized in step 1 with C5-depleted NHS + EDTA; the resulting signal was only 1200 MESF. (**B**) The percentage of dead cells was determined based on uptake of TO-PRO-3. (**A,B**) Representative of five similar experiments. (**C**) Killing of cells under various step 2 conditions. Means and SD are displayed. Representative of three similar experiments [22].

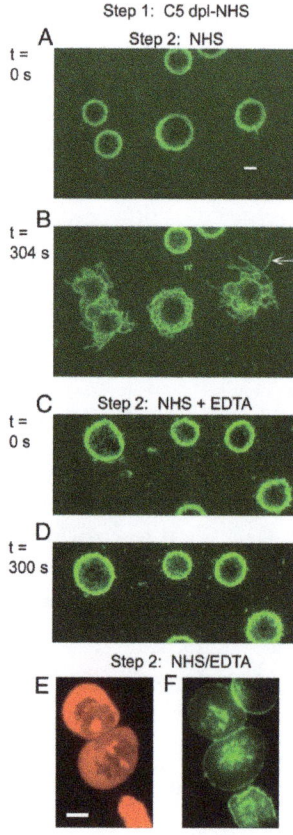

Figure 7. Production of streamers requires Ca^{2+}. OFA-opsonized cells reacted with C5-depleted NHS do not exhibit streaming when they are incubated with NHS + EDTA. (**A–D**) Al488 mAb 3E7 was used to visualize the C3b-opsonized cells, and representative images from spinning disc confocal microscopy (SDCM) movies are displayed at time 0 (**A,C**) and after 304 or 300 s (**B,D**). A streamer in (**B**) is identified by the arrow. Images shown are representative of more than 20 similar experiments. Magnification at 63× in all images. Scale bar = 5 microns. (**E,F**) Fluorescence microscopy (FM) analysis of Al488 OFA-opsonized Daudi cells subjected to the two-step protocol and then stained with PI to identify dead (stained red) cells. Although the cells are dead (**E**) there is no evidence for blebbing or steamers. Magnification at 100×; scale bar = 10 microns. Representative of more than 15 fields examined in two separate experiments. Figures 6 and 7 were originally published in the *European Journal of Immunology*, Vol. 41, Beum, P.V. et al. 2011, Penetration of antibody-opsonized cells by the membrane attack complex of complement promotes Ca^{2+} influx and induces streamers. *Eur. J. Immunol.* pp. 2436–2446, © 2011 Wiley-VCH Verlag GmbH & Co. KGaA, Weinheim [22].

At this point, our research direction was strongly influenced by a general theory as to how toxins kill cells, developed more than 40 years ago by Schanne et al. [55]. They noted that in a first step, toxin could compromise the integrity of cell membranes by a variety of mechanisms that were usually independent of Ca^{2+}. However, they suggested that "the second step of toxin induced killing most likely represents an influx of Ca^{2+} across the damaged plasma membrane ... and represents a final common pathway by which the cells are killed." Indeed, under normal physiological conditions, The external extracellular Ca^{2+} concentration in blood and interstitial fluid is in the millimolar range, but the Ca^{2+} concentration in most nucleated cells is approximately 0.1 uM, and levels above 2 uM are usually lethal [9,56–58]. Therefore, it is quite reasonable to expect that when the plasma membrane of a cell is effectively permeabilized by the MAC "toxin", The cell will then be killed as a consequence of influx of Ca^{2+} and poisoning of many of its major metabolic pathways due to Ca^{2+}-mediated excessive activation of a variety of proteases, endonucleases, and phospholipases [12,14,15].

7. Hexamer-Forming mAbs are More Effective in Activating C

7.1. Cell-Bound Hexamer-Forming mAbs Bind C1q

In a very productive collaboration, we made use of hexamer-forming mAbs that were developed by Prof. Paul Parren and his colleagues at Genmab [16,20,59–62]. We used these mAbs to further study the role of Ca^{2+} entry into cells in the mAb-mediated CDC reaction. These mAbs are modified in the Fc region, which substantially enhances their potential to form hexamers upon binding to cells. The modifications (e.g., E430G) promote much more effective and rapid binding of the classical pathway initiating factor, hexameric C1q, to the mAb-opsonized cells, and thereby increase the CDC potential of a wide range of mAbs. We also note that numerous other strategies are under investigation for increasing the ability of mAbs to promote CDC of tumor cells [26,27,41,63–72]. It will be interesting to compare the efficacy of these strategies if they progress to clinical trials.

We first compared 7D8 (a close analogue of OFA [73]), RTX and the hexamer-forming variants, 7D8-Hx and RTX-Hx. Although approximately comparable amounts of the different CD20 mAbs bind to a given cell, 7D8-Hx and RTX-Hx are considerably more effective at promoting C1q binding and rapid C-mediated killing of the target cells (Figure 8) [16]. We also found that all four mAbs bound to the cells within 1–2 min.

7.2. Four-Color Confocal Microscopy Movies

We next performed a series of kinetic experiments to study CDC-mediated by 7D8-Hx based on four-color confocal microscopy movies. Raji B cells or CLL cells were internally labeled with the green fluorescent Ca^{2+} indicator, Fluo-4, to monitor Ca^{2+} influx. Viable mitochondria were visualized with TMRME (red). The cells were dispersed in NHS containing Alexa-405-labeled anti-C3b/iC3b mAb 3E7 (blue) to follow C3b deposition and TO-PRO-3 (purple) was added to the medium as a live/dead indicator. The screenshots (Figure 9) [16] from the movies of Raji cells reacted with 7D8-Hx demonstrate that many of the cells are opsonized with C3b (binding of blue anti-C3b mAb 3E7) after approximately 90 s. Soon thereafter, enough MAC must have penetrated the cells, because many of them are bright green (indicating influx of Ca^{2+}), but some are still alive, and their mitochondria appear to be alive and intact, based on the viable red TMRME signal (135 and 180 s). We have identified these bright green cells as "transition-state intermediates". They are alive, but are doomed, because lethal amounts of Ca^{2+} had entered the cells. Soon, by 180–270 s, many of the cells are dying or are dead, and this is evident based on three separate criteria: first, most of the Fluo-4 has leaked out of the cells; second, The mitochondria have been poisoned and are no longer stained by TMRME; and third, TO-PRO-3 has entered the cells. Careful inspection of the movies suggested that there was a slight lag (5–10 s) between the coincident leakage of Fluo-4/loss of the TMRME signal, and the final entry of TOPRO-3 into the dead cells. More details on these phenomena can be found in the Figure 9 caption.

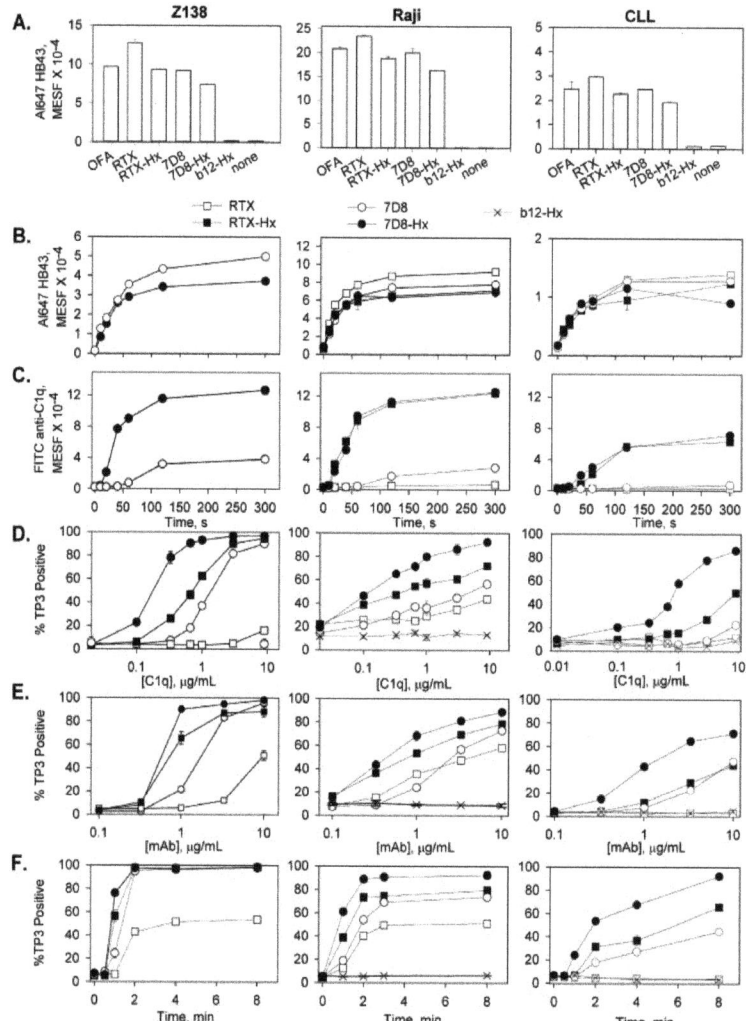

Figure 8. Hexamer-forming CD20 mAbs efficiently utilize small amounts of C1q to mediate CDC. Hexamer-forming CD20 mAbs bind to B cells and promote C1q binding, CDC and efficiently utilize small amounts of C1q to mediate CDC. (**A**) Saturating amounts of mAbs were reacted with cells for 30 min at RT in media, and after two washes, binding was evaluated by development with Al647 mAb HB43 (10 μg/mL, 30 min on ice), specific for human IgG Fc region. All points are in duplicate, and means and SD are displayed. (**B,C**) Kinetics of mAb binding and C1q uptake were determined based on reacting mAbs (10 μg/mL) with cells in 5% NHS for varying times at 37 °C. After washing, development was based on probing with (**B**) Al647 mAb HB43 or (**C**) FITC anti-C1q antibody. (**D**) CDC with 10 μg/mL mAb in 50% C1q-depleted serum supplemented with varying amounts of C1q for 20 min at 37 °C. % TO-PRO-3 (TP3)-positive cells define % CDC. (**E**) Cells were reacted with mAbs at 37 °C for 20 min in 50% NHS, and CDC was evaluated after TO-PRO-3 staining. (**F**) Kinetics of killing were determined after reacting cells with 10 μg/mL mAb in 50% NHS for varying times. (**A–F**) Each graph is representative of 2–4 similar experiments. Results for CLL cells shown in this figure were obtained with cells from four CLL patients. Cytotoxicity for CLL cells reacted in the absence of mAbs, or plus mAb in media, or in heat-inactivated NHS, was less than 6% [16].

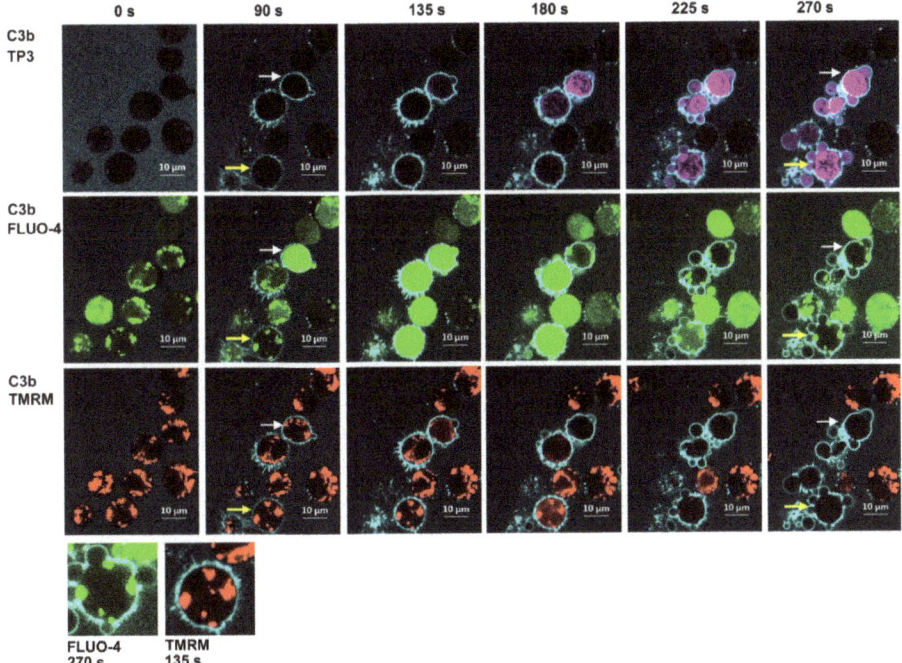

Figure 9. **Four-color confocal fluorescence microscopy analyses of the kinetics of CDC of Raji cells mediated by 7D8-Hx.** Delineation of discrete steps in CDC of Raji cells: four-color confocal fluorescence microscopy analyses of the kinetics of CDC of Raji cells mediated by 7D8-Hx. For clarity, images based on analyses with two colors at advancing times during the reaction are displayed. Upper panel: Al405 mAb 3E7 (C3b/iC3b, light blue) and TO-PRO-3 (dead cells, bright purple). Middle panel: Al405 mAb 3E7 (C3b/iC3b) and Fluo-4 (Ca^{2+}, green). Lower panel: Al405 mAb 3E7 (C3b/iC3b) and TMRM (viable mitochondria red). White arrows mark a representative cell in the transition state at 90 s and dead at 270 s. Yellow arrows identify a cell in which the mitochondria remain viable through the transition-state intermediate. Inset: Amplified image of a single cell at 270 s (Fluo-4) and 135 s (TMRM). Note that the green signal due to Fluo-4 in the dead cell (at 270 s) is localized to places in the live cell in which viable mitochondria (positive TMRM staining) are identified at 135 s. Representative of more than 10 similar experiments [16].

7.3. Kinetics of CDC Monitored by Multicolor HRDI

We also made use of HRDI technology to visualize cells during the CDC process. Figure 10, top panel identifies three distinct populations of cells at the 40 s mark that are either: alive—Fluo-4 very bright (transition-state intermediate) and TMRME positive; and finally dead—Fluo-4 weak, TMRME negative, C3b positive and TOPRO-3 positive [16]. Verification that the *residual* Fluo-4 stain is in the mitochondria (identified with Mitotracker Red) of the cells is demonstrated in Figure 10, bottom panel. It is also noteworthy that there is no noticeable swelling of the dead cells (Figure 10, top panel) at early times, soon after they are killed. This again emphasizes that there is no evidence for an early osmotic burst reaction when the nucleated cells are first killed, in agreement with Papadimitriou et al. [15].

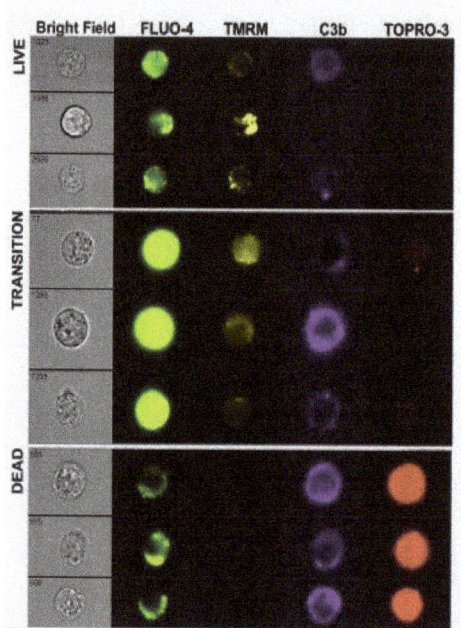
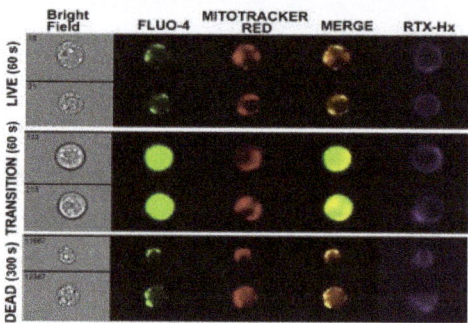

Figure 10. Four-color kinetic analyses by HRDI of the transition-state intermediate. Delineation of discrete steps in CDC: Four-color kinetic analyses by multispectral fluorescence imaging. Top panel: Images of representative 7D8-Hx treated cells that are either alive, in transition, or are dead. Bottom panel: Representative images for cells reacted with Al647 RTX-Hx (E345R) after 60 s (live and transition) or after 300 s (dead). The cells were presumed to be dead by 300 s based on the decrease in the mean Fluo-4 signal. Figures 8–10 are reprinted from Molecular Immunology, Vol. 70, 2016, Lindorfer, M. A. et al. Real-time analysis of the detailed sequence of cellular events in mAb-mediated complement-dependent cytotoxicity of B cell lines and of CLL B cells, pp. 13–23 with permission from Elsevier [16].

We also used HRDI to follow the CDC reaction for Z138 cells. In these experiments, we monitored C9 binding instead of Ca^{2+} influx. We were able to verify that binding of C9 to the Z138 cells followed C3b deposition, and that live cells containing bound C9 could be identified (Figure 11), but we know that these are also "doomed" cells that will soon experience substantial fluxes of Ca^{2+} [20]. In agreement with earlier studies, there is considerable colocalization of cell-bound mAb with deposited C3b, and in addition deposited C3b clearly serves as a "landing site" for binding of C5b-9, based on the colocalization of C3b and C9 (Figure 12). The identification of the transition-state intermediate (very bright homogeneous Fluo-4 signal) raised an interesting question: could we better validate its existence and stabilize it by slowing leakage of Fluo-4 out of the cell? The coincident question raised in these studies centered on the role of C9; is C9 essential to kill the cells as part of the MAC?

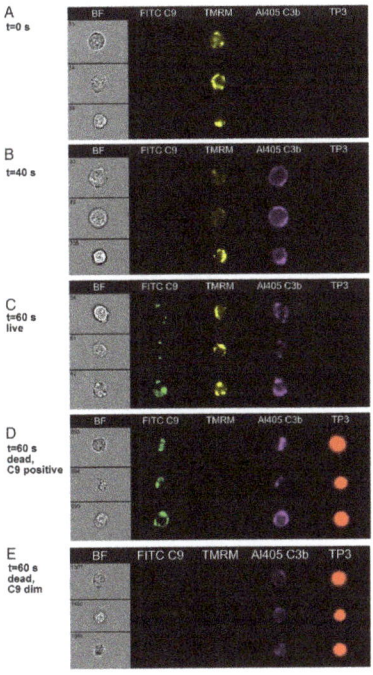

Figure 11. mAb 7D8-Hx mediates CDC of Z138 cells in C9-depleted NHS. Distinct cellular steps in the CDC pathway are illustrated with representative images from an experiment in which Z138 cells were reacted with 7D8-Hx in NHS. (**A**) At zero time, cells are alive (TMRM positive, TP3 negative). (**B**) After 40 s, C3b has deposited, but the cells are still alive, based on the positive TMRM signal and the lack of staining by TP3. (**C,D**) After 60 s, C9 has bound to the cells. Note that both live (**C**) and dead (**D**) (TP3 positive, TMRM negative) C9-positive cells can be seen. (**E**) After 60 s, 8.6% of dead cells are C9 dim [20].

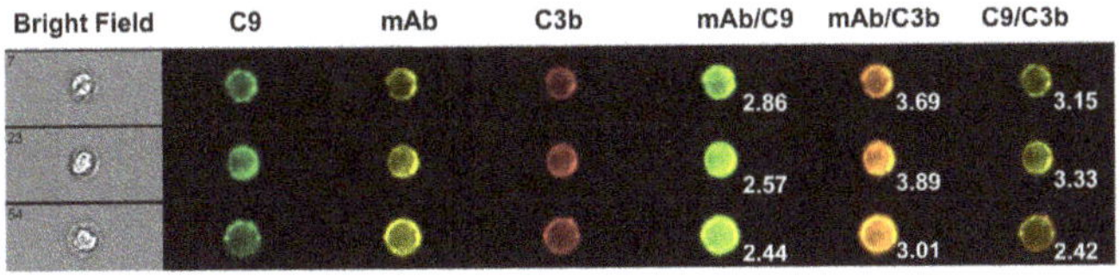

Figure 12. C3b and C9 are colocalized on B cells opsonized with mAb 7D8-Hx. C3b and C9 are colocalized on B cells with opsonizing mAb 7D8-Hx after reaction for brief periods in 50% NHS. Data were obtained based on multispectral high-resolution fluorescence imaging by flow cytometry. CLL cells were reacted with Al546 Hx-7D8 in NHS for 8 min and after two washes were probed with both FITC mAb aE11 and with Al594 3E7 (for C3b/iC3b). Images representative of triple-positive cells are shown. Bright detail similarity score (BDSS) values for the merged images of the individual cells are given. A very high degree of colocalization of Hx-7D8 with C3b is evident, and colocalization of the mAb with C9 is also observed [20].

8. On the Role of C9

We identified small populations of cells that were killed by CDC but did not appear to be stained by C9 [20] (Figure 11, panel E), and we also found that CLL cells and Z138 cells reacted with 7D8-Hx could be killed by CDC in C9-depleted serum. In fact, we reported that the cells could also be killed in sera depleted of Factor B and Factor D (Figure 13). Other mAbs that promote high levels of CDC, including alemtuzumab and W6/32 (Mouse IgG2b, anti-HLA) also were able to mediate CDC in C9-depleted serum, but in all cases mAb-mediated CDC had an absolute requirement for C1q. These findings suggest that the alternative pathway of C (APC) does not appear to be needed to promote effective CDC mediated by the mAbs under investigation. It is generally believed that the APC, based on its inherent exponential amplification loop is responsible for most of the efficacy of C [74,75]. Our findings would suggest this might not be the case for CDC of tumor cells mediated by mAbs, where it appears that the classical pathway (C1q requirement) is key.

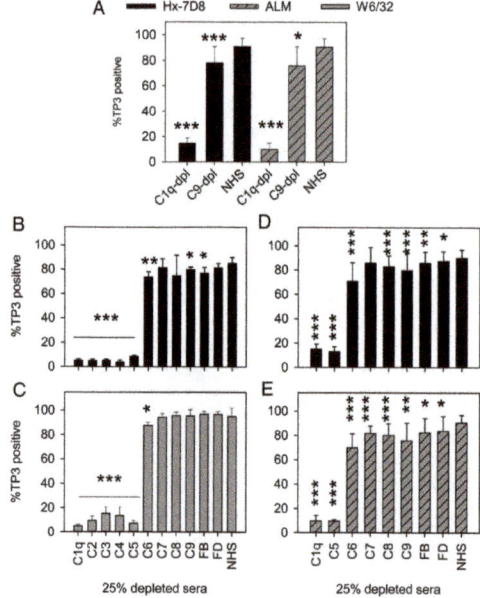

Figure 13. **C9-depleted sera support CDC mediated by several different mAbs.** Sera depleted of one of several terminal (but not upstream) classical pathway complement components support CDC mediated by several different mAbs. (**A**) mAbs Hx-7D8 and ALM promote robust CDC of CLL cells after reaction for 15 min in 25% NHS or C9-dpl sera. The results are the average for duplicate determinations on cells from eight different CLL patients for Hx-7D8 and the average for cells from four of the eight patients for ALM; means and SD are displayed. No CDC is observed if Hx-7D8 or ALM is reacted with CLL cells in C1q-dpl sera. Differences between C1q-dpl and C9-dpl versus NHS are significant, as illustrated. (**B,C**) Both Hx-7D8 and W6/32 mediate CDC of Z138 cells in sera depleted of terminal pathway components or of complement factor B (FB) or complement factor D (FD). $n = 4$–6. Significant differences versus NHS are noted. (**D,E**) Both Hx-7D8 and ALM mediate CDC of CLL cells in sera depleted of terminal pathway components or of FB or FD. The averaged results for duplicate determinations on cells from eight different CLL patients are provided. The results for C1q-dpl, C9-dpl, and NHS are the same as in (**A**), and are repeated to allow for ready inspection and comparison with the other depleted sera. * $p < 0.05$, ** $p < 0.01$, *** $p < 0.001$. Figures 11–13 were originally published in *The Journal of Immunology*. Cook, E. M. et al. 2016, Antibodies that efficiently form hexamers upon antigen binding can induce complement-dependent cytotoxicity under complement-limiting conditions. *J. Immunol.* 197:1762–1775. Copyright © (2016) The American Association of Immunologists, Inc. [20].

The results of the experiments with C9-depleted serum are intriguing, but not definitive because trace amounts of C9 could still be present in the depleted serum. However, The smaller C5b-8 pores that penetrate cells are approximately 3.5 nm in size (pores formed with C5b-9 are 10–11.5 nm) and in principle the C5b-8 pores should be adequate to allow for Ca^{2+} entry and killing of the cell [76]. Therefore, in collaboration with Drs. Paul Morgan and Masashi Mizuno, we used flow cytometry to investigate whether CLL cells could be killed by Ca^{2+} fluxes in serum genetically deficient in C9 [21]. Although we had limited amounts of the C9-deficient serum, we were able to demonstrate that mAb 7D8-Hx promoted substantial CDC of the CLL cells from six different patients (Figure 14). Compared to the reaction in NHS, The CDC kinetics were only slightly slower in the C9-deficient serum. We also asked whether the smaller C5b-8 pores would stabilize the transition-state intermediate (bright green, Fluo-4 very positive) by slowing down exit of Fluo-4 from the cell. Indeed, at the 150 s point, approximately 70% of the cells had been killed, but the net Fluo-4 signal was maximized at this point, indicating that even though most of the cells had been killed due to Ca^{2+} poisoning, The Fluo-4 had not yet leaked out of the cells (Figure 15). The bright green "dead intermediate" was therefore stabilized over a period of approximately 200 s (t = 100 s to 300 s). Due to very limited amounts of C9-deficient serum, we were not able to investigate the reaction with confocal microscopy movies. However, we suggest that further studies with serum from donors genetically deficient in C9 [77] would allow for more comprehensive investigation of these phenomena in the future. For example, it could be quite informative and useful to identify and differentiate tumor cells that are/are not susceptible to CDC in sera lacking C9.

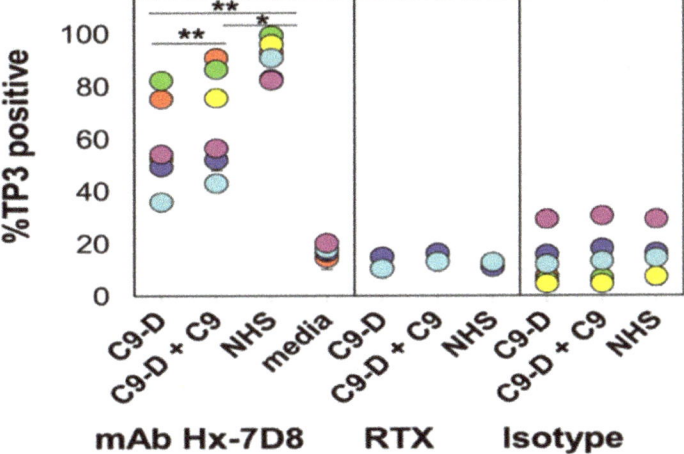

Figure 14. C9-deficient serum can mediate high levels of CDC of CLL cells opsonized with mAb Hx-7D8. C9-deficient (C9-D) serum lacks any detectable C9, but can mediate high levels of lysis of CLL cells reacted with mAb Hx-7D8. The ability of mAb Hx-7D8 to promote CDC in CLL cells from six different patients was evaluated in either: C9-D serum (25%), C9-D serum (25%) supplemented with 18 µg/mL C9, or NHS (25%). Controls included Hx-7D8 reacted with cells in media (4 of 6 CLL cell samples) as well as cells reacted with RTX (2 CLL samples) or an isotype control (Isotype, Hx-b12, 2–4 CLL samples) reacted with CLL cells in all three conditions. Each color represents a different patient (pn); all determinations were in duplicate or triplicate and means and SD are provided. Mean % CDC and SD: 58 ± 17% for CLL cells reacted in C9-D serum; 67 ± 20% for CLL cells reacted in C9-D serum + C9; 91 ± 7% for CLL cells reacted in NHS. * $p < 0.05$; ** $p < 0.01$ [21].

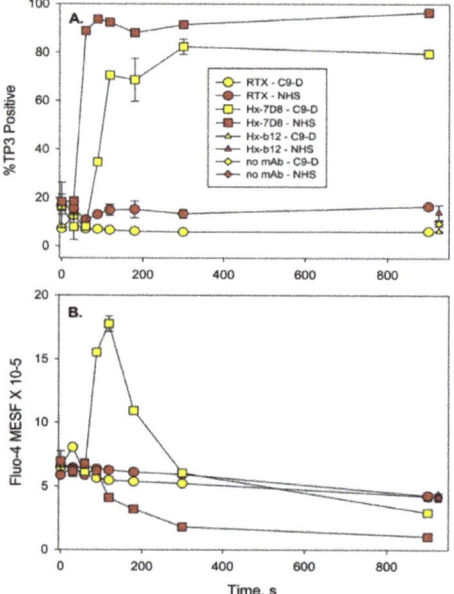

Figure 15. Analysis of CDC and Ca^{2+} fluxes in Fluo-4-loaded CLL cells. (**A**) CDC kinetics mediated by Hx-7D8 in C9-D serum (pn 2014, red circles, Figure 14) were slower and killing peaked at approximately 80%, compared to results in intact NHS where killing reached 95%. CDC mediated by RTX was low under both conditions. (**B**) During CDC mediated by Hx-7D8 (also pn 2014), The Fluo-4 signal is increased considerably and remains substantially elevated for 3 min (indicative of the transition-state intermediate) for CLL cells reacted with Hx-7D8 in C9-D serum. Controls include cells reacted for 900 s in NHS or in C9-D serum, with either the isotype control Hx-b12, or with no mAb. Figures 14 and 15 are reprinted from Clinical Immunology, Vol. 181, 2017, Taylor, R.P. et al. Hexamerization-enhanced CD20 antibody mediates complement-dependent cytotoxicity in serum genetically deficient in C9, pp. 24–28, with permission from Elsevier [21].

9. Ca^{2+} Appears to be the Key: Implications

Our findings, as well as those of the Shin group [10–15], provide compelling evidence that it is the influx of Ca^{2+} into nucleated cells that is the primary cause of cell death in the CDC reaction mediated by anti-tumor mAbs. On this basis, there are several additional strategies that could be employed to bring even more efficacy to this process, based on increasing the flux of lethal amounts of Ca^{2+} into the targeted cell. One possibility is also to stimulate the target cell with other mAbs and/or ligands that promote uptake of Ca^{2+} into the cell. For example, Fifadara reported that mast cells costimulated at the high-affinity receptor for the Fc region of IgE (FcεRI) and chemokine receptor 1 (both of which promote Ca^{2+} fluxes) were not killed, but produced TNTs [78]. Apparently, these cells were "on the edge" of being over-stimulated and killed by Ca^{2+}, but they survived. If these mast cells were reacted with a mAb that only modestly activated C and the Ca^{2+} flux was inadequate, then perhaps synergy in killing could be achieved by coincident treatment with agents that stimulate FcεRI and/or chemokine receptor 1. This proof-of-concept experiment could be extended to target other stimulatory sites on tumor cells that are known to mediate Ca^{2+} entry. Another approach would be to make use of a mAb–drug conjugate. If a Ca^{2+} ionophore (A23187 or ionomycin) [23] could be stably coupled to a C-fixing mAb with no damage to the potential of the mAb to mediate C activation, then the ionophore could independently further increase Ca^{2+} entry into the targeted cell to increase its cell-killing potential. A similar strategy could be based on coupling pore-forming agents such as melittin or perforin to C-fixing anti-tumor mAbs [23]. Indeed, immunoconjugates of melittin have been investigated for cancer immunotherapy [79]. Finally, as we suggested recently, a third strategy would be to develop a C-fixing antibody drug conjugate that blocks the machinery that pumps Ca^{2+} out of cells, thus synergizing with the CDC action of the anti-tumor mAbs [16].

10. The Future

As new and effective C-fixing mAbs are developed for cancer immunotherapy, it is very likely that they will closely follow the patterns we have described here (Table 1). Indeed, in collaboration with investigators at Genmab and Drs. Clive Zent and Richard Burack at the University of Rochester, we recently reported on the properties of CD37 mAbs that contain the E430G hexamer-forming modification [32]. We found that these mAbs promote very high levels (>98%) of CDC of CLL cells taken from newly diagnosed patients. The very high levels of killing are likely due to the fact that most CLL cells express approximately twice as many CD37 epitopes as CD20 epitopes [32,80]. Moreover, based on four-color confocal microscopy real-time movies, we found that upon binding of the CD37-Hx mAb to CLL cells in the presence of NHS, C3b is rapidly colocalized with cell-bound CD37-Hx mAb, and the same pattern of rapid cell killing mediated by Ca^{2+} influx is evident [80]. This includes generation of transition-state intermediates followed by poisoning of mitochondria, leakage of Fluo-4 out of the cell, and finally cell death, all within just a few minutes. We suggest that this cytotoxicity pattern can serve as a "litmus test" for evaluation of the potential of future mAbs intended to be used for cancer immunotherapy based on C-mediated killing.

11. Summary

As illustrated in Figure 16, we have examined and characterized, from the "point of view" of the cell, many of the key steps in the classical complement pathway that are activated when highly effective C-activating mAbs bind to tumor cells. The entire reaction is quite rapid, and both cell lines and primary CLL cells can be killed within just a few minutes due to influx of lethal amounts of Ca^{2+}, clearly not allowing much time for any complex signaling pathways to be activated. The patterns we have described are likely to be quite general, and it may be possible to make use of the lessons we have learned in the development of additional innovative strategies that employ C and mAbs in the treatment of cancer and other diseases as well.

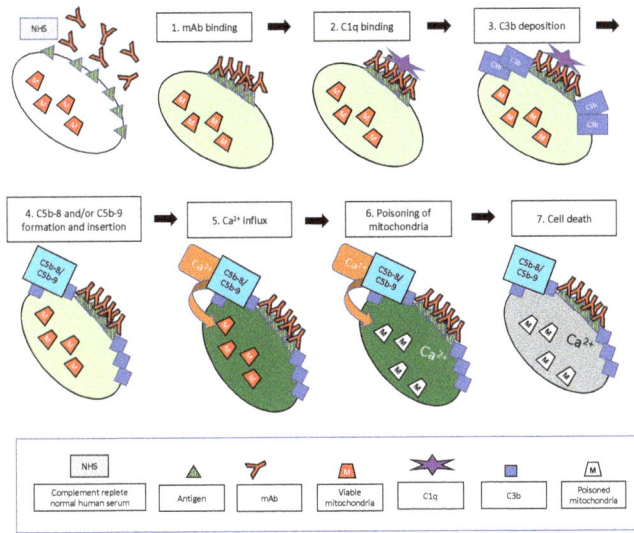

Figure 16. Simplified schematic illustrating the key steps in the CDC reaction that are described in

this review. The reaction takes place at 37 °C in 50% NHS, and the mAb is at a concentration of 10 µg/mL. The target cell is internally labeled with Fluo-4. The pale green color of the cell illustrates the low, physiological levels of cytoplasmic Ca^{+2}. (**1**). Multiple mAbs bind to the cell in proximity, ideally forming hexamers. (**2**). C1q then binds to the mAb hexamers on the cell. (**3**). Downstream, C3b is deposited on the cell, closely associated with bound mAb. (**4**). After sufficient C3b has deposited on the cell, C5b is generated, and C5b-8 and/or C5b-9 assemble close to the sites of C3b deposition. (**5**). The pores formed in the plasma membrane by C5b-8 and/or C5b-9 allow the influx of large amounts of Ca^{2+} and the cell turns bright green (the live, transition-state intermediate). (**6**). Soon thereafter, The Ca^2 in the cell penetrates and poisons the mitochondria. (**7**). This is rapidly followed by cell death. Coincident with cell death, most of the Fluo-4 leaks out of the cell. Not shown are the TNTs that are generated in the cells soon after the initial influx of Ca^{2+}, during steps (**5**) and (**6**). Approximate times for these events are provided in Table 1, and all of the reactions are fast. The hexamer-forming mAbs and C1q are bound to the cell in less than 1 min, and the cells are killed in less than 2 min.

12. Patents

R.P.T. and M.A.L. are listed as co-inventors on a patent that describes the use of hexamer-forming antibodies.

Author Contributions: R.P.T. and M.A.L. wrote and edited this manuscript. All authors have read and agreed to the published version of the manuscript.

Funding: No funding provided for the preparation of this manuscript.

Acknowledgments: The work described herein could never have been accomplished without the enthusiastic participation of the following individuals: Paul Beum, Frank Beurskens, Ricard Burack, Erika Cook, Adam Kennedy, Joanne Lannigan, Monica Liu, Paul Parren, Andrew Pawluczkowycz, Elizabeth Peek, Michael Pokrass, Michael Solga, Janine Schuurman, Jillian Tupitza, Jan van de Winkel, and Clive Zent.

Conflicts of Interest: RPT and MAL have licensed mAbs 3E7 and 7C12 for commercial use through the University of Virginia Licensing and Ventures Group.

Abbreviations

7AAD	7-aminoactinomycin D
Al	Alexa dye
APC	alternative pathway of complement
BDSS	bright detail similarity score
C	complement
CDC	complement-dependent cytotoxicity
CLL	chronic lymphocytic leukemia
EAC	Ehrlich ascites cell
FcεRI	the high-affinity receptor for the Fc region of IgE
FcγR	receptor for the Fc region of IgG
GMF	geometric mean fluorescence
HRDI	high-resolution digital imaging in a flow cytometry environment
MAC	membrane attack complex
mAb	monoclonal antibody
NHS	normal human serum
OFA	ofatumumab
PI	propidium iodide
RTX	rituximab
TNTs	tunneling nanotubules
TMRME	tetramethylrhodamine methyl ester

References

1. Cavaillon, J.M.; Sansonetti, P.; Goldman, M. 100th anniversary of Jules Bordet's Nobel prize: Tribute to a founding father of immunology. *Front. Immunol.* **2019**. [CrossRef] [PubMed]
2. Reis, E.D.; Mastellos, D.C.; Ricklin, D.; Mantovani, A.; Lambris, J.D. Complement in cancer: Untangling an intricate relationship. *Nat. Rev. Immunol.* **2017**. [CrossRef] [PubMed]
3. Ricklin, D.; Mastellos, D.C.; Reis, E.S.; Lambris, J.D. The renaissance of complement therapeutics. *Nat. Rev. Nephrol.* **2018**, *14*, 26–47. [CrossRef] [PubMed]
4. Mastellos, D.C.; Ricklin, D.; Lambris, J.D. Clinical promise of next-generation complement therapeutics. *Nat. Rev. Drug Disc.* **2019**, *18*. [CrossRef] [PubMed]
5. Golay, J.; Taylor, R.P. The role of complement in the mechanism of action of therapeutic anti-cancer mAbs. *Antibodies.* Submitted.
6. Mayer, M.M. Mechanism of cytolysis by complement. *PNAS* **1972**, *69*, 2954–2958. [CrossRef] [PubMed]
7. Ohanian, S.H.; Schlager, S.I. Humoral immune killing of nucleated cells: Mechanisms of complement-mediated attack and target cell defense. *Crit. Rev. Immunol.* **1981**, *1*, 165–209. [PubMed]
8. Walport, M.J. Complement. *N. Engl. J. Med.* **2001**, *344*, 1058–1066. [CrossRef] [PubMed]
9. Morgan, B.P.; Luzio, J.P.; Campbell, A.K. Intracellular Ca^{2+} and cell injury: A paradoxical role of Ca^{2+} in complement membrane attack. *Cell Calcium* **1986**, *7*, 399–411. [CrossRef]
10. Kim, S.H.; Carney, D.F.; Papadimitriou, J.C.; Shin, M.L. Effect of osmotic protection on nucleated cell killing by C5b-9: Cell death is not affected by the prevention of cell swelling. *Mol. Immmunol.* **1989**, *26*, 323–331.
11. Carney, D.F.; Koski, C.L.; Shin, M.L. Elimination of terminal complement intermediates from the plasma membrane of nucleated cells: The rate of disppearance differs for cells carrying C5b-7 or C5b-8 or a mixture of C5b-8 with a limited number of C5b-9. *J. Immunol.* **1985**, *134*, 1804–1809.
12. Kim, S.; Carney, D.F.; Hammer, C.H.; Shin, M.L. Nucleated cell killing by complement: Effects of C5b-9 channel size and extracellular Ca^{2+} on the lytic process. *J. Immunol.* **1987**, *138*, 1530–1536.
13. Carney, D.F.; Lang, T.J.; Shin, M.L. Multiple signal messengers generated by terminal complement complexes and their role in terminal complement complex elimination. *J. Immunol.* **1990**, *145*, 623–629. [PubMed]
14. Papadimitriou, J.C.; Ramm, L.E.; Drachenberg, C.B.; Trump, B.F.; Shin, M.L. Quantitative analysis of adenine nucleotides during the prelytic phase of cell death mediated by C5b-9. *J. Immunol.* **1991**, *147*, 212–217. [PubMed]
15. Papadimitriou, J.C.; Phelps, P.C.; Shin, M.L.; Smith, M.W.; Trump, B.F. Effects of Ca^{2+} deregulation on mitochondrial membrane potential and cell viability in nucleated cells following lytic complement attack. *Cell Calcium* **1994**, *15*, 217–227. [CrossRef]
16. Lindorfer, M.A.; Cook, E.M.; Tupitza, J.C.; Zent, C.S.; Burack, R.; De Jong, R.; Beurskens, F.J.; Schuurman, J.; Parren, P.W.; Taylor, R.P. Real-time analysis of the detailed sequence of cellular events in mAb-mediated complement-dependent cytotoxicity of B-cell lines and of CLL B-cells. *Mol. Immunol.* **2016**, *70*, 13–23. [CrossRef] [PubMed]
17. Pawluczkowycz, A.W.; Beurskens, F.J.; Beum, P.V.; Lindorfer, M.; Van De Winkel, J.G.J.; Parren, P.W.; Taylor, R.P. Binding of submaximal C1q promotes complement-dependent cytotoxicity (CDC) of B cells opsonized with anti-CD20 mAbs ofatumumab (OFA) or rituximab (RTX): Considerably higher levels of CDC are induced by OFA than by RTX. *J. Immunol.* **2009**, *183*, 749–758. [CrossRef] [PubMed]
18. Beum, P.V.; Lindorfer, M.A.; Hall, B.E.; George, T.C.; Frost, K.; Morrissey, P.J.; Taylor, R.P. Quantitative analysis of protein co-localization on B cells opsonized with rituximab and complement using the ImageStream multispectral imaging flow cytometer. *J. Immunol. Methods* **2006**, *317*, 90–99. [CrossRef]
19. Beum, P.V.; Lindorfer, M.A.; Beurskens, F.; Stukenberg, P.; Lokhorst, H.M.; Pawluczkowycz, A.W.; Parren, P.W.; Van De Winkel, J.G.J.; Taylor, R.P. Complement activation on B lymphocytes opsonized with rituximab or ofatumumab produces substantial changes in membrane structure preceding cell lysis. *J. Immunol.* **2008**, *181*, 822–832. [CrossRef]
20. Cook, E.M.; Lindorfer, M.A.; van der Horst, H.; Oostindie, S.; Beurskens, F.J.; Schuurman, J.; Schuurman, J.; Zent, C.S.; Burack, R.; Parren, P.W.H.I.; et al. Antibodies that efficiently form hexamers upon antigen binding can induce complement-dependent cytotoxicity under complement-limiting conditions. *J. Immunol.* **2016**, *197*, 1762–1775. [CrossRef]

21. Taylor, R.P.; Lindorfer, M.A.; Cook, E.M.; Beurskens, F.J.; Schuurman, J.; Parren, P.W.; Zent, C.S.; VanDerMeid, K.R.; Burack, R.; Mizuno, M.; et al. Hexamerization-enhanced CD20 antibody mediates complement-dependent cytotoxicity in serum genetically deficient in C9. *Clin. Immunol.* **2017**, *181*, 24–28. [CrossRef]
22. Beum, P.V.; Lindorfer, M.A.; Peek, E.M.; Stukenberg, P.; De Weers, M.; Beurskens, F.J.; Parren, P.W.; Van De Winkel, J.G.J.; Taylor, R.P. Penetration of antibody-opsonized cells by the membrane attack complex of complement promotes Ca^{2+} influx and induces streamers. *Eur. J. Immunol.* **2011**, *41*, 2436–2446. [CrossRef] [PubMed]
23. Reiter, Y.; Ciobotariu, A.; Jones, J.; Morgan, B.P.; Fishelson, Z. Complement membrane attack complex, perforin, and bacterial exotoxins induce in K562 cells calcium-dependent cross-protection from lysis. *J. Immunol.* **1995**, *155*, 2203–2210. [PubMed]
24. Hörl, S.; Bánki, Z.; Huber, G.; Ejaz, A.; Windisch, D.; Muellauer, B.; Willenbacher, E.; Steurer, M.; Stoiber, H. Reduction of complement factor H binding to CLL cells improves the induction of rituximab-mediated complement-dependent cytotoxicity. *Leukemia* **2013**, *27*, 2200–2208. [CrossRef] [PubMed]
25. Okroj, M.; Holmquist, E.; Nilsson, E.; Anagnostaki, L.; Jirström, K.; Blom, A.M. Local expression of complement factor I in breast cancer cells correlates with poor survival and recurrence. *Cancer Immunol. Immunother.* **2015**, *64*, 467–478. [CrossRef] [PubMed]
26. Bordron, A.; Bagacean, C.; Mohr, A.; Tempescul, A.; Bendaoud, B.; Deshayes, S.; Dalbies, F.; Buors, C.; Saad, H.; Berthou, C.; et al. Resistance to complement activation, cell membrane hypersialytion and relapses in chronic lymphocytic leukemia patients treated with rituximab and chemotherapy. *Oncotarget* **2018**, *9*, 31590–31605. [CrossRef]
27. Fishelson, Z.; Kirschfink, M. Complement C5b-9 and cancer: Mechanisms of cell damage, cancer counteractions, and approaches for intervention. *Front. Immunol.* **2019**. [CrossRef] [PubMed]
28. Geller, A.; Yan, J. The role of membrane bound complement regulatory proteins in tumor development and cancer immunotherapy. *Front. Immunol.* **2019**. [CrossRef] [PubMed]
29. Roumenina, L.T.; Daugan, M.V.; Noe, R.; Petitprez, F.; Vano, Y.-A.; Sanchez-Salas, R.; Becht, E.; Meilleroux, J.; Le Clec'H, B.; A Giraldo, N.; et al. Tumor cells hijack macrophage-produced complement C1q to promote tumor growth. *Cancer Immunol. Res.* **2019**. [CrossRef] [PubMed]
30. Roumenia, L.T.; Daugan, M.V.; Petitprez, F.; Sautes-Fridman, C.; Fridman, W.H. Context-dependentt roles of complement in cancer. *Nat. Rev. Cancer* **2019**, *19*, 1–18. [CrossRef]
31. Beurskens, F.J.; Lindorfer, M.A.; Farooqui, M.; Beum, P.V.; Engelberts, P.; Mackus, W.J.M.; Parren, P.W.; Wiestner, A.; Taylor, R.P. Exhaustion of cytotoxic effector systems may limit monoclonal antibody-based immunotherapy in cancer patients. *J. Immunol.* **2012**, *188*, 3532–3541. [CrossRef]
32. Oostindie, S.C.; Van Der Horst, H.J.; Lindorfer, M.; Cook, E.M.; Tupitza, J.C.; Zent, C.S.; Burack, R.; VanDerMeid, K.R.; Strumane, K.; Chamuleau, M.E.D.; et al. CD20 and CD37 antibodies synergize to activate complement by Fc-mediated clustering. *Haematologica* **2019**, *104*, 1841–1852. [CrossRef] [PubMed]
33. Pokrass, M.J.; Liu, M.F.; Lindorfer, M.A.; Taylor, R.P. Activation of complement by monoclonal antibodies that target cell-associated á2-microglobulin: Implications for cancer immunotherapy. *Mol. Immunol.* **2013**, *56*, 549–560. [CrossRef] [PubMed]
34. Wald, G. Nobel Prize Lecture: The Molecular Basis of Visual Excitation. 1967. Available online: https://www.nobelprize.org/uploads/2018/06/wald-lecture.pdf (accessed on 25 August 2020).
35. Tosic, L.; Sutherland, W.M.; Kurek, J.; Edberg, J.C.; Taylor, R.P. Preparation of monoclonal antibodies to C3b by immunization with C3b(i)-sepharose. *J. Immunol. Methods* **1989**, *120*, 241–249. [CrossRef]
36. Kennedy, A.D.; Solga, M.D.; Schuman, T.; Chi, A.W.; Lindorfer, M.A.; Sutherland, W.M.; Foley, P.L.; Taylor, R.P. An anti-C3b(i) mAb enhances complement activation, C3b(i) deposition, and killing of CD20+ cells by Rituximab. *Blood* **2003**, *101*, 1071–1079. [CrossRef] [PubMed]
37. Edberg, J.C.; Wright, E.; Taylor, R.P. Quantitative analyses of the binding of soluble complement-fixing antibody/dsDNA immune complexes to CR1 on human red blood cells. *J. Immunol.* **1987**, *139*, 3739–3747.
38. Mollnes, T.E.; Lea, T.; Harboe, M.; Tschopp, J. Monoclonal antibodies recognizing a neoantigen of poly(C9) detect the human terminal complement complex in tissue and plasma. *Scand. J. Immunol.* **1985**, *22*, 183–195. [CrossRef] [PubMed]

39. Risitano, A.M.; Notaro, R.; Pascariello, C.; Sica, M.; del Vecchio, L.; Horvath, C.J.; Fridkis-Hareli, M.; Selleri, C.; Lindorfer, M.A.; Taylor, R.P.; et al. The complement receptor 2/factor H fusion protein TT30 protects PNH erythrocytes from complement-mediated hemolysis and C3 fragment opsonization. *Blood* **2012**, *119*, 6307–6316. [CrossRef] [PubMed]
40. Markiewski, M.M.; DeAngelis, R.A.; Benencia, F.; Ricklin-Lichtsteiner, S.K.; Koutoulaki, A.; Gerard, C.; Coukos, G.; Lambris, J.D. Modulation of the antitumor immune response by complement. *Nat. Immunol.* **2008**, *9*, 1225–1235. [CrossRef] [PubMed]
41. Melis, J.P.; Strumane, K.; Ruuls, S.R.; Beurskens, F.J.; Schuurman, J.; Parren, P.W. Complement in therapy and disease: Regulating the complement system with antibody-based therapeutics. *Mol. Immunol.* **2015**, *67*, 117–130. [CrossRef] [PubMed]
42. Cleary, K.L.S.; Chan, H.T.C.; James, S.; Glennis, M.J.; Cragg, M.S. Antibody distance from the cell membrane regulates antibody effector mechanisms. *J. Immunol.* **2017**, *198*, 3999–4011. [CrossRef]
43. Teeling, J.L. Characterization of new human CD20 monoclonal antibodies with potent cytolytic activity against non-Hodgkin's lymphomas. *Blood* **2004**, *104*, 1793–1800. [CrossRef] [PubMed]
44. Teeling, J.L.; Mackus, W.J.M.; Wiegman, L.J.J.M.; Brakel, J.H.N.V.D.; Beers, S.A.; French, R.R.; Van Meerten, T.; Ebeling, S.; Vink, T.; Slootstra, J.W.; et al. The biological activity of human CD20 monoclonal antibodies is linked to unique epitopes on CD20. *J. Immunol.* **2006**, *177*, 362–371. [CrossRef] [PubMed]
45. Hughes-Jones, N.C. The classical pathway. In *Immunobiology of the Complement System*; Ross, G.D., Ed.; Academic Press: Orlando, FL, USA, 1986; pp. 21–44.
46. Okroj, M.; Osterborg, A.; Blom, A.M. Effector mechanisms of anti-CD20 monoclonal antibodies in B cell malignancies. *Cancer Treat. Rev.* **2013**, *39*, 632–639. [CrossRef] [PubMed]
47. Kennedy, A.D.; Beum, P.V.; Solga, M.D.; DiLillo, D.J.; Lindorfer, M.A.; Hess, C.E.; Densmore, J.J.; Williams, M.E.; Taylor, R.P. Rituximab infusion promotes rapid complement depletion and acute CD20 loss in chronic lymphocytic leukemia. *J. Immunol.* **2004**, *172*, 3280–3288. [CrossRef] [PubMed]
48. Williams, M.E.; Densmore, J.J.; Pawluczkowycz, A.W.; Beum, P.V.; Kennedy, A.D.; Lindorfer, M.A.; Hamil, S.H.; Eggleton, J.C.; Taylor, R.P. Thrice-weekly low-dose rituximab decreases CD20 loss via shaving and promotes enhanced targeting in chronic lymphocytic leukemia. *J. Immunol.* **2006**, *177*, 7435–7443. [CrossRef]
49. Grandjean, C.L.; Montalvao, F.; Celli, S.; Michonneau, D.; Breart, B.; Garcia, Z.; Perro, M.; Freytag, O.; Gerdes, C.A.; Bousso, P. Intravital imaging reveals improved Kupffer cell-mediated phagocytosis as a mode of action of glycoengineered anti-CD20 antibodies. *Nat. Sci. Repts.* **2016**, *6*, 34382. [CrossRef]
50. Gül, N.; Babes, L.; Siegmund, K.; Korthouwer, R.; Bögels, M.; Braster, R.; Vidarsson, G.; Hagen, T.L.T.; Kubes, P.; Van Egmond, M. Macrophages eliminate circulating tumor cells after monoclonal antibody therapy. *J. Clin. Investig.* **2014**, *124*, 812–823. [CrossRef]
51. Zent, C.S.; Elliott, M.R. Maxed out macs: Physiologic cell clearance as a function of macrophage phagocytic capacity. *FEBS J.* **2017**, *284*, 1021–1039. [CrossRef]
52. Rustom, A.; Saffrich, R.; Markovic, I.; Walther, P.; Gerdes, H.H. Nanotubular highways for intercellular organelle transport. *Science* **2004**, *303*, 1007–1010. [CrossRef]
53. Dupont, M.; Souriant, S.; Lugo-Villarino, G.; Maridonneau-Parini, I.; Verollet, C. Tunneling nanotubes: Intimate communication between myeloid cells. *Front. Immunol.* **2018**. [CrossRef]
54. Zent, C.S.; Chen, J.B.; Kurten, R.C.; Kaushal, G.P.; Lacy, H.M.; Schichman, S.A. Alemtuzumab (CAMPATH 1H) does not kill chronic lymphocytic leukemia cells in serum free medium. *Leuk. Res.* **2004**, *28*, 495–507. [CrossRef] [PubMed]
55. Schanne, F.A.X.; Kane, A.B.; Young, E.E.; Farber, J.L. Calcium dependence of toxic cell death: A final common pathway. *Science* **1979**, *206*, 700–702. [CrossRef] [PubMed]
56. Bagur, R.; Hajnoczky, G. Intracellular Ca^{2+} sensing: Its role in calcium homeostasis and signaling. *Mol. Cell* **2017**. [CrossRef] [PubMed]
57. Negulescu, P.A.; Shastri, N.; Cahalan, M.D. Intracellular calcium dependence of gene expression in single T lymphocytes. *PNAS* **1994**, *91*, 2873–2877. [CrossRef] [PubMed]
58. Joseph, N.; Reicher, B.; Barda-Saad, M. The calcium feedback loop and T cell activation: How cytoskeleton networks control intracellular calcium flux. *Biochim. Biophys. Acta* **2014**, *1838*, 557–568. [CrossRef]

59. De Jong, R.; Beurskens, F.J.; Verploegen, S.; Strumane, K.; Van Kampen, M.D.; Voorhorst, M.; Horstman, W.; Engelberts, P.J.; Oostindie, S.C.; Wang, G.; et al. A novel platform for the potentiation of therapeutic antibodies based on antigen-dependent formation of IgG hexamers at the cell surface. *PLoS Biol.* **2016**. [CrossRef]
60. Diebolder, C.A.; Beurskens, F.J.; De Jong, R.; Koning, R.A.; Strumane, K.; Lindorfer, M.A.; Voorhorst, M.; Ugurlar, D.; Rosati, S.; Heck, A.; et al. Complement is activated by IgG hexamers assembled at the cell surface. *Science* **2014**, *343*, 1260–1263. [CrossRef]
61. Tammen, A.; Derer, S.; Schwanbeck, R.; Rösner, T.; Kretschmer, A.; Beurskens, F.J.; Schuurman, J.; Parren, P.W.; Valerius, T. Monoclonal antibodies against epidermal growth factor receptor require an ability to kill tumor cells through complement activation by mutations that selectively facilitate the hexamerization of Ig G on opsonized cells. *J. Immunol.* **2017**, *198*, 1585–1594. [CrossRef]
62. Strasser, J.; de Jong, R.N.; Beurskens, F.J.; Wang, G.; Heck, A.J.; Schuurman, J.; Parren, P.W.H.I.; Hinterdorfer, P.; Preiner, J. Unraveling the macromolecular pathways of IgG oliomerization and complement activation on antigenic surfaces. *Nano Lett.* **2019**, *19*, 4787–4796. [CrossRef]
63. Ajona, D.; Hsu, Y.F.; Corrales, L.; Montuenga, L.M.; Pio, R. Down-regulation of human complement factor H sensitizes non-small cell lung cancer cells to complement attack and reduces in vivo tumor growth. *J. Immunol.* **2007**, *178*, 5991–5998. [CrossRef]
64. Derer, S.; Beurskens, F.J.; Rosner, T.; Peipp, M.; Valerius, T. Complement in antibody-based tumor therapy. *Crit. Rev. Immunol.* **2014**, *34*, 199–214. [CrossRef] [PubMed]
65. Mamidi, S.; Cinci, M.; Hasmann, M.; Fehring, V.; Kirschfink, M. Lipoplex mediated silencing of membrane regulators (CD46, CD55 and CD59) enhances complement-dependent anti-tumor activity of trastuzumab and pertuzumab. *Mol. Oncol.* **2013**, *7*, 580–594. [CrossRef] [PubMed]
66. Mamidi, S.; Hone, S.; Kirschfink, M. The complement system in cancer: Ambivalence between tumour destruction and promotion. *Immunobiology* **2017**, *222*, 45–54. [CrossRef] [PubMed]
67. Macor, P.; Tripodo, C.; Zorzet, S.; Piovan, E.; Bossi, F.; Marzari, R.; Amadori, A.; Tedesco, F. In vivo targeting of human neutralizing antibodies against CD55 and CD59 to lymphoma cells increases the antitumor activity of rituximab. *Cancer Res.* **2007**, *67*, 10556–10563. [PubMed]
68. Macor, P.; Secco, E.; Mezzaroba, N.; Zorzet, S.; Durigutto, P.; Gaiotto, T.; De Maso, L.; Biffi, S.; Garrovo, C.; Capolla, S.; et al. Bispecific antibodies targeting tumor-associated antigens and neutralizing complement regulators increase the efficacy of antibody-based immunotherapy in mice. *Leukemia* **2015**, *29*, 406–414. [CrossRef]
69. Kolev, M.; Markiewski, M.M. Targeting complement-mediated immunoregulation for cancer immunotherapy. *Semin. Immunol.* **2018**. [CrossRef]
70. Lindorfer, M.A.; Beum, P.V.; Taylor, R.P. CD20 mAb-Mediated Complement Dependent Cytotoxicity of Tumor Cells is Enhanced by Blocking the Action of Factor I. *Antibodies* **2013**, *2*, 598–616. [CrossRef]
71. Hörl, S.; Bánki, Z.; Huber, G.; Ejaz, A.; Müllauer, B.; Willenbacher, E.; Steurer, M.; Stoiber, H. Complement factor H-derived short consensus repeat 18-20 enhanced complement-dependent cytotoxicity of ofatumumab on chronic lymphocytic leukemia cells. *Haematologica* **2013**, *98*, 1939–1947. [CrossRef]
72. Ge, X.; Wu, L.; Hu, W.; Fernandes, S.; Wang, C.; Li, X.; Brown, J.R.; Qin, X. rILYd4, a human CD59 inhibitor, enhances complement-dependent cytotoxicity of ofatumumab against rituximab-resistant B-cell lymphoma cells and chronic lymphocytic leukemia. *Clin. Cancer Res.* **2011**, *17*, 6702–6711. [CrossRef]
73. Van Meerten, T.; Rozemuller, H.; Hol, S.; Moerer, P.; Zwart, M.; Hagenbeek, A.; Mackus, W.J.; Parren, P.W.; Van De Winkel, J.G.J.; Ebeling, S.B.; et al. HuMab-7D8, a monoclonal antibody directed against the membrane-proximal small loop epitope of CD20, can effectively eliminate CD20 low expressing tumor cells that resist rituximab mediated lysis. *Haematologica* **2010**, *95*, 2063–2071. [CrossRef]
74. Harboe, M.; Mollnes, T.E. The alternative complement pathway revisited. *J. Cell. Mol. Med.* **2008**, *12*, 1074–1084. [CrossRef] [PubMed]
75. Harboe, M.; Ulvund, G.; Vien, L.; Fung, M.; Mollnes, T.E. The quantitative role of alternative pathway amplification in classical pathway induced terminal complement activation. *Clin. Exp. Immunol.* **2004**, *138*, 439–446. [CrossRef] [PubMed]
76. Sharp, T.H.; Koster, A.J.; Gros, P. Heterogeneous MAC initiator and pore structures in a lipid bilayer by phase-plate cryo-electron tomography. *Cell Rep.* **2016**, *15*, 1–8. [CrossRef] [PubMed]

77. Fukumori, Y.; Yoshimura, K.; Ohnokl, S.; Yamaguchl, H.; Akagakl, Y.; Inal, S. A high incidence of C9 deficiency among healthy blood donors in Osaka, Japan. *Int. Immunol.* **1989**, *1*, 1968–1973. [CrossRef] [PubMed]
78. Fifadara, N.H.; Beer, F.; Ono, S.; Ono, S.J. Interaction between activated chemokine receptor 1 and FcɛRI at membrane rafts promotes communication and F-actin-rich cytoneme extensions between mast cells. *Int. Immunol.* **2010**, *22*, 113–128. [CrossRef] [PubMed]
79. Shaw, P.; Kumar, N.; Hammerschmid, D.; Privat-Maldonado, A.; Dewilde, S.; Bogaerts, A. Synergistic effects of melittin and plasma treatment: A promising approach for cancer therapy. *Cancers* **2019**, *11*, 1109. [CrossRef]
80. Taylor, R.; Lindorfer, M.; Oostindie, S.; Cook, E.; Zent, C.; Burack, R.; Beurskens, F.; Schuurman, J.; Breij, E.; Parren, P. Hexamerization-enhanced CD37 and CD20 antibodies synergize in CDC to kill patient-derived CLL cells with unprecedented potency. *Mol. Immmunol.* **2018**, *102*, 218. [CrossRef]

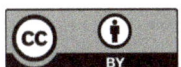 © 2020 by the authors. Licensee MDPI, Basel, Switzerland. This article is an open access article distributed under the terms and conditions of the Creative Commons Attribution (CC BY) license (http://creativecommons.org/licenses/by/4.0/).

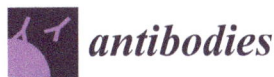

Review

The Role of Complement in Angiogenesis

Maciej M. Markiewski *, Elizabeth Daugherity, Britney Reese and Magdalena Karbowniczek *

Department of Immunotherapeutics and Biotechnology, Jerry H. Hodge School of Pharmacy, Texas Tech University Health Sciences Center, Abilene, TX 79601, USA; Beth.Daugherity@ttuhsc.edu (E.D.); britney.reese@ttuhsc.edu (B.R.)

* Correspondence: maciej.markiewski@ttuhsc.edu (M.M.M.); magdalena.karbowniczek@ttuhsc.edu (M.K.); Tel.: +1-325-696-0430 (M.M.M.); +1-325-696-0435 (M.K.); Fax: +1-325-676-3875 (M.M.M. & M.K.)

Received: 2 October 2020; Accepted: 23 November 2020; Published: 1 December 2020

Abstract: The link of the complement system to angiogenesis has remained circumstantial and speculative for several years. Perhaps the most clinically relevant example of possible involvement of complement in pathological neovascularization is age-related macular degeneration. Recent studies, however, provide more direct and experimental evidence that indeed the complement system regulates physiological and pathological angiogenesis in models of wound healing, retinal regeneration, age-related macular degeneration, and cancer. Interestingly, complement-dependent mechanisms involved in angiogenesis are very much context dependent, including anti- and proangiogenic functions. Here, we discuss these new developments that place complement among other important regulators of homeostatic and pathological angiogenesis, and we provide the perspective on how these newly discovered complement functions can be targeted for therapy.

Keywords: complement; angiogenesis; cancer; ocular pathology

1. Introduction

The complement system plays a key role in innate immunity against pathogens and links the initial innate immune responses with the subsequent adaptive immunity [1,2]. Large quantities of liver-derived complement proteins are always present in plasma and other body fluids as inactive precursors (zymogens), awaiting enzymatic cleavages via one of three canonical pathways: the classical, mannose-binding lectin, or alternative. In addition, the proteolytic enzymes present in inflamed tissues may cleave complement proteins and lead to activation of complement by what was termed the extrinsic pathway [3]. Through the cascade of proteolytic cleavages and protein-to-protein interactions, the protein complexes with enzymatic activity (C3 and C5 convertases), composed of large cleavage fragments, are formed on the activating surfaces [4]. They contribute to the progression and amplification of the complement cascade. The other cleavage fragments, usually smaller, interact with immune cells, including monocytes, macrophages, dendritic cells, granulocytes, NK cells, and B and T lymphocytes. In addition to within the liver, complement proteins are produced locally in immune, neuronal, epithelial, and tumor cells, fibroblasts, osteoblasts, and adipocytes [5]. Small complement cleavage fragments known as anaphylatoxins, C3a, C4a, C5a, in particular C5a, act as potent inflammatory mediators. C3b and C4b function as opsonins that flag pathogens to aid in recognition and phagocytosis by professional phagocytes. C5b-9, known as the terminal complement complex (TCC) or the membrane attack complex (MAC), forms a cytolytic or sublytic pore in the membranes of bacteria or cells. The complement system was originally described to aid (complement) antibodies in killing bacteria, thus the name "complement." However, recent studies have revealed that complement is involved in several immune and inflammatory processes triggered by infection or non-infectious pathologies and contributes to several physiological and pathological process that are not strictly linked to the fight against microbes [6]. This review focuses on the non-immune complement functions associated with angiogenesis.

2. Vasculogenesis and Angiogenesis in Health

New blood vessels are formed through two functionally distinct processes termed vasculogenesis and angiogenesis [7]. *Vasculogenesis* is the formation of the entirely new vasculature during early embryonic development from precursor cells and is pivotal for the development of the cardiovascular system. In this process, mesodermal cells expressing vascular endothelial growth factor receptor 2 (VEGFR-2) are stimulated in a paracrine fashion by VEGF released from endoderm [8]. This stimulation contributes to the conversion of multipotent mesodermal cells to angioblasts or endothelial precursor cells that are located at the periphery of blood islands that emerge from the mesoderm as the earliest vascular structures in embryo. The fusion of the multiple blood islands leads to the formation of the primitive capillary network, which, upon the initiation of blood circulation, converts into the arteriovenous vascular system (Figure 1) [9]. The growth and maturation of this primitive vascular system requires the tight coordination of cell proliferation, differentiation, migration, matrix adhesion, and changes in cell signaling. Although vasculogenesis was initially thought to be exclusively linked to the development of the cardiovascular system in embryo, recent evidence indicates that a similar process may contribute to the creation of new blood vessels in ischemic tissues and tumors. This process has been termed postnatal vasculogenesis [10]. In contrast to de novo formation of blood vessels through vasculogenesis, *angiogenesis* refers to the growth of new capillaries from the existing vasculature (Figure 1) [11]. In adult organisms, endothelial cells remain mostly in the quiescent state and do not proliferate. Therefore, angiogenesis is rarely seen under normal physiological conditions except placental angiogenesis, angiogenesis in ovaries to transform the ovulated follicles into the corpus luteum, and in the uterus to restore the endometrium to be receptive to embryo implantation [12]. In addition, angiogenesis and vasculogenesis are required for wound healing to repair damaged vasculature and accelerate the healing process [13]. This angiogenic response is considered be a part of normal homeostatic regulation, although it occurs as a response to tissue injury.

Complement in Homeostatic Angiogenesis

Wound Healing

Normal (acute) wound healing progresses through several well-orchestrated and, to some extent, overlapping phases that encompass: clotting at the site of injury, an acute inflammatory response and associated recruitment of inflammatory and interstitial cells, the subsequent proliferation of recruited or resident cells, growth of capillaries, extracellular matrix protein deposition, regeneration of parenchymal and non-parenchymal cells, and tissue remodeling [13]. The blood vessel grows within aptly-named granulation tissue, which fills the wound during the repair process. This new vasculature is required to repair damage to the blood vessels and provide nutrients and oxygen to the highly metabolically-active cells in the sites of tissue repair. Both VEGF-mediated sprouting angiogenesis (SA) and vasculogenesis contribute to this process. Bone marrow-derived endothelial progenitors are involved in de novo blood vessel formation through vasculogenesis [13]. Complement effectors generated through complement activation, especially anaphylatoxins, are some of the most potent inflammatory mediators in humans [3]. Therefore, their involvement in the acute inflammatory reactions in wound repair was highly anticipated.

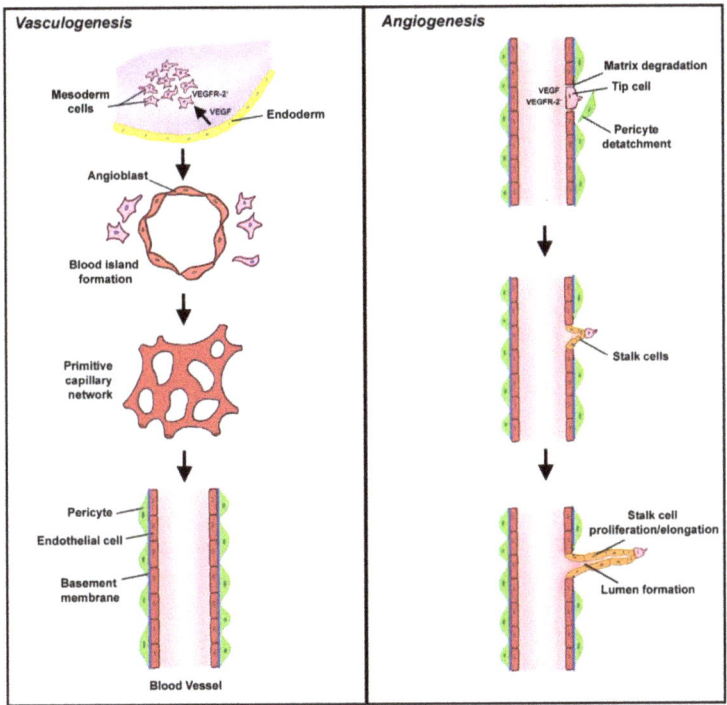

Figure 1. Vasculogenesis vs. angiogenesis. Vasculogenesis in embryos (**left**) is the de novo creation of new vasculature from primitive mesodermal cells that express VEGFR2. VEGF released from neighboring endodermal cells converts these VEGFR2$^+$ cells into angioblasts surrounding the blood islands. These islands fuse to form the primitive vascular network that eventually converts into the arteriovenous system. In contrast, angiogenesis (**right**) is a formation of new vessels from the existing vasculature. The initial steps involve degradation of the extracellular matrix (ECM), detachment of pericytes, and tip formation. The non-proliferating tip endothelial cells move toward proangiogenic factors and are followed by dividing stalk cells. These drawings are based on the figures included in [12,14].

However, in contrast to this anticipation, a recent work demonstrated that complement protein C1q is involved in wound healing vascular changes, independently of complement activation [15]. Although C1q is implicated in the initiation of the classical pathway of complement activation, it also directly regulates function of immune and non-immune cells through binding to the C1q receptors that are expressed on these cells [16], and such interaction of C1q with its reciprocal receptors on endothelial cells may be involved in C1q-mediated angiogenesis. This notion was based on C1q-positive immunohistochemistry staining on endothelial and inflammatory cells of granulation tissue in the healing wound, in the absence of C4 and C3, which are required for the complement activation cascade to proceed [15]. The C1q found in the wounds was likely derived from plasma. However, local generation of C1q was also demonstrated in this study by quantitative PCR and in situ hybridization [15]. In vitro assays with cultured endothelial cells demonstrated the impact of the globular C1q head on the permeability of the endothelial monolayer and proliferation and migration of endothelial cells. Importantly, endothelial cells migrated toward a C1q gradient, suggesting a role of C1q in the tip formation during SA, which is similar to the role of VEGF in this process [15]. Like VEGF, C1q promoted tube formation in the tube formation assay. These proangiogenic C1q properties were further corroborated by the impact of C1q on vessel sprouting in an ex vivo rat aortic ring assay.

Finally, wounds from C1q-deficient mice were less vascular and closed more slowly than in wild-type controls [15]. In contrast, C3 deficiency did not impact wound vasculature suggesting that the canonical complement activation pathways do not play a major role in wound angiogenesis. Adding back C1q to C1q-deficient mice entirely abrogated the effects of C1q deficiency on wound angiogenesis. Topical application of C1q in a rat model of wound healing accelerated the healing process and increased vascularity of the wounds. Overall, this work has demonstrated C1q proangiogenic functions that are independent from complement activation [15].

In contrast, a different study demonstrated that experimental wounds actually heal better in C3, C5 and C5a receptor 1 (C5aR1)-deficient mice than in wild-type controls. The wounds from C3-deficent mice were enriched in mast cells and had better developed vascularity than wounds in wild-type controls. The inflammatory infiltrate of wounds was reduced in C3-deficient mice [17]. Taken together, both studies indicate that properly balanced complement activity is required for smooth wound healing. C1q-mediated angiogenesis seems to be essential for proper wound healing. However, excessive inflammatory infiltrate linked to complement C5a may delay angiogenesis and healing.

3. Vasculogenesis and Angiogenesis in Disease

In contrast to these examples of "beneficial" homeostatic angiogenesis, dysregulated angiogenesis or vascular dysfunction contributes to several common and life-threatening diseases including cancer and diabetes mellitus. In addition to diabetic retinopathy, several other ocular pathologies are associated with aberrant vasculature and angiogenesis. In general, the angiogenic switch is triggered by ischemia followed by hypoxia, as is the case in cancer and other conditions, in which metabolic oxygen demand is higher than the available supply.

3.1. Complement in Pathological Angiogenesis

3.1.1. Cancer

In contrast to normal tissues, exponentially growing tumor mass requires dense and constantly growing vasculature to meet its metabolic demands. Therefore, neoangiogenesis is essential to support tumor growth [18]. Even with robust angiogenesis permanently switched on in tumors, the tumor microenvironment remains hypoxic, and the central portions of solid tumors often become necrotic due lack of sufficient blood and oxygen supply. Hypoxia-induced changes in the tumor microenvironment, soluble factors secreted from tumor cells, and interplay between the resident and recruited components of this microenvironment all contribute to SA in tumors [19]. SA is initiated by several proangiogenic growth factors, including VEGF, produced in the hypoxic and nutrient-deprived tumor microenvironment. Thus, VEGF stimulated endothelial cells leave their quiescent state and proliferate. Matrix metalloproteinases (MMPs) released from activated endothelial or infiltrating cells digest the basement membranes and interstitial stroma allowing endothelial cells to migrate. Migrating frontrunner endothelial cells form a tip that follows the gradient of proangiogenic factors. Tip endothelial cells have low proliferative capacity. However, they are followed by so-called stalk cells, which proliferate and cause the sprout elongation. The vascular lumen is formed between two parallel layers of stalk cells while the sprout elongates (Figure 1). Once tip cells from neighboring sprouts meet, they anastomose to form a new perfused blood vessel. The perfusion causes the maturation and stabilization of these new blood vessels that involves deposition of basement membrane components and establishing pericyte coverage [12]. Paradoxically, VEGF-triggered SA does not lead to well-developed and mature vasculature in tumors. Newly formed tumor blood vessels are convoluted, disorganized and do not have a well-developed endothelial cell lining. Furthermore, pericyte coverage of these newly formed blood vessels is limited. As a result, the vasculature of tumors is leaky and inefficient [20]. To circumvent deficiencies associated with "ineffective" SA, the invading tumor border engulfs normal blood vessels surrounding malignant tissue and incorporates these mature blood vessels into the tumor vasculature. As expected, these co-opted host vessels are functionally different from blood vessels formed through SA. For example, the endothelial cells of co-opted vessels exhibit little proliferative potential. The co-opted vessels, in addition to supplying blood to the tumor, provide the port of entry to the circulation for tumor cells that later give rise to hematogenous metastasis. Therefore, tumor invasion of normal blood vessels in close proximity worsens prognosis [21]. Interestingly, tumor cells can also function as endothelial cells forming vascular channels through the process of vascular mimicry [22]. In addition to a pivotal role of angiogenesis and vascular aberrations in primary tumor sites, the angiogenic switch is required for the progression of small avascular micrometastases to clinically overt rapidly growing lesions, and thus, promotes the wakening of tumor cells from dormancy [23]. The role of complement in cancer has been extensively studied and reviewed in the last decade [24–26]. Overall, it is generally accepted that complement-mediated inflammation supports immune escape of tumors through activation and recruitment of different components of the tumor microenvironment [5].

Primary Tumors

The role of complement in cancer has been postulated for decades, since complement deposition was observed in several common human solid tumors [5,27]. The presence of complement deposits in tumors was seen as an indicator of complement-mediated tumor immune surveillance. The TCC can lyse invading microorganisms through complement-dependent cytotoxicity, and therefore, the TCC was thought to contribute to complement-mediated tumor cell killing. However, more than a decade ago, the protumor functions of complement were discovered [28]. This study linked these tumor-promoting functions to suppression of antitumor immunity through the engagement of C5a with C5aR1 expressed on myeloid-derived suppressor cells (MDSC). Several follow-up studies confirmed these initial findings and discovered new complement-mediated mechanisms contributing to cancer progression. Given the proangiogenic functions of MDSC [29], it is surprising that only a few reports have linked complement to tumor angiogenesis, and in fact, none of them have demonstrated contribution of C5aR1 signaling in these cells to angiogenesis in primary sites.

Perhaps the first study on the role of complement in tumor angiogenesis was the work demonstrating significantly reduced tumor growth and reduced vascularization of tumors from C3 and C5aR1-deficient mice in a transgenic model of ovarian carcinoma [30]. The complete complement deficiencies with both copies of complement gene lost (homozygous mice) had greater impact on tumor growth and vascularization than the partial complement deficiencies in heterozygous mice. The tumor growth and vascular density seemed to be independent from inflammatory infiltrate of tumors, but in ex vivo stimulated immune cells, these correlated with reduced cytokine production including IL-12 and IL-10 produced in macrophages, IL-10 in B cells, and IFN-γ in T cells. In vitro, C5a promoted tube formation (in the tube formation assay) to a similar extent as the VEGF isoforms, which are designated by the number of amino acids in the spliced polypeptide, and this effect was mediated by C5aR1, as the blockade of this receptor by the selective C5aR1 antagonist, PMX53 [31], abrogated this effect. Interestingly, C5a stimulation of human endothelial cells led to increased expression of $VEGF_{165}$ isoform and C5aR1 blockade by PMX53 attenuated tube formation mediated by VEGF, suggesting that the interplay between C5aR1 and VEGF plays a role in complement-dependent regulation of tumor angiogenesis [30]. However, the potential links between VEGF and C5aR1 signaling require further in-depth investigations.

Consistent with the role of C1q in wound healing [15], C1q endothelial positivity by immunohistochemistry was found in histological specimens from melanoma and colon, lung, breast, and pancreatic carcinomas [32]. Conversely, C1s, C4, and C3 were much less abundant or absent in the same specimens, suggesting that C1q deposits were not associated with the activation of the complement cascade. C1q staining was limited to stroma, endothelial cells, and infiltrating leukocytes [32]. A similar pattern of staining was observed in liver metastases of colon carcinoma. In contrast to colon tumors, benign mucosa did not exhibit C1q staining [32]. However, the results of this immunohistochemistry study require cautious interpretation, given that conclusions are based on analysis of only six specimens per cancer. In addition, the analysis does not include adjustments for different histopathological subtypes, grade, and other clinicopathological variables. Furthermore, publicly available data from The Human Protein Atlas indicates C3-positive staining in several common solid tumors (https://www.proteinatlas.org/). In the same study [32], tumor growth was reduced and mouse survival increased in C1q-deficient mice in a syngeneic (B16) model of melanoma. Surprisingly, the authors did not observe the impact of C3 deficiency on the growth of B16 tumors, which was inconsistent with reports documenting the role of C3 in the same murine model of melanoma [33]. Immunohistochemistry of mouse tumors was similar to data from human cancers. The study in bone marrow chimeras suggested that C1q from non-bone marrow-derived cells contributes to the tumor growth in this model. The reduced tumor growth in C1q-deficient mice correlated with reduced vascular density and reduced lung metastatic burden ([32] and Figure 2). Consistently, in a syngeneic model of model of HPV-induced cancer (TC-1), C1q deficiency was linked to morphologically aberrant vasculature in tumors characterized by shorter and disorganized vessels. In contrast, tumor blood vessels from C4-deficienct mice were normal in the same study [34]. In tumor sections obtained from the large cohorts of patients with renal cell carcinoma (RCC), C1q immunofluorescence was mainly detected in infiltrating cells expressing markers of macrophages. However, similar to the healing wounds [15] and specimens of melanoma and colon, lung, breast, and pancreatic carcinomas [32], C1q positivity was also observed in CD31$^+$ cells, suggesting crosstalk of complement with RCC tumor vasculature [34]. However, in contrast to the previous work on C1q functions in tumors [32], C1q in RCC seems to trigger the classical pathway because C1q deposits on tumor cells co-localized with IgG and C4d, and C3 cleavage products were also detected in these tumors [34].

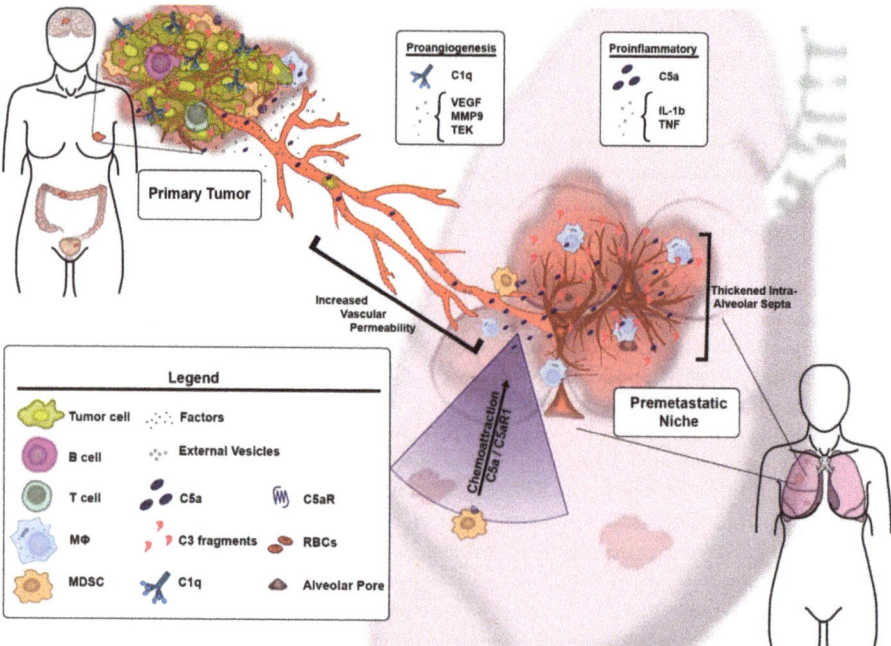

Figure 2. Overview of the role of complement in cancer-associated angiogenesis. C1q, C3 and C5aR1 were implicated in angiogenesis in primary tumors in cancer models and patients. In the premetastatic niches, angiogenesis seems to be regulated by MDSC activated and recruited to these niches through C5aR1-mediated signaling. MDSC secrete proangiogenic and proinflammatory factors contributing to this process.

The contribution of complement to RCC is also evident from the most recent research, which demonstrated the striking association of several complement genes and proteins with prognosis and response to immune checkpoint inhibitors. This study has also shown reduced vascular density in C3aR-deficient and wild-type mice treated with C5aR1 and C3aR inhibitors in a mouse model of RCC. Consistently, several proangiogenic factors were downregulated in complement-deficient or wild-type mice treated with complement inhibitors [35].

Premetastatic Niche

A recent study documented the role of complement in cancer metastasis and, specifically, C5aR1-mediated recruitment of MDSC to the premetastatic niche with the impact of this recruitment on CD8$^+$T cell mediated antitumor immunity and lung and liver metastatic burden [36]. The premetastatic niche represents a stage during the metastatic progression of cancer, in which tumors in primary sites induce changes in metastasis-targeted distal organs prior to the arrival of very first tumor cells. These changes are thought to be related to the factors secreted from tumors or delivered through the external vesicle cargo. However, complement was not linked to the premetastatic niche prior to the paper by Vadrevu et al. [36]. Therefore, this work added complement activation in the premetastatic niche as a source of additional mediators promoting metastasis (Figure 2). In a model of metastatic breast cancer, the deposition of C3 cleavage fragments, indicating complement activation, was found in the lungs starting from day 4 after injecting tumor cells into the mammary fat pad and before the arrival of tumor cells to this organ. Significant inflammatory infiltration and thickening of intra-alveolar septa reflecting pneumonitis, that was named premetastatic pneumonia, was also present at this stage [25,36]. The vast majority of infiltrating cells were identified as MDSC and their recruitment was mediated by C5a/C5aR1 [36]. Because MDSC are proangiogenic in primary tumor sites [29,37], it is conceivable that they may actually initiate angiogenesis in the premetastatic niche. Although vascular changes such as increased permeability are well-defined for the premetastatic niche [38], in general, angiogenic switching is thought to be limited to the progression of dormant micrometastases to clinically overt lesions and not triggered prior to the arrival of tumor cells [39,40]. Despite several proangiogenic factors and cells being implicated in the premetastatic niche [38,41,42], the studies documenting "true" angiogenesis at this stage of cancer are limited [38]. The transcriptomic analysis of the mouse lungs, at the stages of premetastatic niche, confirmed upregulation of pathways associated with activation of myeloid cells that can be potentially linked to angiogenesis [43]. Transcriptomic data were corroborated by gene expression profiling showing upregulation of the well-established regulators of SA including different forms of *Vegf*, *Vegfr1* and *Vegfr2*, and *Tek* genes [43]. Tek, for example, plays a key role in tip formation during SA [44]. Other factors that are linked to SA, inflammation, and changes in vascular permeability included upregulation of *IL-1b*, *Tnf* and *Mmp9* genes [43]. Importantly, IL-1β and TNF are important in activating and recruiting myeloid cells to tumors. These cells regulate angiogenesis in an MMP9-dependent fashion [45]. The upregulation of proangiogenic factors correlated well with key morphological hallmarks of angiogenesis such as increased vascular density in the interalveolar septa of the premetastatic lungs, endothelial cell proliferation, and increased vascular permeability. The increased vascular permeability was caused by reduced pericyte coverage [43]. The activation of endothelial cells was further confirmed by upregulation of TGF-β1 accessory receptor (CD105), known also as endoglin [43], because endoglin protein is rarely expressed on the quiescent endothelial cells and is a marker of tumor angiogenesis [46]. A causative role of MDSC in premetastatic angiogenesis was supported by the MDSC-depletion studies which showed a reduction in vascular density in the premetastatic lungs because of this depletion. Blockade of C5aR1 with PMX53 or genetic C5aR1 deficiency resulted in reduced vascular density in the lung premetastatic niche and was associated with overall downregulation of proangiogenic pathways, therefore implicating C5a/C5aR1 in regulation of premetastatic angiogenesis. As anticipated, reduced angiogenesis in C5aR1 deficiency or blockade correlated with reduced infiltration of the lungs by MDSC [43]. Overall, this study provides (1) preliminary evidence for angiogenesis in the premetastatic niches, which may explain a lack of dormancy in some aggressive malignancies that manifest with rapid development of metastasis even when the primary tumor site cannot be identified [47], and (2) implicates complement in premetastatic angiogenesis through the regulation of MDSC (Figure 2). Thus, the complement-MDSC crosstalk is important for both suppression of antitumor $CD8^+$ T cells [36] and angiogenesis in the premetastatic niche [43].

3.1.2. Ocular Pathologies

Age-Related Macular Degeneration

Age-related macular degeneration (AMD) is the leading etiology of irreversible vision loss in the elderly, which is caused by the progressive degeneration of the photoreceptor cells in the center of the retina, known as the macula [48]. The morphological hallmark of disease is the accumulation of waste products of retinal metabolism known as drusen underneath the retinal pigmented epithelium (RPE), which is adjacent to photoreceptors and provides structural and functional support for these photoreceptors (Figure 3). RPE sits on the basement membrane that separates these cells from capillaries in the choroid, a vascular layer in the eye There are two major forms of AMD: (1) neovascular (wet AMD, 10–15%) and (2) geographic atrophy (dry AMD, 85–90%) [49,50]. In wet AMD, which may start suddenly and progresses rapidly, the abnormal blood vessels sprout from the choroid into the retina as a consequence of VEGF secretion from RPE (choroidal neovascularization) [51]. These blood vessels are fragile and leaky. When they rupture, the resulting hemorrhage into the retina can cause blindness (Figure 3). The importance of VEGF-dependent neovascularization for the pathophysiology of wet AMD triggered the approval of anti-VEGF agents for treatment of this condition. After 2 years of treatment with an anti-VEGF agent, more than 95% of patients can expect to remain within 3 lines of their baseline visual acuity on a standard eye testing chart, and up to 40% can expect an improvement of 3 lines in the affected eye over baseline [52,53]. Dry AMD progresses slowly and causes some degree of visual impairment including, sometimes, complete blindness (Figure 3). However, the magnitude of visual impairment is lower in dry than in wet AMD which progresses inevitably and rapidly to blindness when left untreated [48]. Both forms of AMD appear to be linked to the proinflammatory factors that are produced by stressed RPE or inflammatory cells, including macrophages, infiltrating the retina [50]. In both patients and mouse models, early deposition of complement components C3 and C5 is observed in retina, suggesting a contributing role of complement in AMD (Figure 3). The presence of C3a and C5a in drusen of patients with AMD and in animal models of AMD further points to the pivotal role of complement activation in AMD pathogenesis [54,55]. Because C3a and C5a, but in particular C5a, are potent inflammatory mediators that activate and recruit leukocytes to inflammatory sites [3], it is likely that these mediators enhance the proinflammatory and proangiogenic environment in the retina of patients with AMD. Further evidence for the role of complement in AMD is the strong associations of several complement genetic variants with an enhanced risk of AMD, as demonstrated by large family-based studies and a genome-wide association study. This work led to the discovery of the complement factor H gene variant (*CFH*; Tyr402His) that is strongly associated with higher AMD prevalence [56]. Furthermore, common genetic variants in or near complement genes *CFH*, *C2*, *CFB*, *C3* and *CFI* explain almost 40–60% of the heritability of AMD [57]. The remaining heritable AMD cases could possibly be linked to the rare genetic variants. Several of these variants are linked to complement genes including *CFH* and *CFI* [49]. The functional significance of genetic alterations in complement genes for mechanisms behind AMD remain to be established. However, since risk of AMD is often associated with genetic variants of genes for complement regulators (*CFH* and *CFI*) and, at least, some of these variants associate with impaired function of these regulators, it is conceivable that the excessive complement activation contributes to AMD. This notion is consistent with the concept of a harmful role of the highly proinflammatory retinal milieu in AMD.

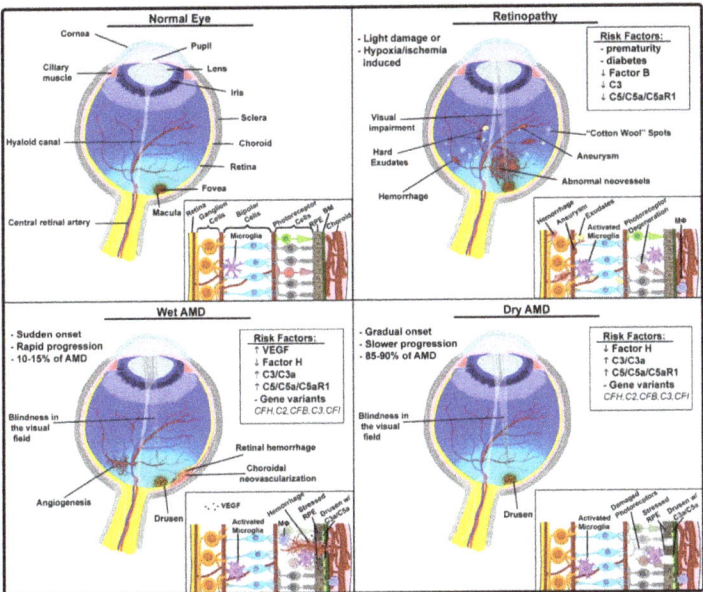

Figure 3. Ocular pathologies with complement involvement. Anatomy and histology of normal eye (**upper left**); proliferative retinopathies (**upper right**): the process of neovascularization leads to formation of blood vessels that are fragile and leaky, increased permeability or rupture of newly formed blood vessels and subsequent hemorrhage cause impairment or loss of vision, in mouse models of these retinopathies, complement seems to have a protective role; wet AMD (**lower left**) and dry AMD (**lower right**): in both forms, excessive complement activation and subsequent generation of complement effectors (C3a and C5a) has been implicated; frequently AMD is linked to *FH* polymorphism; in wet AMD, VEGF-driven neovascularization, possibly also regulated by complement, leads to severe impairment or loss of vision.

Thus, restoring factor H function and, consequently, inhibiting the alternative pathway may offer a new therapeutic avenue for AMD. A study utilizing a mouse model of AMD-laser induced choroidal neovascularization (CNV) explored the impact of the deficiency in complement factor B, which is required for the alternative pathway, on vascular changes. In addition, the effect of treatment with a recombinant complement receptor 2 (CR2)-*N*-terminal factor H domain construct (CR2-FH) on vasculature was tested in the same model. The *N*-terminus of mouse factor H contains the alternative pathway inhibitory domain whereas CR2 was used to target the factor H fragment to complement cleavage fragments. After induction of choroidal neovascularization by laser photocoagulation, mice were treated with CR2-FH, which significantly reduced CNV to the extent observed in factor B-deficient mice. Reduced CNV correlated with reduced damage to the retina [58].

Proliferative Retinopathies

Proliferative retinopathies are often associated with neovascularization of the retina resulting from vascular dysfunction, vessel loss, and hypoxia. Newly formed blood vessels are, however, dysfunctional and leaky, and therefore, they lead to impairment and, eventually, vision loss (Figure 3). These vascular alterations contribute to pathogenesis of common retinopathies, including diabetic retinopathy and retinopathy of prematurity, which all cause impaired vision in millions of patients in the USA [59,60]. From 2010 to 2050, the number of Americans with diabetic retinopathy is expected to nearly double from 7.7 million to 14.6 million according to Center for Disease Control and Prevention. In contrast to its harmful role in a model of AMD, the alternative pathway of complement activation appears to prune neovessels in oxygen-induced retinopathy (OIR) mouse models, thereby reducing severity of disease [60]. Factor B-deficient mice had a significantly higher number of neovessels than wild-type controls in the OIR model, and these neovessels persisted longer in these mice during the resolution phase, in which vasculature normalizes. However, eventually neovessels disappeared in these mice, indicating that the alternative pathway is not the only player in the process of retinal neovascularization [60]. Although the number of neovessels was higher in retinas of factor B-deficient mice, the proliferation of endothelial cells remained at the level of wild-type controls, indicating that the removal of neovessels is affected in these mice rather than neovessel formation [60]. These findings are consistent with the similar expression of *Vegf* isoforms and *Vegfr2*, which are key factors inducing endothelial cell proliferation, despite the loss of factor B [60]. Furthermore, immunofluorescence in wild-type mice demonstrated deposition of factor B in neovessels but not in normal vasculature, indicating that neovessels specifically induce complement activation. Factor B deposits were present during neovessel formation and the resolution phase and correlated with apoptosis of endothelial cells. The reduced expression of complement regulator CD55, known as decay accelerating factor, which inhibits both the classical and alternative pathway C3 convertases, appears to render neovessels vulnerable to complement-mediated removal [60].

Like factor B knockouts in the OIR model, C3-deficient mice displayed increased neovascularization in the model of retinopathy of prematurity (ROP) and in an in vivo matrix plug assay [59]. In addition, C5 neutralization by monoclonal antibody, C5aR1 blockade by PMX53, and C5aR1 deficiency led to increased vascularization of retina in ROP [59]. The mechanisms of complement-mediated inhibition of pathological angiogenesis involved regulation of macrophages through C5aR1 signaling. Stimulation of this receptor in macrophages induced antiangiogenic phenotypes in these cells that were associated with the increased expression and secretion of antiangiogenic soluble VEGFR1. Consistent with these findings, macrophage depletion reversed phenotypes associated with complement deficiencies [59].

4. Targeting Complement-Mediated Angiogenesis

Complement-dependent vascular alterations discussed here contribute to the most common human diseases that are associated with significant morbidity and mortality. Diabetes mellitus with subsequent cardiovascular complications and cancer are leading causes of mortality world-wide [61]. Despite the preclinical evidence of complement involvement in these pathologies and availability of therapeutics targeting complement, complement-based therapies for these common diseases have not entered the clinic [62]. However, some complement-based therapies were or are currently being tested in clinical trials. Perhaps, the most tested application for complement therapeutics is in AMD. Therapeutics targeting C3, Factor D, Properdin, C5 and CD59 were or are being tested in clinical trials for AMD [62,63]. Moreover, a C5aR1 antibody (IPH5401) entered a phase I clinical trial in combination with anti-PDL1, durvulumab, in patients with selected advanced solid tumors (NCT03665129). The expected study completion is June 2021. These recent developments have promise for more complement-based therapies for common human diseases. The limited progress in targeting complement-mediated vascular aberrations in the clinic can be associated with a relative paucity of studies documenting the role of complement in pathological angiogenesis, some conflicting data on the pro- vs. antiangiogenic role of complement, and limited interest of industry in targeting complement pathways for therapy. In cancer, the additional hurdles include uncertainty as to which of the complement-dependent mechanisms of cancer progression should be specifically targeted for therapy and determining which cancer patients will benefit most from complement-based interventions [35].

Author Contributions: Conceptualization, M.M.M. and M.K.; writing-original draft preparation, reviewing, and editing, M.M.M., E.D., B.R., and M.K.; visualization E.D. and B.R.; supervision, M.M.M. and M.K.; funding acquisition, M.M.M. All authors have read and agreed to the published version of the manuscript.

Funding: This work was funded by the National Institute of Health (RO1CA190209 to M.M.).

Conflicts of Interest: The authors declare no conflict of interest.

Abbreviations

TCC—terminal complement complex, MAC—membrane attack complex, VEGF—vascular endothelial growth factor, VEGFR—vascular growth factor receptor, ECM—extracellular matrix, SA—sprouting angiogenesis, C5aR1—C5a receptor 1, C3aR—C3a receptor, MMPs—matrix metalloproteinases, MDSC—myeloid-derived suppressor cells, IL—interleukin, INF—interferon, PMX53—C5aR1 inhibitor, HPV—human papilloma virus, TC-1—mouse tumor cell line, RCC—renal cell carcinoma, AMD—age-related macular degeneration, RPE—retinal pigmented epithelium, CNV—choroidal neovascularization, OIR—oxygen-induced retinopathy, and ROP—retinopathy of prematurity.

References

1. Ricklin, D.; Reis, E.S.; Lambris, J.D. Complement in disease: A defence system turning offensive. *Nat. Rev. Nephrol.* **2016**, *12*, 383–401. [CrossRef]
2. Ricklin, D.; Lambris, J.D. Complement in Immune and Inflammatory Disorders: Pathophysiological Mechanisms. *J. Immunol.* **2013**, *190*, 3831–3838. [CrossRef] [PubMed]
3. Markiewski, M.M.; Lambris, J.D. The Role of Complement in Inflammatory Diseases From Behind the Scenes into the Spotlight. *Am. J. Pathol.* **2007**, *171*, 715–727. [CrossRef] [PubMed]
4. Walport, M.J. Complement. First of two parts. *N. Engl. J. Med.* **2001**, *344*, 1058–1066. [CrossRef] [PubMed]
5. Kolev, M.; Markiewski, M.M. Targeting complement-mediated immunoregulation for cancer immunotherapy. *Semin. Immunol.* **2018**, *37*, 85–97. [CrossRef] [PubMed]
6. Ricklin, D.; Hajishengallis, G.; Yang, K.; Lambris, J.D. Complement: A key system for immune surveillance and homeostasis. *Nat. Immunol.* **2010**, *11*, 785–797. [CrossRef] [PubMed]
7. Risau, W.; Flamme, I. Vasculogenesis. *Annu. Rev. Cell Dev. Biol.* **1995**, *11*, 73–91. [CrossRef]
8. Flamme, I.; Breier, G.; Risau, W. Vascular Endothelial Growth Factor (VEGF) and VEGF Receptor 2(flk-1) are Expressed during Vasculogenesis and Vascular Differentiation in the Quail Embryo. *Dev. Biol.* **1995**, *169*, 699–712. [CrossRef]
9. Risau, W.; Sariola, H.; Zerwes, H.G.; Sasse, J.; Ekblom, P.; Kemler, R.; Doetschman, T. Vasculogenesis and angiogenesis in embryonic-stem-cell-derived embryoid bodies. *Development* **1988**, *102*, 471–478.
10. Asahara, T.; Kawamoto, A. Endothelial progenitor cells for postnatal vasculogenesis. *Am. J. Physiol. Cell Physiol.* **2004**, *287*, C572–C579. [CrossRef]
11. Folkman, J. Tumor angiogenesis: Therapeutic implications. *N. Engl. J. Med.* **1971**, *285*, 1182–1186. [CrossRef] [PubMed]
12. Eelen, G.; Treps, L.; Li, X.; Carmeliet, P. Basic and Therapeutic Aspects of Angiogenesis Updated. *Circ. Res.* **2020**, *127*, 310–329. [CrossRef]
13. Eming, S.A.; Martin, P.; Tomic-Canic, M. Wound repair and regeneration: Mechanisms, signaling, and translation. *Sci. Transl. Med.* **2014**, *6*, 265sr6. [CrossRef] [PubMed]
14. ten Dijke, P.; Arthur, H.M. Extracellular control of TGFbeta signalling in vascular development and disease. *Nat. Rev. Mol. Cell Biol.* **2007**, *8*, 857–869. [CrossRef] [PubMed]
15. Bossi, F.; Tripodo, C.; Rizzi, L.; Bulla, R.; Agostinis, C.; Guarnotta, C.; Munaut, C.; Baldassarre, G.; Papa, G.; Zorzet, S.; et al. C1q as a unique player in angiogenesis with therapeutic implication in wound healing. *Proc. Natl. Acad. Sci. USA* **2014**, *111*, 4209–4214. [CrossRef]
16. Ghebrehiwet, B.; Geisbrecht, B.V.; Xu, X.; Savitt, A.G.; Peerschke, E.I. The C1q Receptors: Focus on gC1qR/p33 (C1qBP, p32, HABP-1)1. *Semin. Immunol.* **2019**, *45*, 101338. [CrossRef]
17. Rafail, S.; Kourtzelis, I.; Foukas, P.G.; Markiewski, M.M.; DeAngelis, R.A.; Guariento, M.; Ricklin, D.; Grice, E.A.; Lambris, J.D. Complement Deficiency Promotes Cutaneous Wound Healing in Mice. *J. Immunol.* **2015**, *194*, 1285–1291. [CrossRef]
18. Folkman, J. Tumor Angiogenesis: A Possible Control Point in Tumor Growth. *Ann. Intern. Med.* **1975**, *82*, 96–100. [CrossRef]
19. Krock, B.L.; Skuli, N.; Simon, M.C. Hypoxia-Induced Angiogenesis: Good and Evil. *Genes Cancer* **2011**, *2*, 1117–1133. [CrossRef]
20. Nagy, J.A.; Chang, S.-H.; Dvorak, A.M.; Dvorak, H.F. Why are tumour blood vessels abnormal and why is it important to know? *Br. J. Cancer* **2009**, *100*, 865–869. [CrossRef]

21. Kuczynski, E.A.; Vermeulen, P.B.; Pezzella, F.; Kerbel, R.S.; Reynolds, A.R. Vessel co-option in cancer. *Nat. Rev. Clin. Oncol.* **2019**, *16*, 469–493. [CrossRef] [PubMed]
22. Maniotis, A.J.; Folberg, R.; Hess, A.; Seftor, E.A.; Gardner, L.M.; Pe'Er, J.; Trent, J.M.; Meltzer, P.S.; Hendrix, M.J.C. Vascular Channel Formation by Human Melanoma Cells in Vivo and in Vitro: Vasculogenic Mimicry. *Am. J. Pathol.* **1999**, *155*, 739–752. [CrossRef]
23. Giancotti, F.G. Mechanisms Governing Metastatic Dormancy and Reactivation. *Cell* **2013**, *155*, 750–764. [CrossRef] [PubMed]
24. Reis, E.S.; Mastellos, D.C.; Ricklin, D.; Mantovani, A.; Lambris, J.D. Complement in cancer: Untangling an intricate relationship. *Nat. Rev. Immunol.* **2018**, *18*, 5–18. [CrossRef]
25. Kochanek, D.M.; Ghouse, S.M.; Karbowniczek, M.; Markiewski, M.M. Complementing Cancer Metastasis. *Front. Immunol.* **2018**, *9*, 1629. [CrossRef]
26. Roumenina, L.T.; Daugan, M.V.; Petitprez, F.; Sautès-Fridman, C.; Fridman, W.H. Context-dependent roles of complement in cancer. *Nat. Rev. Cancer* **2019**, *19*, 698–715. [CrossRef]
27. Markiewski, M.M.; Lambris, J.D. Is complement good or bad for cancer patients? A new perspective on an old dilemma. *Trends Immunol.* **2009**, *30*, 286–292. [CrossRef]
28. Markiewski, M.M.; DeAngelis, R.A.; Benencia, F.; Ricklin-Lichtsteiner, S.K.; Koutoulaki, A.; Gerard, C.; Coukos, G.; Lambris, J.D. Modulation of the antitumor immune response by complement. *Nat. Immunol.* **2008**, *9*, 1225–1235. [CrossRef]
29. Gabrilovich, D.I. Myeloid-Derived Suppressor Cells. *Cancer Immunol. Res.* **2017**, *5*, 3–8. [CrossRef]
30. Nunez-Cruz, S.; Gimotty, P.A.; Guerra, M.W.; Connolly, D.C.; Wu, Y.-Q.; DeAngelis, R.A.; Lambris, J.D.; Coukos, G.; Scholler, N. Genetic and Pharmacologic Inhibition of Complement Impairs Endothelial Cell Function and Ablates Ovarian Cancer Neovascularization. *Neoplasia* **2012**, *14*, 994-IN1. [CrossRef]
31. Monk, P.N.; Scola, A.-M.; Madala, P.; Fairlie, D.P. Function, structure and therapeutic potential of complement C5a receptors. *Br. J. Pharmacol.* **2007**, *152*, 429–448. [CrossRef] [PubMed]
32. Bulla, R.; Tripodo, C.; Rami, D.; Ling, G.S.; Agostinis, C.; Guarnotta, C.; Zorzet, S.; Durigutto, P.; Botto, M.; Tedesco, F. C1q acts in the tumour microenvironment as a cancer-promoting factor independently of complement activation. *Nat. Commun.* **2016**, *7*, 10346. [CrossRef] [PubMed]
33. Wang, Y.; Sun, S.-N.; Liu, Q.; Yu, Y.-Y.; Guo, J.; Wang, K.; Xing, B.-C.; Zheng, Q.-F.; Campa, M.J.; Patz, E.F.; et al. Autocrine Complement Inhibits IL10-Dependent T-cell-Mediated Antitumor Immunity to Promote Tumor Progression. *Cancer Discov.* **2016**, *6*, 1022–1035. [CrossRef] [PubMed]
34. Roumenina, L.T.; Daugan, M.V.; Noe, R.; Petitprez, F.; Vano, Y.A.; Sanchez-Salas, R.; Becht, E.; Meilleroux, J.; Le Clec'H, B.; Giraldo, N.A.; et al. Tumor cells hijack macrophage-produced complement C1q to promote tumor growth. *Cancer Immunol. Res.* **2019**, *7*, 1091–1105. [CrossRef] [PubMed]
35. Reese, B.; Silwal, A.; Daugherity, E.; Daugherity, M.; Arabi, M.; Daly, P.; Paterson, Y.; Woolford, L.; Christie, A.; Elias, R.; et al. Complement as Prognostic Biomarker and Potential Therapeutic Target in Renal Cell Carcinoma. *J. Immunol.* **2020**, *205*, 3218–3229. [CrossRef]
36. Vadrevu, S.K.; Chintala, N.K.; Sharma, S.K.; Sharma, P.; Cleveland, C.; Riediger, L.; Manne, S.; Fairlie, D.P.; Gorczyca, W.; Almanza, O.; et al. Complement C5a Receptor Facilitates Cancer Metastasis by Altering T-Cell Responses in the Metastatic Niche. *Cancer Res.* **2014**, *74*, 3454–3465. [CrossRef]
37. Talmadge, J.E.; Gabrilovich, D.I. History of myeloid-derived suppressor cells. *Nat. Rev. Cancer* **2013**, *13*, 739–752. [CrossRef]
38. Liu, Y.; Cao, X. Characteristics and Significance of the Pre-metastatic Niche. *Cancer Cell* **2016**, *30*, 668–681. [CrossRef]
39. Gao, D.; Nolan, D.J.; Mellick, A.S.; Bambino, K.; McDonnell, K.; Mittal, V. Endothelial Progenitor Cells Control the Angiogenic Switch in Mouse Lung Metastasis. *Science* **2008**, *319*, 195–198. [CrossRef]
40. Welti, J.; Loges, S.; Dimmeler, S.; Carmeliet, P. Recent molecular discoveries in angiogenesis and antiangiogenic therapies in cancer. *J. Clin. Investig.* **2013**, *123*, 3190–3200. [CrossRef]
41. Kaplan, R.N.; Rafii, S.; Lyden, D. Preparing the "Soil": The Premetastatic Niche. *Cancer Res.* **2006**, *66*, 11089–11093. [CrossRef] [PubMed]
42. Sceneay, J.; Chow, M.T.; Chen, A.; Halse, H.M.; Wong, C.S.F.; Andrews, D.M.; Sloan, E.K.; Parker, B.S.; Bowtell, D.D.; Smyth, M.J.; et al. Primary Tumor Hypoxia Recruits CD11b+/Ly6Cmed/Ly6G+ Immune Suppressor Cells and Compromises NK Cell Cytotoxicity in the Premetastatic Niche. *Cancer Res.* **2012**, *72*, 3906–3911. [CrossRef] [PubMed]

43. Ghouse, S.M.; Vadrevu, S.K.; Manne, S.; Reese, B.; Patel, J.; Patel, B.; Silwal, A.; Lodhi, N.; Paterson, Y.; Srivastava, S.K.; et al. Therapeutic Targeting of Vasculature in the Premetastatic and Metastatic Niches Reduces Lung Metastasis. *J. Immunol.* **2020**, *204*, 990–1000. [CrossRef]
44. Koblizek, T.I.; Weiss, C.; Yancopoulos, G.D.; Deutsch, U.; Risau, W. Angiopoietin-1 induces sprouting angiogenesis in vitro. *Curr. Biol.* **1998**, *8*, 529–532. [CrossRef]
45. Voronov, E.; Carmi, Y.; Apte, R.N. The role IL-1 in tumor-mediated angiogenesis. *Front. Physiol.* **2014**, *5*, 114. [CrossRef]
46. Nassiri, F.; Cusimano, M.D.; Scheithauer, B.W.; Rotondo, F.; Fazio, A.; Yousef, G.M.; Syro, L.V.; Kovacs, K.; Lloyd, R.V. Endoglin (CD105): A review of its role in angiogenesis and tumor diagnosis, progression and therapy. *Anticancer Res.* **2011**, *31*, 2283–2290.
47. Noone, A.-M.; Cronin, K.A.; Altekruse, S.F.; Howlader, N.; Lewis, D.R.; Petkov, V.I.; Penberthy, L. Cancer Incidence and Survival Trends by Subtype Using Data from the Surveillance Epidemiology and End Results Program, 1992–2013. *Cancer Epidemiol. Biomark. Prev.* **2017**, *26*, 632–641. [CrossRef]
48. Wong, W.L.; Su, X.; Li, X.; Cheung, C.M.G.; Klein, B.E.K.; Cheng, C.-Y.; Wong, T.Y. Global prevalence of age-related macular degeneration and disease burden projection for 2020 and 2040: A systematic review and meta-analysis. *Lancet Glob. Health* **2014**, *2*, e106–e116. [CrossRef]
49. Geerlings, M.J.; De Jong, E.K.; Hollander, A.I.D. The complement system in age-related macular degeneration: A review of rare genetic variants and implications for personalized treatment. *Mol. Immunol.* **2017**, *84*, 65–76. [CrossRef]
50. Ambati, J.; Fowler, B.J. Mechanisms of Age-Related Macular Degeneration. *Neuron* **2012**, *75*, 26–39. [CrossRef]
51. Apte, R.S.; Chen, D.S.; Ferrara, N. VEGF in Signaling and Disease: Beyond Discovery and Development. *Cell* **2019**, *176*, 1248–1264. [CrossRef] [PubMed]
52. Holz, F.G.; Dugel, P.U.; Weissgerber, G.; Hamilton, R.; Silva, R.; Bandello, F.; Larsen, M.; Weichselberger, A.; Wenzel, A.; Schmidt, A.; et al. Single-Chain Antibody Fragment VEGF Inhibitor RTH258 for Neovascular Age-Related Macular Degeneration: A Randomized Controlled Study. *Ophthalmology* **2016**, *123*, 1080–1089. [CrossRef] [PubMed]
53. Ammar, M.J.; Hsu, J.; Chiang, A.; Ho, A.C.; Regillo, C.D. Age-related macular degeneration therapy: A review. *Curr. Opin. Ophthalmol.* **2020**, *31*, 215–221. [CrossRef] [PubMed]
54. Nozaki, M.; Raisler, B.; Sakurai, E.; Sarma, J.; Barnum, S.; Lambris, J.; Chen, Y.; Zhang, K.; Ambati, B.; Baffi, J.; et al. Drusen complement components C3a and C5a promote choroidal neovascularization. *Proc. Natl. Acad. Sci. USA* **2006**, *142*, 201. [CrossRef]
55. Zhou, J.; Jang, Y.P.; Kim, S.R.; Sparrow, J.R. Complement activation by photooxidation products of A2E, a lipofuscin constituent of the retinal pigment epithelium. *Proc. Natl. Acad. Sci. USA* **2006**, *103*, 16182–16187. [CrossRef]
56. Klein, R.; Zeiss, C.; Chew, E.; Tsai, J.; Sackler, R.; Haynes, C.; Henning, A.; SanGiovanni, J.; Manne, S.; Mayne, S.; et al. Complement factor H polymorphism in age-related macular degeneration. *Science* **2005**, *140*, 352. [CrossRef]
57. Fritsche, L.G.; Fariss, R.N.; Stambolian, D.; Abecasis, G.R.; Curcio, C.A.; Swaroop, A. Age-Related Macular Degeneration: Genetics and Biology Coming Together. *Annu. Rev. Genom. Hum. Genet.* **2014**, *15*, 151–171. [CrossRef]
58. Rohrer, B.; Long, Q.; Coughlin, B.; Wilson, R.B.; Huang, Y.; Qiao, F.; Tang, P.H.; Kunchithapautham, K.; Gilkeson, G.S.; Tomlinson, S. A targeted inhibitor of the alternative complement pathway reduces angiogenesis in a mouse model of age-related macular degeneration. *Investig. Ophthalmol. Vis. Sci.* **2009**, *50*, 3056–3064. [CrossRef]
59. Langer, H.F.; Chung, K.-J.; Orlova, V.V.; Choi, E.Y.; Kaul, S.; Kruhlak, M.J.; Alatsatianos, M.; DeAngelis, R.A.; Roche, P.A.; Magotti, P.; et al. Complement-mediated inhibition of neovascularization reveals a point of convergence between innate immunity and angiogenesis. *Blood* **2010**, *116*, 4395–4403. [CrossRef]
60. Sweigard, J.H.; Yanai, R.; Gaissert, P.; Saint-Geniez, M.; Kataoka, K.; Thanos, A.; Stahl, G.L.; Lambris, J.D.; Connor, K.M. The alternative complement pathway regulates pathological angiogenesis in the retina. *FASEB J.* **2014**, *28*, 3171–3182. [CrossRef]
61. Leon, B.M. Diabetes and cardiovascular disease: Epidemiology, biological mechanisms, treatment recommendations and future research. *World J. Diabetes* **2015**, *6*, 1246–1258. [CrossRef] [PubMed]

62. Ricklin, D.; Mastellos, D.C.; Lambris, J.D. Therapeutic targeting of the complement system. *Nat. Rev. Drug Discov.* **2019**, *1*, 10–1038. [CrossRef] [PubMed]
63. Park, D.H.; Connor, K.M.; Lambris, J.D. The Challenges and Promise of Complement Therapeutics for Ocular Diseases. *Front. Immunol.* **2019**, *10*, 1007. [CrossRef] [PubMed]

Publisher's Note: MDPI stays neutral with regard to jurisdictional claims in published maps and institutional affiliations.

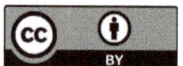 © 2020 by the authors. Licensee MDPI, Basel, Switzerland. This article is an open access article distributed under the terms and conditions of the Creative Commons Attribution (CC BY) license (http://creativecommons.org/licenses/by/4.0/).

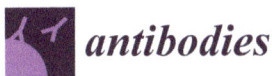

Review

Complement and Cancer—A Dysfunctional Relationship?

Joshua M. Thurman *, Jennifer Laskowski and Raphael A. Nemenoff

Division of Nephrology and Hypertension, University of Colorado Anschutz Medical Campus, Aurora, CO 80045, USA; Jennifer.laskowski@cuanschutz.edu (J.L.); raphael.nemenoff@cuanschutz.edu (R.A.N.)
* Correspondence: joshua.thurman@cuanschutz.edu; Tel.: +1-303-724-7584

Received: 11 August 2020; Accepted: 3 November 2020; Published: 5 November 2020

Abstract: Although it was long believed that the complement system helps the body to identify and remove transformed cells, it is now clear that complement activation contributes to carcinogenesis and can also help tumors to escape immune-elimination. Complement is activated by several different mechanisms in various types of cancer, and complement activation fragments have multiple different downstream effects on cancer cells and throughout the tumor microenvironment. Thus, the role of complement activation in tumor biology may vary among different types of cancer and over time within a single tumor. In multiple different pre-clinical models, however, complement activation has been shown to recruit immunosuppressive myeloid cells into the tumor microenvironment. These cells, in turn, suppress anti-tumor T cell immunity, enabling the tumor to grow. Based on extensive pre-clinical work, therapeutic complement inhibitors hold great promise as a new class of immunotherapy. A greater understanding of the role of complement in tumor biology will improve our ability to identify those patients most likely to benefit from this treatment and to rationally combine complement inhibitors with other cancer therapies.

Keywords: complement; cancer; immunity; myeloid cells; therapeutics

1. Introduction

It was long assumed that the complement cascade contributes to the immunosurveillance of cancers, helping the body to recognize and eliminate transformed cells. In 2008, however, Markiewski and colleagues reported that mice with targeted deletion of the genes for C3 or C4 are protected from cancer in an implantation model [1]. This landmark study revealed that complement activation can promote tumor growth in some settings. Since then, studies from many different research groups have confirmed and expanded on these findings. It is now clear that the complement cascade is activated in many tumors, and that this component of the innate immune system plays a complex role in carcinogenesis and anti-tumor immunity. The mechanisms of complement activation seem to vary among different types of cancer, and the cancer cells themselves often play an active role in modulating complement activation within the tumor microenvironment (TME). For example, various types of cancer express proteins that both activate and inhibit the complement cascade within the TME.

2. How Does Carcinogenesis Occur?

Cancer is a disease of dysregulated growth. While our knowledge of cancer dates back centuries, it has been more challenging to actually define the critical properties of cancer. Starting in the 1980s, studies identified several somatic mutations as critical to the disease. These included activating mutations in drivers of proliferation, designated as oncogenes, and loss of function mutations in tumor suppressor genes. These mutations result in the development of the "transformed" phenotype. Transformed cells acquire new features such as the loss of contact inhibition and the ability to grow in suspension. The biological consequences of these mutations were formally characterized as the "Hallmarks of Cancer" in a seminal review by Hanahan and Weinberg in 2000 [2]. However, solid tumors originate in specific organs and are surrounded by a variety of non-transformed cells. The surrounding cell populations and stroma have been designated as the TME. The TME includes vascular cells, inflammatory and immune cells, fibroblasts, and extracellular matrix. While the initial focus on the transformed epithelial cell did not consider the TME as a driver of cancer progression, it has become apparent that the interactions between cancer cells and the TME are critical. Studies performed in the first decade of this century identified important features of the TME that regulate anti-tumor immunity and cancer metabolism and define additional "Hallmarks" of cancer [3].

A current view of cancer development needs to take into account the complexity of the interactions between cancer cells and the TME, as well as how these interactions change in a spatiotemporal fashion. Thus, epithelial cells undergo initial somatic mutations resulting in activation of oncogenic signaling or loss of tumor suppressor function. This results in increased "fitness" of these cells, giving them a survival advantage. Additional mutations occur which lead to improved cell-autonomous fitness and/or altered interactions with the surrounding TME. Thus, targeting these interactions therapeutically has become a major focus of research.

Additional complexity in this setting is the degree of heterogeneity observed in human tumors. This is reflected by differences in mutational status and metabolic qualities of cancer cells within the same tumor. This variability makes the development of novel therapeutic approaches particularly challenging. Developing rational combinations of therapeutic agents to target this heterogeneity is often limited by the fact that most preclinical models of cancer fail to recapitulate these critical features of human disease.

3. Cancer, Inflammation, and Immunity

The immune system has a complex relationship with carcinogenesis. Chronic inflammation is strongly linked with the risk for many cancers, and it is generally associated with the promotion of tumor progression and metastasis. Cancer-causing inflammation can be produced by infections [4,5], environmental irritants [6,7], and autoimmune diseases [8]. For example, chronic viral infections, such as the human papillomavirus, are associated with the development of head and neck cancers. Chronic pancreatitis, hepatitis, and inflammatory bowel disease are strongly predictive of pancreatic, hepatocellular, and colon cancer, respectively. Perhaps most notably, cigarette smoking leads to the development of chronic lung inflammation and chronic obstructive pulmonary disease (COPD), and it is a major contributor to lung cancer. The immune response in these diverse settings probably contributes to genomic instability, cellular proliferation, and remodeling in the target tissues. Tissue-specific mechanisms are also undoubtedly important, however, as some organs are particularly susceptible to inflammation-associated cancers. Inflammatory changes also occur within the TME of cancers after they have formed, even in tumors for which inflammation is not an initial predisposing factor. As a result, essentially all tumors engage with the immune system as they develop and grow.

Inflammatory responses within tumors induce the recruitment of myeloid cells, including neutrophils and macrophages. Myeloid cells are initially recruited to the site of tumors as a result of specific molecules produced by the cancer cells, including cytokines, growth factors, and other molecules that attract myeloid cells and modulate their phenotype [9,10]. Macrophages are the most abundant leukocyte subtype in the TME, and they continually infiltrate the tumor [11]. This process appears to depend on the trafficking of monocytes from the bone marrow in response to specific chemokines produced by the cancer cells, such as (C-C motif) ligand 2 (CCL2). These innate immune cells are critical to the general response to injury and acute infection and act to eliminate infections and promote healing. Similar to what is seen during infection, the initial phenotype of myeloid cells in the TME is generally proinflammatory, designated as M1 macrophages and N1 neutrophils. The phenotypes of these cells become altered in the setting of chronic inflammation, however. Similarly, cross-talk between cancer cells and myeloid cells eventually results in modulation to alternatively activated phenotypes, designated as M2 or N2 [12]. These cells then actually promote tumor progression through the production of growth factors and proangiogenic cytokines which, in turn, signal back to the cancer cells. While this model is definitely an oversimplification, it serves as a framework for understanding the interactions between the cancer cells and these innate immune cell populations.

Cancer cells express mutated or aberrantly expressed proteins on their cell surface. These so-called neoantigens can be recognized by the adaptive immune system (CD8 and CD4 T cells) potentially leading to immune elimination. However, cancer cells can evade immune attack through multiple mechanisms. A model for this, designated as immunoediting, was proposed several years ago by Schreiber and colleagues [13]. This model comprises three stages of interaction with the immune system. Initially, tumor cells can be eliminated by the immune system; however, responses of the tumor lead to an equilibrium where the tumors are not eliminated but held in check by the immune system. Eventually, through the activation of additional cancer cell-autonomous and non-autonomous mechanisms, the cancers evade immune attack and escape.

Numerous mechanisms control these events. Cancer cells can develop additional mutations that target antigen-presentation pathways, thus becoming invisible to the immune system. Alternatively, myeloid cells within the TME can undergo phenotypic modulation, acquiring anti-inflammatory properties [14]. The cells can then inhibit CD4 T cells and block CD8 T cell-mediated killing. Finally, a variety of pathways that regulate the immune system under non-cancerous conditions can be co-opted by cancer cells to block T cell function. Prominent among these are immune checkpoints expressed on the surface of cancer cells and other cell types which block T cell activation and lead to an "exhausted" T cell phenotype [15]. Targeting these pathways through the use of checkpoint inhibitors can result in T cell reactivation and tumor regression. These agents have been approved in a variety of cancers and have revolutionized the treatment of many types of cancer [16,17]. For several reasons that are only partially understood, however, the majority of patients either do not respond to these agents or develop resistance.

A major challenge, therefore, is the development of rational combinations of therapies that will increase the number of responders as well as the duration of the response to treatment. In particular, targeting inflammation and the cross-talk between innate and adaptive immunity could enhance the ability of the immune system to eliminate tumors.

4. The Role of the Complement System in Carcinogenesis

The complement system is a cascade of proteins that form part of the innate immune system. Complement factors circulate as inactive precursor proteins (zymogens) that are cleaved and activated by three different pathways: the classical, lectin, and alternative [18]. Activation of these pathways generates soluble fragments (C3a and C5a, or the "anaphylatoxins") and also covalently fixes protein fragments (C3 and C4 fragments) on the surface of target cells. Immune cells express specific receptors for the anaphylatoxins and C3 fragments and this interaction links complement activation fragments with modulation of immune cell function. Consequently, complement activation has strong effects on innate and adaptive immunity. Full complement activation also generates multimeric complexes that form pores in target cells. In the literature, this is variably referred to as the membrane attack complex (MAC), the terminal complement complex, or C5b-9.

Complement activation is traditionally regarded as proceeding through three different pathways: the classical, lectin, and alternative pathways. The classical and lectin pathways are activated by specific proteins that activate these cascades after binding to target ligands. IgG and IgM bound to target antigens activate the classical pathway, and mannose-binding lectin bound to target sugars activates the lectin pathway [19]. The alternative pathway is spontaneously activated in plasma through a process called "tickover". It is also secondarily activated by the classical and lectin pathways, thereby amplifying their effects.

4.1. Complement Activation as a Cause of Cancer

Carcinogenesis involves several steps, including the acquisition of a series of mutations that give a cell growth or survival advantages ("initiation") and proliferation and/or decreased death of the transformed cells ("promotion") [20]. The immune system is integrally involved with both of these stages of carcinogenesis. In most inflammatory settings, complement activation occurs as part of a broader immune response, so it is difficult to distinguish the effects of complement activation from those of other components of the immune system. Nevertheless, we recently published a study showing that chronic complement activation in the liver causes cancer [21]. Mice with targeted deletion of the gene for factor H, a key complement regulatory protein, have spontaneous complement activation within the liver [21]. As the mice aged, they developed hepatocellular carcinoma at a greater rate than control mice, whereas complement deficient mice did not. Although the experiments did not determine which stage(s) of tumorigenesis complement directly affects, it did demonstrate that, at least in the liver, chronic complement activation is sufficient to cause tumor formation.

There is a rationale for suspecting that the complement system plays a part in tumor initiation (Figure 1). Activated macrophages [22] and neutrophils [23] produce reactive oxygen species and reactive nitrogen intermediates, molecules that can cause DNA mutations [24]. C3a and C5a are strongly chemotactic for these cells and induce the cells to undergo oxidative burst. Thus, complement activation within inflamed tissues is probably integrally involved in these initiation events [25]. In support of this, Bonavita and colleagues studied the role of pentraxin-3 (PTX3) in models of chemically induced sarcomas and skin carcinomas [26]. PTX3 is expressed by many types of cancers, and it can bind to circulating factor H, tethering this inhibitor to cells and suppressing complement activation within the TME. The authors found that PTX3-deficient mice were susceptible to chemically induced sarcomas and skin carcinomas, presumably because inadequate control of complement activation increases carcinogenesis in affected tissues. Furthermore, complement deficiency reversed this tumorigenic effect. The authors also noted that PTX3-deficient mice developed a greater degree of DNA damage and a higher number of P53 mutations at early timepoints compared to wild-type mice, further supporting the conclusion that complement-mediated inflammation contributes to genomic instability and cancer initiation.

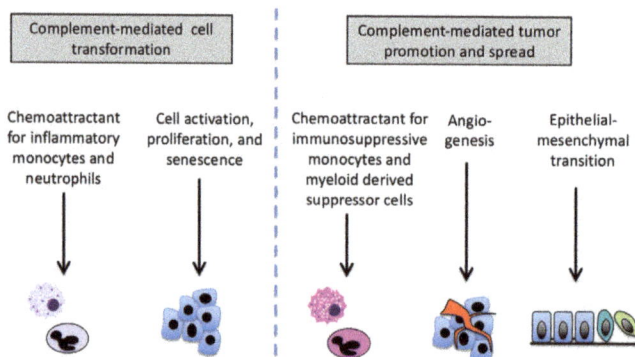

Figure 1. Possible roles for complement in tumor initiation and promotion. Complement activation is a frequent component of the acute inflammatory response. Complement fragments are chemotactic for myeloid cells, and also elicit the production of chemokines by epithelial cells. This contributes to inflammatory injury. Complement also directly stimulates cell activation and proliferation in target tissues. Once cancers have developed, complement fragments protect the tumor from immune-elimination by attracting immune-suppressive myeloid cells into the tumor microenvironment. Complement fragments may be involved with angiogenesis, which supports the expanding tumor mass. It may also trigger epithelial-mesenchymal transition, which contributes to tissue remodeling and tumor spread.

Once cells have acquired cancer-causing mutations, the promotion of the nascent tumor requires the proliferation and survival of the transformed cells [27,28]. This involves pro-mitotic signals as well as angiogenic signals to support the expanding tumor, processes that have been linked to inflammatory cytokines. The complement system may indirectly contribute to this process by inducing the production of cytokines and chemokines [29]. Furthermore, in vitro experiments have also shown that C3a and/or C5a directly stimulate cancer cell proliferation [30–32]. Consistent with these mitogenic effects on cancer cells, studies in non-cancer models have also shown that C3a and C5a induce survival and proliferation of cells during tissue regeneration [33–35]. In addition to C3a and C5a, the insertion of MAC in tumor cell membranes can stimulate cell proliferation [36] and induce chemokine and metalloprotease production by the cells [37]. These findings support a role for complement activation in tumor promotion.

Regions of hypoxia develop in solid tumors as they expand, and angiogenesis becomes essential for all tumor growth. Complement is frequently activated within ischemic tissues, and hypoxia induces some cell types, including non-small cell lung cancer cells, to decrease expression of complement regulatory proteins in vitro [38]. Thus, complement may be preferentially activated in hypoxic regions of a tumor. Complement activation has been linked with angiogenesis [39], raising the possibility that the complement activation provides a link between tissue hypoxia and the production of angiogenic signals. A comprehensive analysis of the mutational landscape in tumors revealed that there is cross-talk between the complement system and hypoxic signals in some cancers [40]. Nevertheless, in one study of non-small cell lung cancer, the C5a blockade did not have a detectable effect on vascular density within tumors [41].

4.2. Complement as a Mechanism of Immune Evasion

The study by Markiewski and colleagues used an implantation model of cancer [1]. Because the mice were injected with cells that were already transformed, the study implicated complement in the growth of existing tumors rather than in cancer initiation per se. In that study, the investigators showed that the generation of C5a attracted myeloid-derived suppressor cells (MDSCs) to the tumor, which reduced the anti-tumor response of CD8 T cells. Complement activation in that model, therefore, is analogous to an immune checkpoint insofar as it suppresses the immune-elimination of cancers (Figure 1). Over the subsequent 12 years, additional pre-clinical studies have reported a similar role for complement activation in promoting the growth of other types of cancer, including lung [42], squamous cell [43], melanoma [44], colon [45], and ovarian cancer [30]. Many other effects of complement on cancer cells and the TME have been identified, but the pattern of inducing myeloid cells to suppress the adaptive immune system has been generalizable across tumor types.

Studies in multiple different types of cancer have also confirmed that the pro-tumorigenic effects of complement are mediated by immunosuppressive myeloid cells, such as MDSCs [1,41,46]. The anaphylatoxins generally have pro-inflammatory effects, but studies in solid organ transplant models have shown that C5a can also attract immunosuppressive myeloid cells into tissues [47]. It is not clear whether it is the context or the duration of complement signaling that determines whether the net effect is pro or anti-inflammatory. Interestingly, studies have revealed that both C3a and C5a contribute to the immunosuppressive effect of complement within tumors [42,44]. Furthermore, C3 produced by stellate cells in the liver affects dendritic cell maturation and attracts MDSCs, facilitating the growth of hepatocellular carcinoma [48]. Another study of stellate cells indicated that this immunomodulatory effect is caused by the iC3b fragment [49]. Thus, multiple different complement activation fragments seem to interact with myeloid cells in the TME, helping the tumor to evade immune-elimination.

Complement activation may also play a role in protective anti-tumor immune responses. For example, it has been shown to be involved in the formation of tertiary lymphoid structures (TLS), which are structures consisting of B and T cells as well as dendritic cells. Interactions between these cells result in strong immune activation, and the presence of these structures is associated with a good response to immunotherapy in multiple cancers [50]. Complement activation in the setting of chemotherapy has been shown to promote a subset of B cells that regulate the formation of these structures [51].

Distinct from systemic production of complement, recent studies have identified key functional roles for intracellular production of complement, specifically in human CD4+ T cells [52,53]. Activation of T cells is associated with translocation of intracellular C3a and C3b to the cell surface, where these fragments regulate T cell activation and metabolism through the engagement of the C3a receptor (C3aR) and the regulatory protein CD46, respectively. These data would indicate that in the setting of cancer progression complement activation in cancer cells and T cells play opposing roles, with cancer cell complement mediating immunosuppression and T cell complement mediating T cell activation. Further research is required to dissect out the relevant importance of these pathways in specific malignancies. One complication in studying the T cell intracellular complement pathway is the fact that CD46 is not expressed in mice, making it difficult to assess this pathway in preclinical models.

4.3. Complement Activation and Metastatic Spread of Cancer

Beyond its effects on carcinogenesis and tumor growth, there is also experimental evidence that the complement cascade increases the invasiveness and metastatic potential of cancer [recently reviewed in [41]]. Complement activation has been linked to the metastatic potential of colon cancer [54] as well as leptomeningeal metastases of cancer cells [55]. The effect of complement fragments on metastases may be due to their direct effects on cancer cells as well as their effect on tissue remodeling in the TME and metastatic niche. C5a, for example, directly induces epithelial-mesenchymal transformation (EMT) of hepatocellular carcinoma [56] and gastric cancer cells [57], and can induce expression of metalloproteinases [58]. Conversely, the C5a receptor blockade reduces some hallmarks of EMT [59]. Work in animal models has also shown that the C5a blockade reduces metastasis of colon and lung cancers by regulating immune responses and the premetastatic niche [46,54].

5. Cancer as a Cause of Complement Activation

Complement activation contributes to the development of cancer by the mechanisms discussed above, but the reverse is true too: tumors actively promote complement activation within the TME (Figure 1). Inflammatory cells and molecules are present within the TME of essentially all cancers, regardless of their tissue of origin [60]. The adaptive immune response to cancer cells is a function of tumor immunogenicity, which is determined by both the antigenic burden in the cancer and the host immune system [61]. Inflammation can cause DNA damage, but DNA damage can cause the production of mutant proteins that are antigenic and elicit an immune response [62]. Cancer cells that cannot evade the immune system will be eliminated, so the cancer must either stop producing the target antigen, downregulate MHC, or suppress the immune response to the tumor antigen through immunoediting [63,64]. Although the anti-tumor immunity is primarily executed by CD4 T cells, CD8 T cells, and natural killer (NK) T cells, B cells are also seen within the TME of some tumors, and patients often develop IgG that is specifically reactive with tumor antigens [65,66]. This can serve as a link between the adaptive immune response to a tumor with complement activation within the TME.

There is evidence of classical pathway activation in several animal models of cancer. The growth of TC-1 tumors was significantly reduced in mice with targeted deletion of C4 (classical and lectin pathway deficient), but tumor growth was not affected by the deletion of factor B (alternative pathway deficient) [1]. Similarly, studies in non-small cell lung cancer showed that IgM and C4 are deposited in both a mouse model and in human samples, pointing to the involvement of the classical pathway in this type of cancer [42]. Furthermore, tumor growth was not affected by factor B deficiency in this model. A study using the TC-1 cell line also found that C1q was required for tumor growth, further supporting the involvement of the classical pathway [67]. C1q deposits are seen in human lung, colon, breast, and pancreatic adenocarcinoma, as well as melanoma [68]. Because patients so frequently develop antibodies against tumor antigens, it is logical that classical pathway activation would be a frequent occurrence. In a mouse model of melanoma, however, investigators have also shown that C1q contributes to tumor growth in a complement-independent fashion [68]. Studies in models of systemic lupus erythematosus, an autoimmune disease, revealed that C1q directly affects the CD8 T cell response to antigens independent of the classical pathway [69]. In that study, C1q-deficient CD8 T cells displayed greater reactivity against autoantigens and viruses. Such an effect could also potentially modulate anti-tumor immunity.

In addition to the adaptive B cell response to foreign antigens, natural antibodies are produced by B-1 cells in the absence of an antigenic stimulus and often react with carbohydrate epitopes [70]. Tumor cells frequently display abnormal post-translational modifications, including altered glycosylation patterns. Natural antibodies can bind to carbohydrate epitopes, and they have been found to react to glycans displayed on the surface of cancer cells [71]. Interestingly, a hybridoma generated from a patient with signet-ring cell carcinoma of the stomach reacts specifically with an N-linked carbohydrate on CD55 [72]. CD55 is a cell surface complement regulatory protein that protects cancer cells from complement-mediated lysis and contributes to chemoresistance of the cells [51]. Antibodies that bind to neo-epitopes displayed on the surface of CD55 could activate the classical pathway on the target cell while simultaneously impairing complement regulation by CD55 on the cell surface.

Although the requirement of C4 expression for tumor growth could also reflect a role for the lectin pathway in the TC-1 model, there is less published evidence for specific involvement of this pathway in cancer models. However, one recent study found that certain species of gut fungi can migrate to the pancreas and foster the development of pancreatic ductal adenocarcinoma [73]. MBL was required for tumor growth in this model, indicating that the lectin pathway activation was probably involved. This study also showed that signaling through the C3a receptor was necessary for tumor growth.

Although several studies have found that an intact alternative pathway is not necessary for tumor growth [1,42], it is notable that alternative pathway proteins are expressed by most tumors [74]. The alternative pathway also amplifies complement activation that is initiated through the other pathways, so this pathway may contribute to tumor growth by increasing the overall magnitude and duration of complement activation, even if it is not essential for the reaction. Our recent study using factor H deficient mice showed that chronic alternative pathway activation in the liver is sufficient to cause HCC [21]. However, it is possible that the liver—as the source of the alternative proteins factor B and C3—may be uniquely susceptible to alternative pathway-mediated injury.

It is striking that cancer cells and other cells within the TME synthesize complement proteins [74]. Several inflammatory cytokines induce parenchymal cells to produce complement proteins, and the transcription factor twists basic helix-loop-helix transcription factor 1 (TWIST1) has been identified as a key regulator of the expression of C3 by cancer cells [75]. Although high levels of complement proteins are already present in plasma, studies in organ transplantation revealed the importance of locally produced proteins in activation within tissues [76]. Similarly, studies in cancer models have revealed that complement proteins produced by the cancer cells, themselves, contribute to tumor growth in vivo despite the expression of the same proteins by the host [30].

Various proteases are also able to directly activate complement proteins, potentially bypassing the conventional initiation mechanisms and convertases. The cathepsins, for example, are a family of serine proteases that are upregulated and secreted by many different types of cancer [77], and cathepsin L can cleave C3 into C3a and C3b [52]. Human melanoma cells express cathepsin L and cleavage of C3 by the protease is associated with growth and metastasis [78]. Similarly, thrombin is capable of directly cleaving complement C5 [79]. Cancer cells can, directly and indirectly, activate thrombin [80], providing a mechanism for the direct generation of the terminal complement components. Additional cancer-associated proteases capable of activating complement proteins have also been identified, including prostate-specific antigen [81].

6. Complement Regulatory Proteins

In addition to the many molecules that activate the complement pathways, the body also expresses a family of proteins that inhibit activation of the cascade [82]. Some soluble regulators circulate in plasma and other body fluids, as well as regulators expressed on the outer membrane of all cells. The various regulatory proteins inhibit complement activation by distinct mechanisms and at different sites within the cascade.

All cancer cells express cell surface complement regulators, and most cancer cells express more than one of the proteins. The cell surface regulators CD46, CD55, and CD59, for example, are all expressed by squamous cell cancers [83] and uveal melanomas [84]. Multiple studies have also shown that cancer cells overexpress complement regulators compared to the corresponding tissue of origin [85–87]. For years, the presumption was that overexpression of the complement regulatory proteins is a mechanism by which cancer cells evade complement-mediated elimination. In support of this, functional studies in which expression of the proteins is knocked down with small interfering RNA (siRNA) have confirmed that the regulatory proteins protect the cells from lysis [88]. Expression levels of the regulatory proteins have also been shown to correlate with complement activation with the tumor and with patient outcomes [89,90]. Interestingly, cancer cells frequently overexpress factor H, and factor H-like protein 1 (FHL-1), soluble proteins that are already present at high concentrations in plasma [91]. Studies have shown that factor H is expressed by ovarian, squamous, and colon cancer cells [92,93]. Knockdown of factor H production can reduce tumor cell survival, proliferation, and migration in vivo [94,95]. Although liver-derived factor H and FHL-1 is almost certainly present in the TME, production of these proteins by cancer cell may ensure that local concentrations are sufficient to protect the cells. Cancer cells can also express non-complement proteins, such as osteopontin, that bind to factor H, holding it within the TME [96].

Several studies have linked the expression of complement regulatory proteins by tumors with adverse clinical outcomes [97,98]. In patients with breast cancer, for example, the expression of CD59 was associated with lung metastasis and shorter [98]. Similarly, in cholangiocarcinoma higher expression of CD55 is associated with shorter survival [97]. Unsurprisingly, being able to control complement activation gives a cancer cell a survival advantage, but this does lead to a paradox. On the one hand, complement activation supports tumor growth in many contexts, yet cancer cells also actively express proteins that inhibit the complement system. It is noteworthy, however, that the expression of complement regulatory proteins by cancer cells is quite heterogeneous, and cells within the same tumor can express different repertoires of regulatory proteins [99]. Expression of these proteins is also dynamic, changing in response to local conditions such as hypoxia and inflammatory cytokines [100,101]. One model to account for these data would suggest that regulatory proteins protect cancer cells from the deleterious effects of complement, such as lysis through the MAC complex while allowing the pro-tumorigenic effects mediated by C3a/C5a to act on the TME leading to immunosuppression. Thus, complement activation may have opposing effects on tumor growth, and the effects may fluctuate depending on time and location within the tumor. Furthermore, while complement activation may destroy a limited number of cells within the tumor mass, the immunosuppressive effects of C3a and C5a may suppress the immune system throughout the TME (Figure 2).

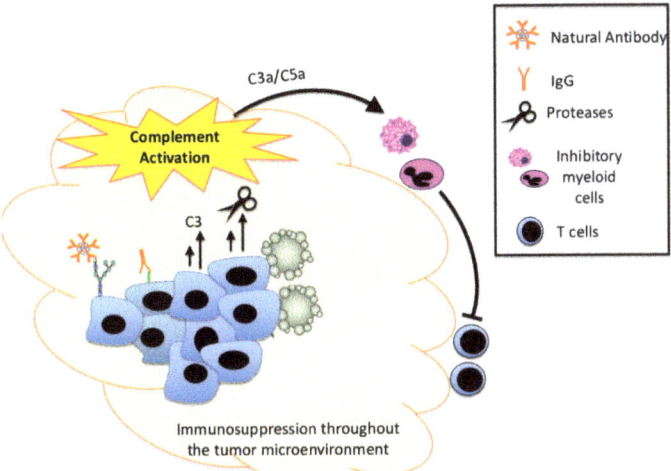

Figure 2. Mechanisms by which cancer cells activate complement to control the tumor microenvironment. Tumor cells actively promote complement activation by several mechanisms. The natural antibody binds to glycans on the cell surface, and IgG binds to tumor neoepitopes. Cancer cells also produced complement proteins, such as C3, which fuels local activation. Cancer cells can also release proteases, such as cathepsin L, which directly activate complement proteins. Complement activation within tumors likely causes apoptosis and necrosis of some target cells, but it also produces C3a and C5a which recruit inhibitory myeloid cells into the tumor microenvironment. These myeloid cells suppress the anti-tumor function of CD4 and CD8 T cells.

7. Complement Inhibitors as Cancer Treatment

As outlined above, complement inhibitory drugs are effective for reducing tumor size in multiple different pre-clinical cancer models [1,41,42,44,102–104]. Inhibitory anti-C5 antibodies have been approved for several non-malignant diseases [105,106], and many additional complement inhibitory agents are in development [107]. Some of the new drugs block all activation, some selectively block the various activation pathways, and others target specific complement fragments and receptors. Thus, shortly there will likely be a range of therapeutic options for blocking the complement system. C3 fragments clearly play a role in tumor biology, but multiple studies have shown that C5aR antagonism is an effective cancer treatment. Several C5a antagonists are currently in clinical development for other indications, so this approach is already feasible.

If complement inhibitors are to be used to treat cancer, then it will be important to understand: (1) which types of cancer are responsive to this approach, (2) when in the course of the disease is complement inhibition most effective, and (3) which components of the complement system contribute to tumor growth. Furthermore, based on the experience with immune checkpoint inhibitors, complement inhibitory drugs will be most effective when combined with other therapies. The efficacy of including complement inhibitors in combination therapy likely depends on the treatments with which they are paired. For example, the efficacy of monoclonal antibodies often involves complement-mediated cytotoxicity. Consequently, the use of complement inhibitors could undermine the efficacy of these drugs. Indeed, some drugs impair the ability of cancer cells to regulate the complement cascade, thereby increasing complement activation on the cell surface. These agents have been used as a means of sensitizing tumors to monoclonal antibody treatments [108].

The combination of anti-complement drugs with immune checkpoint inhibitors may also represent a special case. In many studies, complement blockade has been shown to affect existing tumors via its effects on myeloid cell recruitment and polarization. This, in turn, enhances the anti-tumor effects of

T cells. Complement inhibition and immune checkpoint inhibition, therefore, have similar, and possibly redundant, effects on anti-tumor immunity. However, preclinical studies also suggest that these drugs work by different mechanisms and can have additive effects on tumor size [104,109]. Indeed, a clinical trial is currently underway in which an anti-C5aR antibody is being combined with a PD-L1 antagonist for the treatment of solid tumors (NCT03665129; the type of cancer has not been disclosed). Finally, the development of novel targeted complement inhibitors might represent a therapeutic strategy to selectively regulate complement at the site of the tumor, without the adverse effects that might occur with systemic complement inhibition. Several fusion proteins have been developed which need to be tested in appropriate preclinical models [110].

8. Conclusions

One of the most unexpected and powerful discoveries in complement research is the critical role of this system in cancer biology. Although the full range of effects that complement fragments have on cancer initiation and tumor growth are not yet known, a frequent finding is that complement inhibition increases anti-tumor immunity and reduces tumor size. This is, in many respects, analogous to checkpoint inhibition. Many different complement inhibitors are in clinical development, and this class of drugs holds great promise for the treatment of cancer. Based on what is currently known about the role of complement in carcinogenesis, there is reason to suspect that complement inhibition can reduce the risk of tumor initiation in patients with some chronic inflammatory diseases, and it can slow the growth and spread of many types of cancer.

The optimal use of complement inhibitory drugs will entail a greater understanding of the role of complement activation in specific types of cancer, as well as the potential and limitations of combining complement inhibitory drugs with various other cancer therapies. Studies have shown that cancer cells express many different proteins that promote and inhibit complement activation, highlighting a complex interaction between cancer cells and complement proteins that may vary over time and throughout the tumor. Although disentangling all the details of this relationship will be challenging, many of the tools developed for complement research in other fields are being applied to cancer models. Furthermore, activation of the complement system generates several tissue bound and soluble biomarkers, which may provide accurate methods by which complement activation within a tumor can be monitored in the clinic.

Funding: This research was funded by National Institutes of Health Grant numbers DK113586, DK076690, CA225840, CA236222, the Department of Defense Grant LR180050 (JMT), and a grant from LUNGevity.

Conflicts of Interest: JMT receives royalties from Alexion Pharmaceuticals, Inc. and is a consultant for Q32 Bio, Inc., a company developing complement inhibitors. He also holds stock and will receive royalty income from Q32 Bio, Inc. The funders had no role in the writing of the manuscript.

References

1. Markiewski, M.M.; DeAngelis, R.A.; Benencia, F.; Ricklin-Lichtsteiner, S.K.; Koutoulaki, A.; Gerard, C.; Coukos, G.; Lambris, J.D. Modulation of the antitumor immune response by complement. *Nat. Immunol.* **2008**, *9*, 1225–1235. [CrossRef] [PubMed]
2. Hanahan, D.; Weinberg, R.A. The hallmarks of cancer. *Cell* **2000**, *100*, 57–70. [CrossRef]
3. Hanahan, D.; Weinberg, R.A. Hallmarks of cancer: The next generation. *Cell* **2011**, *144*, 646–674. [CrossRef] [PubMed]
4. De Martel, C.; Franceschi, S. Infections and cancer: Established associations and new hypotheses. *Crit. Rev. Oncol./Hematol.* **2009**, *70*, 183–194. [CrossRef] [PubMed]
5. Karin, M. Nuclear factor-kappaB in cancer development and progression. *Nature* **2006**, *441*, 431–436. [CrossRef] [PubMed]
6. Takahashi, H.; Ogata, H.; Nishigaki, R.; Broide, D.H.; Karin, M. Tobacco smoke promotes lung tumorigenesis by triggering IKKbeta- and JNK1-dependent inflammation. *Cancer Cell* **2010**, *17*, 89–97. [CrossRef]

7. Doerner, S.K.; Reis, E.S.; Leung, E.S.; Ko, J.S.; Heaney, J.D.; Berger, N.A.; Lambris, J.D.; Nadeau, J.H. High-Fat Diet-Induced Complement Activation Mediates Intestinal Inflammation and Neoplasia, Independent of Obesity. *Mol. Cancer Res.* **2016**, *14*, 953–965. [CrossRef]
8. Waldner, M.J.; Neurath, M.F. Colitis-associated cancer: The role of T cells in tumor development. *Semin. Immunopathol.* **2009**, *31*, 249–256. [CrossRef] [PubMed]
9. Franklin, R.A.; Liao, W.; Sarkar, A.; Kim, M.V.; Bivona, M.R.; Liu, K.; Pamer, E.G.; Li, M.O. The cellular and molecular origin of tumor-associated macrophages. *Science* **2014**, *344*, 921–925. [CrossRef]
10. Colegio, O.R.; Chu, N.-Q.; Szabo, A.L.; Chu, T.; Rhebergen, A.M.; Jairam, V.; Cyrus, N.; Brokowski, C.E.; Eisenbarth, S.C.; Phillips, G.M.; et al. Functional polarization of tumour-associated macrophages by tumour-derived lactic acid. *Nature* **2014**, *513*, 559–563. [CrossRef] [PubMed]
11. Murray, P.J. Nonresolving macrophage-mediated inflammation in malignancy. *FEBS J.* **2018**, *285*, 641–653. [CrossRef] [PubMed]
12. Allavena, P.; Sica, A.; Solinas, G.; Porta, C.; Mantovani, A. The inflammatory micro-environment in tumor progression: The role of tumor-associated macrophages. *Crit. Rev. Oncol./Hematol.* **2008**, *66*, 1–9. [CrossRef] [PubMed]
13. Schreiber, R.D.; Old, L.J.; Smyth, M.J. Cancer immunoediting: Integrating immunity's roles in cancer suppression and promotion. *Science* **2011**, *331*, 1565–1570. [CrossRef]
14. Woo, S.R.; Corrales, L.; Gajewski, T.F. Innate immune recognition of cancer. *Annu. Rev. Immunol.* **2015**, *33*, 445–474. [CrossRef] [PubMed]
15. Wherry, E.J. T cell exhaustion. *Nat. Immunol.* **2011**, *12*, 492–499. [CrossRef]
16. Pardoll, D.M. The blockade of immune checkpoints in cancer immunotherapy. *Nat. Rev. Cancer* **2012**, *12*, 252–264. [CrossRef]
17. Topalian, S.L.; Drake, C.G.; Pardoll, D.M. Immune checkpoint blockade: A common denominator approach to cancer therapy. *Cancer Cell* **2015**, *27*, 450–461. [CrossRef]
18. Walport, M.J. Complement. First of two parts. *N. Engl. J. Med.* **2001**, *344*, 1058–1066. [CrossRef]
19. Merle, N.S.; Church, S.E.; Fremeaux-Bacchi, V.; Roumenina, L.T. Complement System Part I—Molecular Mechanisms of Activation and Regulation. *Front. Immunol.* **2015**, *6*, 262. [CrossRef]
20. Coussens, L.M.; Werb, Z. Inflammation and cancer. *Nature* **2002**, *420*, 860–867. [CrossRef]
21. Laskowski, J.; Renner, B.; Pickering, M.C.; Serkova, N.J.; Smith-Jones, P.M.; Clambey, E.T.; Nemenoff, R.A.; Thurman, J.M. Complement factor H-deficient mice develop spontaneous hepatic tumors. *J. Clin. Investig.* **2020**. [CrossRef]
22. Coussens, L.M.; Raymond, W.W.; Bergers, G.; Laig-Webster, M.; Behrendtsen, O.; Werb, Z.; Caughey, G.H.; Hanahan, D. Inflammatory mast cells up-regulate angiogenesis during squamous epithelial carcinogenesis. *Genes Dev.* **1999**, *13*, 1382–1397. [CrossRef]
23. Fridlender, Z.G.; Albelda, S.M. Tumor-associated neutrophils: Friend or foe? *Carcinogenesis* **2012**, *33*, 949–955. [CrossRef] [PubMed]
24. Kraus, S.; Arber, N. Inflammation and colorectal cancer. *Curr. Opin. Pharmacol.* **2009**, *9*, 405–410. [CrossRef]
25. Guglietta, S.; Chiavelli, A.; Zagato, E.; Krieg, C.; Gandini, S.; Ravenda, P.S.; Bazolli, B.; Lu, B.; Penna, G.; Rescigno, M. Coagulation induced by C3aR-dependent NETosis drives protumorigenic neutrophils during small intestinal tumorigenesis. *Nat. Commun.* **2016**, *7*, 11037. [CrossRef]
26. Bonavita, E.; Gentile, S.; Rubino, M.; Maina, V.; Papait, R.; Kunderfranco, P.; Greco, C.; Feruglio, F.; Molgora, M.; LaFace, I.; et al. PTX3 is an extrinsic oncosuppressor regulating complement-dependent inflammation in cancer. *Cell* **2015**, *160*, 700–714. [CrossRef]
27. Guerra, C.; Schuhmacher, A.J.; Cañamero, M.; Grippo, P.J.; Verdaguer, L.; Pérez-Gallego, L.; Dubus, P.; Sandgren, E.P.; Barbacid, M. Chronic pancreatitis is essential for induction of pancreatic ductal adenocarcinoma by K-Ras oncogenes in adult mice. *Cancer Cell* **2007**, *11*, 291–302. [CrossRef] [PubMed]
28. Sieweke, M.H.; Thompson, N.L.; Sporn, M.B.; Bissell, M.J. Mediation of wound-related Rous sarcoma virus tumorigenesis by TGF-beta. *Science* **1990**, *248*, 1656–1660. [CrossRef] [PubMed]
29. Thurman, J.M.; Lenderink, A.M.; Royer, P.A.; Coleman, K.E.; Zhou, J.; Lambris, J.D.; Nemenoff, R.A.; Quigg, R.J.; Holers, V.M. C3a is required for the production of CXC chemokines by tubular epithelial cells after renal ishemia/reperfusion. *J. Immunol.* **2007**, *178*, 1819–1828. [CrossRef]

30. Cho, M.S.; Vasquez, H.G.; Rupaimoole, R.; Pradeep, S.; Wu, S.; Zand, B.; Han, H.-D.; Rodriguez-Aguayo, C.; Bottsford-Miller, J.; Huang, J.; et al. Autocrine effects of tumor-derived complement. *Cell Rep.* **2014**, *6*, 1085–1095. [CrossRef] [PubMed]
31. Fan, Z.; Qin, J.; Wang, D.; Geng, S. Complement C3a promotes proliferation, migration and stemness in cutaneous squamous cell carcinoma. *J. Cell. Mol. Med.* **2019**, *23*, 3097–3107. [CrossRef]
32. Lu, Y.; Hu, X.B. C5a stimulates the proliferation of breast cancer cells via Akt-dependent RGC-32 gene activation. *Oncol. Rep.* **2014**, *32*, 2817–2823. [CrossRef]
33. Lara-Astiaso, D.; Izarra, A.; Estrada, J.C.; Albo, C.; Moscoso, I.; Samper, E.; Moncayo-Arlandi, J.; Solano, A.; Bernad, A.; Diez-Juan, A. Complement anaphylatoxins C3a and C5a induce a failing regenerative program in cardiac resident cells. Evidence of a role for cardiac resident stem cells other than cardiomyocyte renewal. *Springerplus.* **2012**, *1*, 63. [CrossRef]
34. Daveau, M.; Benard, M.; Scotte, M.; Schouft, M.-T.; Hiron, M.; Francois, A.; Salier, J.-P.; Fontaine, M. Expression of a functional C5a receptor in regenerating hepatocytes and its involvement in a proliferative signaling pathway in rat. *J. Immunol.* **2004**, *173*, 3418–3424. [CrossRef]
35. Strey, C.W.; Markiewski, M.; Mastellos, D.; Tudoran, R.; Spruce, L.A.; Greenbaum, L.E.; Lambris, J.D. The proinflammatory mediators C3a and C5a are essential for liver regeneration. *J. Exp. Med.* **2003**, *198*, 913–923. [CrossRef]
36. Vlaicu, S.I.; Tegla, C.A.; Cudrici, C.D.; Danoff, J.; Madani, H.; Sugarman, A.; Niculescu, F.; Mircea, P.A.; Rus, V.; Rus, H. Role of C5b-9 complement complex and response gene to complement-32 (RGC-32) in cancer. *Immunol. Res.* **2013**, *56*, 109–121. [CrossRef]
37. Towner, L.D.; Wheat, R.A.; Hughes, T.R.; Morgan, B.P. Complement Membrane Attack and Tumorigenesis: A systems biology approach. *J. Biol. Chem.* **2016**, *291*, 14927–14938. [CrossRef]
38. Okroj, M.; Corrales, L.; Stokowska, A.; Pio, R.; Blom, A.M. Hypoxia increases susceptibility of non-small cell lung cancer cells to complement attack. *Cancer Immunol. Immunother. CII* **2009**, *58*, 1771–1780. [CrossRef]
39. Kurihara, R.; Yamaoka, K.; Sawamukai, N.; Shimajiri, S.; Oshita, K.; Yukawa, S.; Tokunaga, M.; Iwata, S.; Saito, K.; Chiba, K.; et al. C5a promotes migration, proliferation, and vessel formation in endothelial cells. *Inflamm. Res.* **2010**, *59*, 659–666. [CrossRef]
40. Olcina, M.M.; Balanis, N.G.; Kim, R.K.; Aksoy, B.A.; Kodysh, J.; Thompson, M.J.; Hammerbacher, J.; Graeber, T.G.; Giaccia, A.J. Mutations in an Innate Immunity Pathway Are Associated with Poor Overall Survival Outcomes and Hypoxic Signaling in Cancer. *Cell Rep.* **2018**, *25*, 3721–3732.e6. [CrossRef]
41. Corrales, L.; Ajona, D.; Rafail, S.; Lasarte, J.J.; Riezu-Boj, J.I.; Lambris, J.D.; Rouzaut, A.; Pajares, M.J.; Montuenga, L.M.; Pio, R. Anaphylatoxin C5a creates a favorable microenvironment for lung cancer progression. *J. Immunol.* **2012**, *189*, 4674–4683. [CrossRef]
42. Kwak, J.W.; Laskowski, J.; Li, H.Y.; McSharry, M.V.; Sippel, T.R.; Bullock, B.L.; Johnson, A.M.; Poczobutt, J.M.; Neuwelt, A.J.; Malkoski, S.P.; et al. Complement Activation via a C3a Receptor Pathway Alters CD4(+) T Lymphocytes and Mediates Lung Cancer Progression. *Cancer Res.* **2018**, *78*, 143–156. [CrossRef]
43. Medler, T.R.; Murugan, D.; Horton, W.; Kumar, S.; Cotechini, T.; Forsyth, A.M.; Leyshock, P.; Leitenberger, J.J.; Kulesz-Martin, M.; Margolin, A.A.; et al. Complement C5a Fosters Squamous Carcinogenesis and Limits T Cell Response to Chemotherapy. *Cancer Cell* **2018**, *34*, 561–578.e6. [CrossRef]
44. Nabizadeh, J.A.; Manthey, H.D.; Steyn, F.J.; Chen, W.; Widiapradja, A.; Akhir, F.N.M.; Boyle, G.M.; Taylor, S.M.; Woodruff, T.M.; Rolfe, B.E. The Complement C3a Receptor Contributes to Melanoma Tumorigenesis by Inhibiting Neutrophil and CD4+ T Cell Responses. *J. Immunol.* **2016**, *196*, 4783–4792. [CrossRef] [PubMed]
45. Downs-Canner, S.; Magge, D.; Ravindranathan, R.; O'Malley, M.E.; Francis, L.; Liu, Z.; Guo, Z.S.; Obermajer, N.; Bartlett, D.L. Complement Inhibition: A Novel Form of Immunotherapy for Colon Cancer. *Ann. Surg. Oncol.* **2016**, *23*, 655–662. [CrossRef]
46. Vadrevu, S.K.; Chintala, N.K.; Sharma, S.K.; Sharma, P.; Cleveland, C.; Riediger, L.; Manne, S.; Fairlie, D.P.; Gorczyca, W.; Almanza, O.; et al. Complement c5a receptor facilitates cancer metastasis by altering T-cell responses in the metastatic niche. *Cancer Res.* **2014**, *74*, 3454–3465. [CrossRef]
47. Llaudo, I.; Fribourg, M.; Medof, M.E.; Conde, P.; Ochando, J.; Heeger, P.S. C5aR1 regulates migration of suppressive myeloid cells required for costimulatory blockade-induced murine allograft survival. *Am. J. Transplant.* **2019**, *19*, 633–645. [CrossRef]

48. Xu, Y.; Huang, Y.; Xu, W.; Zheng, X.; Yi, X.; Huang, L.; Wang, Y.; Wu, K. Activated Hepatic Stellate Cells (HSCs) Exert Immunosuppressive Effects in Hepatocellular Carcinoma by Producing Complement C3. *OncoTargets Ther.* **2020**, *13*, 1497–1505. [CrossRef]
49. Hsieh, C.-C.; Chou, H.-S.; Yang, H.-R.; Lin, F.; Bhatt, S.; Qin, J.; Wang, L.; Fung, J.J.; Qian, S.; Lu, L. The role of complement component 3 (C3) in differentiation of myeloid-derived suppressor cells. *Blood* **2013**, *121*, 1760–1768. [CrossRef]
50. Sautes-Fridman, C.; Petitprez, F.; Calderaro, J.; Fridman, W.H. Tertiary lymphoid structures in the era of cancer immunotherapy. *Nat. Rev. Cancer* **2019**, *19*, 307–325. [CrossRef]
51. Lu, Y.; Zhao, Q.; Liao, J.-Y.; Song, E.; Xia, Q.; Pan, J.; Li, Y.; Li, J.; Zhou, B.; Ye, Y.; et al. Complement Signals Determine Opposite Effects of B Cells in Chemotherapy-Induced Immunity. *Cell* **2020**, *180*, 1081–1097.e24. [CrossRef]
52. Liszewski, M.K.; Kolev, M.; Le Friec, G.; Leung, M.; Bertram, P.G.; Fara, A.F.; Subias, M.; Pickering, M.C.; Drouet, C.; Meri, S.; et al. Intracellular complement activation sustains T cell homeostasis and mediates effector differentiation. *Immunity* **2013**, *39*, 1143–1157. [CrossRef]
53. West, E.E.; Kunz, N.; Kemper, C. Complement and human T cell metabolism: Location, location, location. *Immunol. Rev.* **2020**, *295*, 68–81. [CrossRef]
54. Piao, C.; Zhang, W.-M.; Li, T.-T.; Zhang, C.-C.; Qiu, S.; Liu, Y.; Liu, S.; Jin, M.; Jia, L.-X.; Song, W.-C.; et al. Complement 5a stimulates macrophage polarization and contributes to tumor metastases of colon cancer. *Exp. Cell Res.* **2018**, *366*, 127–138. [CrossRef]
55. Boire, A.; Zou, Y.; Shieh, J.; Macalinao, D.G.; Pentsova, E.; Massague, J. Complement Component 3 Adapts the Cerebrospinal Fluid for Leptomeningeal Metastasis. *Cell* **2017**, *168*, 1101–1113.e13. [CrossRef]
56. Hu, W.H.; Hu, Z.; Shen, X.; Dong, L.Y.; Zhou, W.Z.; Yu, X.X. C5a receptor enhances hepatocellular carcinoma cell invasiveness via activating ERK1/2-mediated epithelial-mesenchymal transition. *Exp. Mol. Pathol.* **2016**, *100*, 101–108. [CrossRef]
57. Kaida, T.; Nitta, H.; Kitano, Y.; Yamamura, K.; Arima, K.; Izumi, D.; Higashi, T.; Kurashige, J.; Imai, K.; Hayashi, H.; et al. C5a receptor (CD88) promotes motility and invasiveness of gastric cancer by activating RhoA. *Oncotarget* **2016**, *7*, 84798–84809. [CrossRef]
58. Nitta, H.; Wada, Y.; Kawano, Y.; Murakami, Y.; Irie, A.; Taniguchi, K.; Kikuchi, K.; Yamada, G.; Suzuki, K.; Honda, J.; et al. Enhancement of human cancer cell motility and invasiveness by anaphylatoxin C5a via aberrantly expressed C5a receptor (CD88). *Clin. Cancer Res.* **2013**, *19*, 2004–2013. [CrossRef]
59. Gu, J.; Ding, J.-Y.; Lu, C.; Lin, Z.-W.; Chu, Y.; Zhao, G.-Y.; Guo, J.; Ge, D. Overexpression of CD88 predicts poor prognosis in non-small-cell lung cancer. *Lung Cancer* **2013**, *81*, 259–265. [CrossRef]
60. Coussens, L.M.; Zitvogel, L.; Palucka, A.K. Neutralizing tumor-promoting chronic inflammation: A magic bullet? *Science* **2013**, *339*, 286–291. [CrossRef]
61. Blankenstein, T.; Coulie, P.G.; Gilboa, E.; Jaffee, E.M. The determinants of tumour immunogenicity. *Nat. Rev. Cancer* **2012**, *12*, 307–313. [CrossRef] [PubMed]
62. Rodier, F.; Coppé, J.-P.; Patil, C.K.; Hoeijmakers, W.A.M.; Muñoz, D.P.; Raza, S.R.; Freund, A.; Campeau, E.; Davalos, A.R.; Campisi, J. Persistent DNA damage signalling triggers senescence-associated inflammatory cytokine secretion. *Nat. Cell Biol.* **2009**, *11*, 973–979. [CrossRef]
63. Dunn, G.P.; Koebel, C.M.; Schreiber, R.D. Interferons, immunity and cancer immunoediting. *Nat. Rev. Immunol.* **2006**, *6*, 836–848. [CrossRef] [PubMed]
64. Shankaran, V.; Ikeda, H.; Bruce, A.T.; White, J.M.; Swanson, P.E.; Old, L.J.; Schreiber, R.D. IFNgamma and lymphocytes prevent primary tumour development and shape tumour immunogenicity. *Nature* **2001**, *410*, 1107–1111. [CrossRef]
65. Garaud, S.; Zayakin, P.; Buisseret, L.; Rulle, U.; Silina, K.; De Wind, A.; Eyden, G.V.D.; Larsimont, D.; Willard-Gallo, K.; Linē, A. Antigen Specificity and Clinical Significance of IgG and IgA Autoantibodies Produced in situ by Tumor-Infiltrating B Cells in Breast Cancer. *Front. Immunol.* **2018**, *9*, 2660. [CrossRef] [PubMed]
66. Liu, W.; Peng, B.; Lu, Y.; Xu, W.; Qian, W.; Zhang, J.Y. Autoantibodies to tumor-associated antigens as biomarkers in cancer immunodiagnosis. *Autoimmun. Rev.* **2011**, *10*, 331–335. [CrossRef]
67. Roumenina, L.T.; Daugan, M.V.; Noe, R.; Petitprez, F.; Vano, Y.A.; Sanchez-Salas, R.; Becht, E.; Meilleroux, J.; Le Clec'H, B.; A Giraldo, N.; et al. Tumor Cells Hijack Macrophage-Produced Complement C1q to Promote Tumor Growth. *Cancer Immunol. Res.* **2019**, *7*, 1091–1105. [CrossRef]

68. Bulla, R.; Tripodo, C.; Rami, D.; Ling, G.S.; Agostinis, C.; Guarnotta, C.; Zorzet, S.; Durigutto, P.; Botto, M.; Tedesco, F. C1q acts in the tumour microenvironment as a cancer-promoting factor independently of complement activation. *Nat. Commun.* **2016**, *7*, 10346. [CrossRef]

69. Ling, G.S.; Crawford, G.; Buang, N.; Bartok, I.; Tian, K.; Thielens, N.M.; Bally, I.; Harker, J.A.; Ashton-Rickardt, P.G.; Rutschmann, S.; et al. C1q restrains autoimmunity and viral infection by regulating CD8(+) T cell metabolism. *Science* **2018**, *360*, 558–563. [CrossRef]

70. Ehrenstein, M.R.; Notley, C.A. The importance of natural IgM: Scavenger, protector and regulator. *Nat. Rev. Immunol.* **2010**, *10*, 778–786. [CrossRef]

71. Vollmers, H.P.; Brandlein, S. Natural antibodies and cancer. *New Biotechnol.* **2009**, *25*, 294–298. [CrossRef]

72. Hensel, F.; Hermann, R.; Schubert, C.; Abe, N.; Schmidt, K.; Franke, A.; Shevchenko, A.; Mann, M.; Müller-Hermelink, H.K.; Vollmers, H.P. Characterization of glycosylphosphatidylinositol-linked molecule CD55/decay-accelerating factor as the receptor for antibody SC-1-induced apoptosis. *Cancer Res.* **1999**, *59*, 5299–5306.

73. Aykut, B.; Pushalkar, S.; Chen, R.; Li, Q.; Abengozar, R.; Kim, J.I.; Shadaloey, S.A.; Wu, D.; Preiss, P.; Verma, N.; et al. The fungal mycobiome promotes pancreatic oncogenesis via activation of MBL. *Nature* **2019**, *574*, 264–267. [CrossRef]

74. Roumenina, L.T.; Daugan, M.V.; Petitprez, F.; Sautes-Fridman, C.; Fridman, W.H. Context-dependent roles of complement in cancer. *Nat. Rev. Cancer* **2019**, *19*, 698–715. [CrossRef]

75. Cho, M.S.; Rupaimoole, R.; Choi, H.J.; Noh, K.; Chen, J.; Hu, Q.; Sood, A.K.; Afshar-Kharghan, V. Complement Component 3 Is Regulated by TWIST1 and Mediates Epithelial-Mesenchymal Transition. *J. Immunol.* **2016**, *196*, 1412–1418. [CrossRef]

76. Pratt, J.R.; Basheer, S.A.; Sacks, S.H. Local synthesis of complement component C3 regulates acute renal transplant rejection. *Nat. Med.* **2002**, *8*, 582–587. [CrossRef]

77. Gocheva, V.; Joyce, J.A. Cysteine cathepsins and the cutting edge of cancer invasion. *Cell Cycle* **2007**, *6*, 60–64. [CrossRef]

78. Frade, R.; Rodrigues-Lima, F.; Huang, S.; Xie, K.; Guillaume, N.; Bar-Eli, M. Procathepsin-L, a proteinase that cleaves human C3 (the third component of complement), confers high tumorigenic and metastatic properties to human melanoma cells. *Cancer Res.* **1998**, *58*, 2733–2736. [CrossRef]

79. Krisinger, M.J.; Goebeler, V.; Lu, Z.; Meixner, S.C.; Myles, T.; Pryzdial, E.L.; Conway, E.M. Thrombin generates previously unidentified C5 products that support the terminal complement activation pathway. *Blood* **2012**, *120*, 1717–1725. [CrossRef] [PubMed]

80. Reddel, C.J.; Tan, C.W.; Chen, V.M. Thrombin Generation and Cancer: Contributors and Consequences. *Cancers* **2019**, *11*, 100. [CrossRef]

81. Manning, M.L.; Williams, S.A.; Jelinek, C.A.; Kostova, M.B.; Denmeade, S.R. Proteolysis of complement factors iC3b and C5 by the serine protease prostate-specific antigen in prostatic fluid and seminal plasma. *J. Immunol.* **2013**, *190*, 2567–2574. [CrossRef] [PubMed]

82. Schmidt, C.Q.; Lambris, J.D.; Ricklin, D. Protection of host cells by complement regulators. *Immunol. Rev.* **2016**, *274*, 152–171. [CrossRef]

83. Ravindranath, N.M.; Shuler, C. Expression of complement restriction factors (CD46, CD55 & CD59) in head and neck squamous cell carcinomas. *J. Oral Pathol. Med.* **2006**, *35*, 560–567.

84. Goslings, W.R.; Blom, D.J.; De Waard-Siebinga, I.; Van Beelen, E.; Claas, F.H.; Jager, M.J.; Gorter, A. Membrane-bound regulators of complement activation in uveal melanomas. CD46, CD55, and CD59 in uveal melanomas. *Investig. Ophthalmol. Visual Sci.* **1996**, *37*, 1884–1891.

85. Bjorge, L.; Vedeler, C.A.; Ulvestad, E.; Matre, R. Expression and function of CD59 on colonic adenocarcinoma cells. *Eur. J. Immunol.* **1994**, *24*, 1597–1603. [CrossRef]

86. Simpson, K.L.; Jones, A.; Norman, S.; Holmes, C.H. Expression of the complement regulatory proteins decay accelerating factor (DAF, CD55), membrane cofactor protein (MCP, CD46) and CD59 in the normal human uterine cervix and in premalignant and malignant cervical disease. *Am. J. Pathol.* **1997**, *151*, 1455–1467.

87. Murray, K.P.; Mathure, S.; Kaul, R.; Khan, S.; Carson, L.F.; Twiggs, L.B.; Martens, M.G.; Kaul, A. Expression of complement regulatory proteins-CD 35, CD 46, CD 55, and CD 59-in benign and malignant endometrial tissue. *Gynecol. Oncol.* **2000**, *76*, 176–182. [CrossRef]

88. Geis, N.; Zell, S.; Rutz, R.; Li, W.; Giese, T.; Mamidi, S.; Schultz, S.; Kirschfink, M. Inhibition of membrane complement inhibitor expression (CD46, CD55, CD59) by siRNA sensitizes tumor cells to complement attack in vitro. *Curr. Cancer Drug Targets* **2010**, *10*, 922–931. [CrossRef]
89. Blok, V.T.; Daha, M.R.; Tijsma, O.M.; Weissglas, M.G.; van den Broek, L.J.; Gorter, A. A possible role of CD46 for the protection in vivo of human renal tumor cells from complement-mediated damage. *Lab. Investig.* **2000**, *80*, 335–344. [CrossRef] [PubMed]
90. Surowiak, P.; Materna, V.; Maciejczyk, A.; Kaplenko, I.; Spaczyński, M.; Dietel, M.; Lage, H.; Zabel, M. CD46 expression is indicative of shorter revival-free survival for ovarian cancer patients. *Anticancer Res.* **2006**, *26*, 4943–4948.
91. Ajona, D.; Castaño, Z.; Garayoa, M.; Zudaire, E.; Pajares, M.J.; Martínez, A.; Cuttitta, F.; Montuenga, L.M.; Pio, R. Expression of complement factor H by lung cancer cells: Effects on the activation of the alternative pathway of complement. *Cancer Res.* **2004**, *64*, 6310–6318. [CrossRef] [PubMed]
92. Wilczek, E.; Rzepko, R.; Nowis, D.; Legat, M.; Golab, J.; Glab, M.; Gorlewicz, A.; Konopacki, F.; Mazurkiewicz, M.; Śladowski, D.; et al. The possible role of factor H in colon cancer resistance to complement attack. *Int. J. Cancer* **2008**, *122*, 2030–2037. [CrossRef] [PubMed]
93. Junnikkala, S.; Hakulinen, J.; Jarva, H.; Manuelian, T.; Bjørge, L.; Bützow, R.; Zipfel, P.F.; Meri, S. Secretion of soluble complement inhibitors factor H and factor H-like protein (FHL-1) by ovarian tumour cells. *Br. J. Cancer* **2002**, *87*, 1119–1127. [CrossRef] [PubMed]
94. Ajona, D.; Hsu, Y.F.; Corrales, L.; Montuenga, L.M.; Pio, R. Down-regulation of human complement factor H sensitizes non-small cell lung cancer cells to complement attack and reduces in vivo tumor growth. *J. Immunol.* **2007**, *178*, 5991–5998. [CrossRef]
95. Riihilä, P.; Nissinen, L.; Farshchian, M.; Kivisaari, A.; Ala-Aho, R.; Kallajoki, M.; Grénman, R.; Meri, S.; Peltonen, S.; Peltonen, J.; et al. Complement factor I promotes progression of cutaneous squamous cell carcinoma. *J. Investig. Dermatol.* **2015**, *135*, 579–588. [CrossRef]
96. Fedarko, N.S.; Fohr, B.; Robey, P.G.; Young, M.F.; Fisher, L.W. Factor H binding to bone sialoprotein and osteopontin enables tumor cell evasion of complement-mediated attack. *J. Biol. Chem.* **2000**, *275*, 16666–16672. [CrossRef]
97. Meng, Z.W.; Liu, M.C.; Hong, H.J.; Du, Q.; Chen, Y.L. Expression and prognostic value of soluble CD97 and its ligand CD55 in intrahepatic cholangiocarcinoma. *Tumour Biol.* **2017**, *39*. [CrossRef]
98. Ouyang, Q.; Zhang, L.; Jiang, Y.; Ni, X.; Chen, S.; Ye, F.; Du, Y.; Huang, L.; Ding, P.; Wang, N.; et al. The membrane complement regulatory protein CD59 promotes tumor growth and predicts poor prognosis in breast cancer. *Int. J. Oncol.* **2016**, *48*, 2015–2024. [CrossRef]
99. Niehans, G.A.; Cherwitz, D.L.; Staley, N.A.; Knapp, D.J.; Dalmasso, A.P. Human carcinomas variably express the complement inhibitory proteins CD46 (membrane cofactor protein), CD55 (decay-accelerating factor), and CD59 (protectin). *Am. J Pathol.* **1996**, *149*, 129–142.
100. Bjorge, L.; Jensen, T.S.; Ulvestad, E.; Vedeler, C.A.; Matre, R. The influence of tumour necrosis factor-alpha, interleukin-1 beta and interferon-gamma on the expression and function of the complement regulatory protein CD59 on the human colonic adenocarcinoma cell line HT29. *Scand. J. Immunol.* **1995**, *41*, 350–356. [CrossRef]
101. Spiller, O.B.; Criado-Garcia, O.; Rodriguez De Cordoba, S.; Morgan, B.P. Cytokine-mediated up-regulation of CD55 and CD59 protects human hepatoma cells from complement attack. *Clin. Exp. Immunol.* **2000**, *121*, 234–241. [CrossRef]
102. Janelle, V.; Langlois, M.P.; Tarrab, E.; Lapierre, P.; Poliquin, L.; Lamarre, A. Transient Complement Inhibition Promotes a Tumor-Specific Immune Response through the Implication of Natural Killer Cells. *Cancer Immunol. Res.* **2014**, *2*, 200–206. [CrossRef]
103. Wang, X.; Schoenhals, J.E.; Li, A.; Valdecanas, D.R.; Ye, H.; Zhang, F.; Tang, C.; Tang, M.; Liu, C.-G.; Liu, X.; et al. Suppression of Type I IFN Signaling in Tumors Mediates Resistance to Anti-PD-1 Treatment That Can Be Overcome by Radiotherapy. *Cancer Res.* **2017**, *77*, 839–850. [CrossRef] [PubMed]
104. Ajona, D.; Ortiz-Espinosa, S.; Moreno, H.; Lozano, T.; Pajares, M.J.; Agorreta, J.; Bértolo, C.; Lasarte, J.J.; Vicent, S.; Hoehlig, K.; et al. A Combined PD-1/C5a Blockade Synergistically Protects against Lung Cancer Growth and Metastasis. *Cancer Discov.* **2017**, *7*, 694–703. [CrossRef]

105. Rondeau, E.; Scully, M.; Ariceta, G.; Barbour, T.; Cataland, S.; Heyne, N.; Miyakawa, Y.; Ortiz, S.; Swenson, E.; Vallee, M.; et al. The long-acting C5 inhibitor, Ravulizumab, is effective and safe in adult patients with atypical hemolytic uremic syndrome naive to complement inhibitor treatment. *Kidney Int.* **2020**, *97*, 1287–1296. [CrossRef] [PubMed]
106. Rother, R.P.; Rollins, S.A.; Mojcik, C.F.; Brodsky, R.A.; Bell, L. Discovery and development of the complement inhibitor eculizumab for the treatment of paroxysmal nocturnal hemoglobinuria. *Nat. Biotechnol.* **2007**, *25*, 1256–1264. [CrossRef]
107. Mastellos, D.C.; Ricklin, D.; Lambris, J.D. Clinical promise of next-generation complement therapeutics. *Nat. Rev. Drug Discov.* **2019**, *18*, 707–729. [CrossRef] [PubMed]
108. Fishelson, Z.; Donin, N.; Zell, S.; Schultz, S.; Kirschfink, M. Obstacles to cancer immunotherapy: Expression of membrane complement regulatory proteins (mCRPs) in tumors. *Mol. Immunol.* **2003**, *40*, 109–123. [CrossRef]
109. Wang, Y.; Sun, S.-N.; Liu, Q.; Yu, Y.-Y.; Guo, J.; Wang, K.; Xing, B.-C.; Zheng, Q.-F.; Campa, M.J.; Patz, E.F.; et al. Autocrine Complement Inhibits IL10-Dependent T-cell-Mediated Antitumor Immunity to Promote Tumor Progression. *Cancer Discov.* **2016**, *6*, 1022–1035. [CrossRef]
110. Tomlinson, S.; Thurman, J.M. Tissue-targeted complement therapeutics. *Mol. Immunol.* **2018**, *102*, 120–128. [CrossRef]

Publisher's Note: MDPI stays neutral with regard to jurisdictional claims in published maps and institutional affiliations.

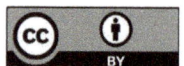

© 2020 by the authors. Licensee MDPI, Basel, Switzerland. This article is an open access article distributed under the terms and conditions of the Creative Commons Attribution (CC BY) license (http://creativecommons.org/licenses/by/4.0/).

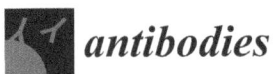

Article

An Immunoregulatory Role for Complement Receptors in Murine Models of Breast Cancer

Fazrena Nadia Md Akhir [1,2,†,‡], Mohd Hezmee Mohd Noor [3,‡,§], Keith Weng Kit Leong [1,∥], Jamileh A. Nabizadeh [1], Helga D. Manthey [1], Stefan E. Sonderegger [1], Jenny Nga Ting Fung [1], Crystal E. McGirr [1], Ian A. Shiels [3], Paul C. Mills [3], Trent M. Woodruff [2,¶] and Barbara E. Rolfe [1,*,¶]

1. Australian Institute for Bioengineering and Nanotechnology, The University of Queensland, St Lucia, QLD 4072, Australia; fazrena@utm.my (F.N.M.A.); Keith_Leong@immunol.a-star.edu.sg (K.W.K.L.); j.nabizadeh@uq.edu.au (J.A.N.); h.manthey@uq.edu.au (H.D.M.); s.sonderegger@uq.edu.au (S.E.S.); j.fung1@uq.edu.au (J.N.T.F.); c.mcgirr@uq.edu.au (C.E.M.)
2. School of Biomedical Sciences, The University of Queensland, St Lucia, QLD 4072, Australia; t.woodruff@uq.edu.au
3. School of Veterinary Science, The University of Queensland, Gatton, QLD 4343, Australia; hezmee@upm.edu.my (M.H.M.N.); ian.shiels@uq.edu.au (I.A.S.); p.mills@uq.edu.au (P.C.M.)
* Correspondence: b.rolfe@uq.edu.au; Tel.: +61-7-3346-3856
† Current address: Malaysia-Japan International Institute of Technology (MJIIT), Universiti Teknologi Malaysia, Jalan Sultan Yahya Petra, Kuala Lumpur 54100, Malaysia.
‡ These authors contributed equally.
§ Current address: Fakulti Perubatan Veterinar, Universiti Putra, Malaysia.
∥ Current address: Singapore Immunology Network (SIgN), Agency for Science, Technology and Research (A*STAR), Singapore.
¶ Joint senior authors.

Citation: Akhir, F.N.M.; Noor, M.H.M.; Leong, K.W.K.; Nabizadeh, J.A.; Manthey, H.D.; Sonderegger, S.E.; Fung, J.N.T.; McGirr, C.E.; Shiels, I.A.; Mills, P.C.; et al. An Immunoregulatory Role for Complement Receptors in Murine Models of Breast Cancer. *Antibodies* 2021, 10, 2. https://doi.org/10.3390/antib10010002

Received: 28 September 2020
Accepted: 7 December 2020
Published: 8 January 2021

Publisher's Note: MDPI stays neutral with regard to jurisdictional claims in published maps and institutional affiliations.

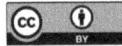

Copyright: © 2021 by the authors. Licensee MDPI, Basel, Switzerland. This article is an open access article distributed under the terms and conditions of the Creative Commons Attribution (CC BY) license (https://creativecommons.org/licenses/by/4.0/).

Abstract: The complement system has demonstrated roles in regulating tumor growth, although these may differ between tumor types. The current study used two murine breast cancer models (EMT6 and 4T1) to investigate whether pharmacological targeting of receptors for complement proteins C3a (C3aR) and C5a (C5aR1) is protective in murine breast cancer models. In contrast to prior studies in other tumor models, treatment with the selective C5aR1 antagonist PMX53 had no effect on tumor growth. However, treatment of mice with a dual C3aR/C5aR1 agonist (YSFKPMPLaR) significantly slowed mammary tumor development and progression. Examination of receptor expression by quantitative polymerase chain reaction (qPCR) analysis showed very low levels of mRNA expression for either *C3aR* or *C5aR1* by EMT6 or 4T1 mammary carcinoma cell lines compared with the J774 macrophage line or bone marrow-derived macrophages. Moreover, flow cytometric analysis found no evidence of C3aR or C5aR1 protein expression by either EMT6 or 4T1 cells, leading us to hypothesize that the tumor inhibitory effects of the dual agonist are indirect, possibly via regulation of the anti-tumor immune response. This hypothesis was supported by flow cytometric analysis of tumor infiltrating leukocyte populations, which demonstrated a significant increase in T lymphocytes in mice treated with the C3aR/C5aR1 agonist. These results support an immunoregulatory role for complement receptors in primary murine mammary carcinoma models. They also suggest that complement activation peptides can influence the anti-tumor response in different ways depending on the cancer type, the host immune response to the tumor and levels of endogenous complement activation within the tumor microenvironment.

Keywords: complement C5a; complement C3a; complement receptors; mammary carcinoma; immunoregulation; tumor infiltrating leukocytes

1. Introduction

Breast cancer is the most common cancer diagnosed in women world-wide, accounting for 25% of all cancers and 15% of cancer deaths in women [1]. Despite significant advances in understanding the underlying biology, some forms of disease remain resistant to current treatments—in particular, triple-negative breast cancers [2]. Chronic inflammation is linked to the development and progression of many cancers [3,4]. As powerful mediators of inflammation, complement proteins have been implicated for a role in tumorigenesis [5], with elevated complement regulatory proteins and activation fragments identified as biomarkers and prognostic indicators for many cancers, including breast cancer [6–8].

Comprising more than 40 plasma- and membrane-bound proteins, the overall function of the complement system is to regulate inflammation, facilitate immune defense mechanisms and maintain tissue homeostasis [9]. The complement system has long been recognized to contribute to anti-tumor defense mechanisms via complement-dependent cytotoxicity (CDC) [10] and antibody-dependent cell-mediated cytotoxicity (ADCC) [11]. The upregulation of complement inhibitory proteins is thought to be an important mechanism by which cancer cells evade complement-mediated destruction [12–14]. There is also increasing evidence of a role for the complement activation products C3a and C5a in regulating tumor growth and metastasis. C3a and C5a are small polypeptides with 36% homology [15]. C5a is one of the most potent inflammatory proteins and chemoattractant for neutrophils, monocytes and macrophages [16]. It binds two specific receptors, C5a receptor (CD88/C5aR1) and C5a receptor-like 2 (C5L2/C5aR2), of which the former (G-protein coupled C5aR1) is thought to be the predominant driver of biological activity [17,18]. C3a binds a single receptor, C3aR1, which like C5aR1 is a G-protein-coupled receptor expressed primarily by cells of myeloid origin [15]. Originally thought to have similar pro-inflammatory effects to C5a, C3a is now known to exert a range of apparently contradictory immunomodulatory functions—attenuating neutrophil mobilization in response to injury [19] but inducing production of pro-inflammatory cytokines [20].

Kim and co-workers [21] were the first to show a direct role for complement C5a in regulating breast cancer growth, demonstrating that over-expression by EMT6 mammary tumor cells protected against tumor growth in mice. Tumor inhibitory effects of complement proteins were confirmed by Bandini et al., who showed in an autochthonous mammary carcinoma model that Her2/neu-driven carcinogenesis is accelerated in C3-deficient mice [22]. Conversely, Vadrevu and co-workers found no effect of C5aR1 deficiency on primary tumor growth, but metastatic tumor burden was reduced in the murine 4T1 breast cancer model [23]. Moreover, C5a-C5aR1 signaling has been associated with cancer progression and poor prognosis in breast cancer patients [8,23]. Tumor-promoting effects of C5a have also been reported in other murine cancer models, including cervical [24], lung [25], ovarian [26] and melanoma [27]. Less is known about the role of C3a in tumor growth, although our laboratory and others have demonstrated that inhibition of C3aR signaling inhibits the growth of murine melanoma, colon, breast [28], intestinal [29] and lung cancer [30]. Whilst most of these studies have identified indirect (immune-mediated) mechanisms responsible for regulating tumor growth, tumor-intrinsic effects have also been reported [21,31]. Other effects are also possible. For example, there is evidence that C5a promotes vascularization of ovarian tumors [26], while C3a has been demonstrated to promote leptomeningeal metastasis by disrupting the blood-cerebrospinal fluid barrier [32].

To further explore the effects of the complement receptors in mammary cancer, we used two syngeneic murine mammary carcinoma models: EMT6, which is weakly estrogen receptor (ER)-positive [33], and 4T1, a model of triple-negative breast cancer [34]. Mice were treated with a selective C5aR1 antagonist (AcF-[OPdChaWR]; PMX53) [35], which has been demonstrated to effectively reduce C5a-mediated inflammatory responses in animal disease models [36–38], including murine melanoma [27], cervical [24] and lung [25] cancers. Because there are no selective agonists for mouse C5aR1 suitable for in vivo application, and native C3a and C5a proteins are highly susceptible to proteolysis by serum carboxypeptidases [39], mice were treated with a dual C3aR/C5aR1 agonist (YSFKPMPLaR; EP54) [40]. Although we found no effect of C5aR1 inhibition on tumor growth, treatment with the dual C3aR/C5aR1 agonist inhibited tumor development and progression. The results suggest that the anti-tumor effects are indirect, possibly due to enhancement of the T lymphocyte-mediated anti-tumor response.

2. Materials and Methods

2.1. Drugs

The dual C3aR/C5aR1 agonist YSFKPMPLaR (EP54) and the cyclic peptide C5aR1 antagonist AcF-[OP(D-Cha)WR] (PMX53) were synthesized in-house using previously described methods [41–43]. Drugs for injection were diluted in either 5% glucose or 0.9% saline.

2.2. Cell Culture

Tumorigenic mouse mammary carcinoma EMT6 (ATCC *CRL-2755*) and 4T1 (ATCC *CRL-2539*) as well as J774A.1 macrophage (ATCC TIB-67) cell lines were obtained from the American Type Cell Culture Collection. EMT6 cells were maintained in Waymouths medium (Invitrogen, Carlsbad, CA, USA) containing 10% heat-inactivated fetal calf serum (FCS; Moregate, Brisbane, QLD, Australia). 4T1 and J774 cells were grown in RPMI 1640 medium (Invitrogen) + 10% FCS.

Bone marrow-derived macrophages (BMDM) were prepared by flushing femurs of 8- to 12-week-old mice with phosphate buffered saline (PBS). Bone marrow cells were seeded onto untreated culture plates and cultured for 7 days in RPMI + 10% FCS containing mouse colony stimulating factor (mCSF)-1 (50 ng/mL; BioLegend, San Diego, CA, USA). All cells were maintained at 37 °C in an atmosphere of 5% CO_2 in air (Invitrogen).

2.3. Animals

Female BALB/c mice (Monash Animal Services, Melbourne, Aust), 6–8 weeks of age, were housed 4/cage in the UQBR animal facility, University of Queensland, with lighting schedules of a 12 h light/dark cycle, and water and standard rodent diet provided ad libitum. All procedures were approved by the University of Queensland Animal Ethics Committee Guidelines and conformed to the *Australian Code of Practice for the Care and Use of Animals for Scientific Purposes* (8th Edition, 2013).

Tumor Cell Injections and Drug Treatments

BALB/c mice (bodyweight approximately 20–25 g; n = 7–8 animals/group) were lightly anesthetized with isofluorane (1.5% in oxygen) and the left mammary fat pad injected with 0.5×10^6 of either EMT6 or 4T1 cells in a total volume of 0.05 mL serum-free medium. Mice commenced daily sub-cutaneous (s.c.) injections with EP54 (1 or 3 mg/kg bodyweight), PMX53 (1 mg/kg bodyweight) or vehicle only (5% glucose or 0.9% saline solution), either from the time of tumor injection (day 0) or once tumors became palpable (approximately day 7). These drug doses were previously shown to be effective in other mouse models of disease [43,44].

Mice were monitored daily and once tumors became palpable (at approximately day 7), tumor areas were measured daily by the same individual using digital Vernier calipers. Since it was not possible to measure tumor height accurately, and area measurements have been shown to correlate well with the mass of small tumors [45], tumor width and length were measured, and tumor areas calculated [46]. Once the largest tumor area had reached approximately 200 mm^2, mice in all groups were euthanized and tumors removed from each mouse. Excised tumors were weighed, then processed for flow cytometric analysis.

2.4. RNA Extraction and Quantitative Polymerase Chain Reaction (qPCR)

Total RNA was isolated from EMT6, 4T1 mammary carcinoma cells (n = 3), BMDM (n = 3) and J774 macrophages (n = 2) using the RNeasy plus Mini Kit (Qiagen, Hilden, Germany). RNA quality was determined and quantified by spectrophotometer (Nanodrop ND1000; Thermo Scientific, Waltham, MA, USA). Total RNA (1 µg) was then converted to cDNA using the iScript™ cDNA synthesis kit (Bio-Rad, Hercules, CA, USA). Taqman probes for *C3* (Mm01232779_m1), *Hc* (*C5*; Mm00439275_m1), *C3aR* (Mm02620006_s1) and *C5ar1* (Mm00500292_s1) (Applied Biosystems, Foster City, CA, USA) were used to amplify the target genes. Relative target gene expression to reference gene hypoxanthine guanine phosphoribosyl transferase (*Hprt*; Mm03024075_m1) was determined using the formula: $2^{-\Delta CT}$, where $\Delta CT = (Ct_{(Target\ gene)} - Ct_{(Hprt)})$.

2.5. Calcium Mobilization Assay

Cells were seeded at 3×10^4 cells/well into 96-well, black-walled, clear-bottom plates (Nunc™, Thermo Fisher Scientific) and allowed to attach overnight. Cells were loaded with Fluo-4 dye (Invitrogen), then transferred to a FlexStation III microplate reader (Molecular Devices, San Jose, CA, USA) before addition of EP54 (5×10^{-4} to 5×10^{-9} mol/L), and changes in fluorescence ($\lambda ex = 485$ nm; $\lambda em = 525$ nm) were measured at 3 s intervals.

2.6. Flow Cytometric Analysis

EMT6, 4T1 and J774 cells were detached from culture dishes by trypsinization or aspiration with ice-cold Dulbecco's phosphate buffered saline (D-PBS; Ca and Mg free). Single cell suspensions were prepared from excised tumors by mechanical disaggregation, followed by filtration through 70 μm nylon cell strainers, and resuspended ($0.5–2.0 \times 10^6$ cells/mL) in calcium- and magnesium-free PBS containing 0.1% bovine serum albumin and 0.1% sodium azide (PBA). Cells were dispensed into 96-well plates ($0.5–2.0 \times 10^5$ viable cells/well) and pre-incubated with anti-CD16/32 (2.4G2; BioLegend) for 15 min to block Fc receptors. Cultured cells were incubated with fluorescein isothiocyanate (FITC)-conjugated rat anti-mouse C3aR (14D4; Hycult, Uden, NL, USA) or control Ig for 1 h. Cells from excised tumors were incubated with fluorophore-conjugated rat monoclonal antibodies for mouse surface leukocyte markers: CD45, CD11b, F4/80, Gr-1, CD25, CD3, CD4 and CD8a (all from BioLegend). To identify regulatory T cells (Tregs), cells were surface-stained, then fixed and permeabilized (FoxP3 Fix/Perm kit; BioLegend) for intracellular staining with anti-Foxp3 (BioLegend). To identify Th1, Th2 and Th17 subsets, cells were stimulated with phorbol 12-myristate 13-acetate (PMA; 50 ng/mL; Sigma) and ionomycin (10^{-6} M; Sigma) in the presence of Brefeldin A (5 μg/mL; BioLegend) for 4 h at 37 °C, surface-stained with anti-CD3 and CD4, then fixed, permeabilized and stained with antibodies to intracellular cytokines interleukin (IL)-4, interferon (IFN)-γ or IL-17A (BioLegend). Cell viability was determine using DRAQ7 (Cell Signaling, Danvers, MA, USA). Cells were analyzed on an Accuri C6 or LSR Fortessa X-20 flow cytometer (BD Biosciences, Franklin Lakes, NJ, USA) followed by data analysis with FlowJo software (Tree Star, Inc., Ashland, OR, USA). Gating strategies are shown in Supplementary Figure S1.

2.7. Statistical Analysis

All experiments were performed a minimum of two times, and values expressed as mean ± standard deviation (SD). Tumor growth was analyzed by two-way analysis of variance (ANOVA). All other data were analyzed using unpaired Student's *t*-test, or one-way ANOVA followed by Dunnett's multiple comparison tests and Bonferroni post-test (GraphPad Software Inc., San Diego, CA, USA). A *p*-value of <0.05 was considered significant.

3. Results

3.1. Effects of Pharmacological Modulation of C3aR/C5aR1 Signaling on Mammary Carcinoma Growth in Mice

To determine the influence of C3aR/C5aR1 signaling on tumor development, mice were injected with EMT6 mammary carcinoma cells. On the same day (day 0), mice commenced daily injections with either C5aR1 antagonist, PMX53 (1 mg/kg/day), dual C3aR/C5aR1 agonist, EP54 (1 mg/kg/day) or vehicle (control). Tumors became palpable at approximately day 7 (Figure 1A). Caliper measurements showed that PMX53 had no significant effect on the growth of EMT6 tumors, but tumor growth was slowed by EP54 treatment ($p < 0.01$; Figure 1A). Excised tumor weight at day 14 was also significantly reduced in mice treated with EP54 (0.07 ± 0.05 g) compared with the control group (0.25 ± 0.1 g; $p < 0.01$; Figure 1A'). Health assessment scores showed that treatment with EP54 was associated with significantly less deterioration in general health of the mice and there was no significant change in body weight for any group: body weights for EP54-treated mice were 19.1 ± 1.6 g on day 1 and 19.2 ± 1.4 g at day 14 post-tumor induction, compared with 19.9 ± 1.7 g and 19.5 ± 2.2 g respectively, for the control (vehicle-treated) group. The reduction in tumor growth was not significantly enhanced by a higher dose of EP54 (3 mg/kg/day; data not shown), indicating that a dose of 1 mg/kg/day is sufficient.

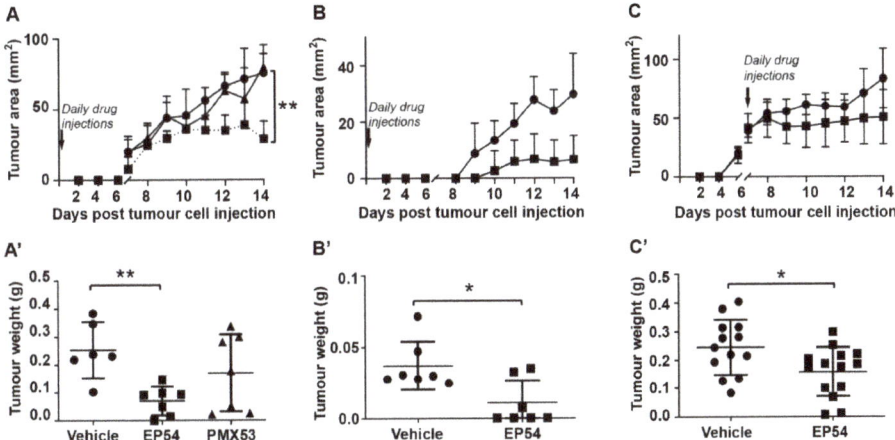

Figure 1. Effect of pharmacological modulation of C3aR/C5aR1 signaling on growth of murine mammary carcinomas. Tumor areas (mm^2) (**A–C**) and excised tumor weights (g) at the end of trial (day 14) (**A'–C'**) in female BALB/c mice injected with (**A,A'**) EMT6 tumor cells and treated by daily sub-cutaneous (s.c.) injection with vehicle alone (5% dextrose, ●), dual C3aR/C5aR1 agonist (EP54; 1 mg/kg/day, ■) or C5a antagonist (PMX53; 1 mg/kg/day, ▲), commencing day 0. (**B,B'**) 4T1 tumor cells treated by daily s.c. injection with vehicle alone or EP54 (1 mg/kg/day), commencing day 0. (**C,C'**) Established EMT6 tumors treated by daily injection of EP54 from day 7 after tumor cell injection. Data expressed as mean ± standard deviation (SD). Results are representative of two separate experiments ($n = 6$–7/group); ** $p < 0.01$; * $p < 0.05$.

A similar trend was observed in mice injected with 4T1 tumors (Figure 1B,B'), with EP54 treatment slowing tumor growth ($p < 0.01$; Figure 1B). Excised tumor weights in the EP54-treated group (0.011 ± 0.016 g) were also significantly lower than the control group (0.037 ± 0.017 g; $p < 0.05$) (Figure 1B'). Having shown that EP54 treatment inhibits tumor initiation, we next investigated its effect on established EMT6 tumors. For these experiments, mice were injected with EMT6 cells, and once tumors were established (day 7), daily s.c. injections of EP54 (1 mg/kg/day) or saline alone (vehicle control) were commenced. As shown in Figure 1C,C', tumor growth was significantly slowed ($p < 0.01$), and excised tumor weights were smaller in EP54-treated mice (0.16 ± 0.09 g) compared with the control group (0.24 ± 0.1 g; $p < 0.05$). For all experiments, there were no signs of drug toxicity, and mice showed no significant changes in bodyweight.

3.2. Expression of Complement Receptors C5aR1 (CD88) and C3aR by EMT6 and 4T1 Mammary Carcinoma Cell Lines

Having established that C3a/C5aR1 agonism is effective in inhibiting mammary tumor growth in mice, we next explored possible mechanisms responsible for the anti-tumor effects. Since Kim and co-workers [21] suggested that C5a may act directly on tumor cells, we first investigated receptor expression by cultured EMT6 and 4T1 cells. Analysis by qPCR showed that both cell lines expressed mRNA for *C3aR* and *C5aR1*, but at levels 600–750-fold lower than J774 cells and 300–500 times lower than BMDMs. Neither cell line expressed *Hc* (C5), but *C3* expression by EMT6 cells was more than 7-fold higher than J774 macrophages and 30-fold higher than BMDM (Figure 2A). Flow cytometric analysis found no detectable expression of C3aR or C5aR1 protein by either tumor cell line, whereas J774 macrophages and BMDM expressed high levels of both receptors (Figure 2B).

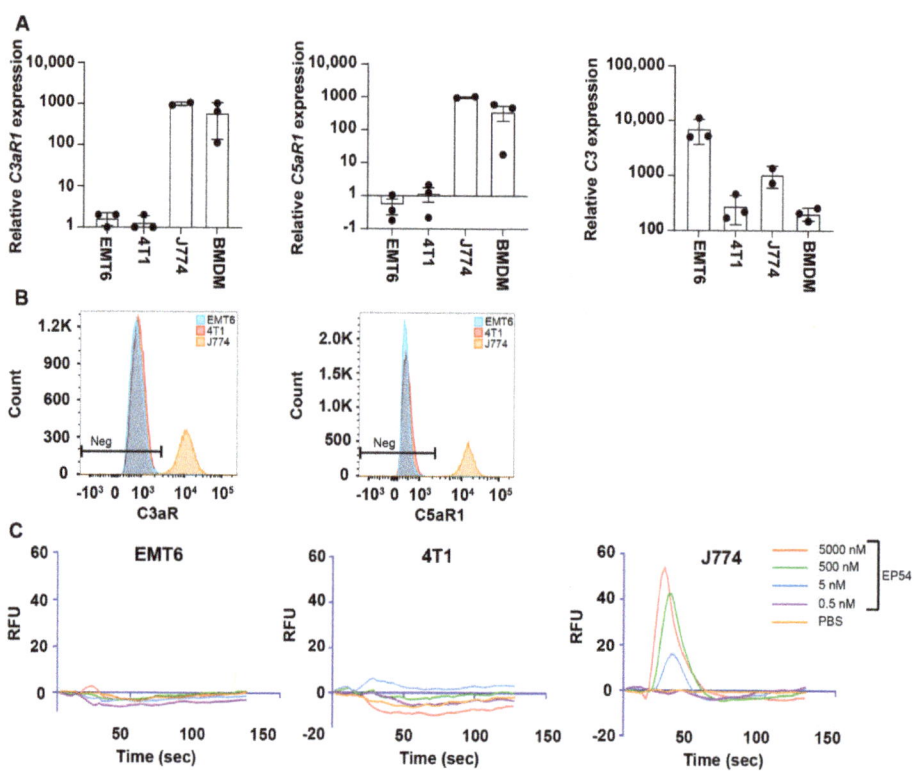

Figure 2. Complement receptor expression by mouse mammary carcinoma cell lines. (**A**) Quantitative polymerase chain reaction (qPCR) analysis shows relative expression of mRNA for *C3aR1*, *C5aR1* and *C3* by cultured EMT6 (n = 3) and 4T1 (n = 3) mammary carcinoma cell lines compared to J774 macrophages (n = 2) and bone marrow-derived macrophages (BMDM; n = 3). Data are normalized to the reference gene, *Hprt*, and expression is shown relative to J774 cells (mean ± SD). (**B**) Flow cytometric analysis shows C3aR and C5aR1 expression by EMT6 and 4T1 cell lines compared with J774 macrophages. (**C**) Dose-response to dual C3aR/C5aR1 agonist EP54 and phosphate buffered saline (PBS; negative control) for EMT6 and 4T1 mouse mammary carcinoma cells and J774 macrophages (positive control). Intracellular calcium levels were measured in real time using Fluo-4 dye, with change in relative fluorescence units (RFU) indicative of intracellular calcium flux. RFU was measured for 160 s with drug addition at 15 s. Results are representative of data collected from three separate experiments.

Although we found very low or undetectable expression of C3aR and C5aR1 by either EMT6 or 4T1 cell lines, we investigated whether these cells might be capable of signal transduction in response to the dual C3aR/C5aR1 agonist, EP54. Although EP54 elicited a dose-dependent calcium response in J774 macrophages, it failed to mobilize intracellular calcium in either EMT6 or 4T1 cells (Figure 2C). Similarly, neither EP54 (10 μmol/L), recombinant mouse C3a (100 nmol/L) nor recombinant C5a (10 nmol/L) activated mitogen activated protein kinase (MAPK) signaling, as indicated by the inability to induce the phosphorylation of extracellular signal-regulated kinases (ERK) 1/2 (data not shown).

3.3. Leukocyte Response to Pharmacological Modulation of C3aR/C5aR1 in Tumor-Bearing Mice

Having found no evidence of receptor expression or signal activation by mammary carcinoma tumor cells, we next investigated whether EP54 may be acting on immune cells. Differential blood counts revealed that treatment with EP54 (1 mg/kg/day) resulted in a slight but significant increase in circulating leukocytes to $13.08 \pm 0.42 \times 10^6$ cells/mL compared with $12.19 \pm 0.01 \times 10^6$ cells/mL in vehicle-treated (control) mice ($p < 0.05$). There was no difference in neutrophil or monocyte numbers between groups, but lymphocytes were significantly increased in mice receiving EP54 ($11.48 \pm 0.51 \times 10^6$ cells/mL) compared with vehicle-treated control mice ($9.91 \pm 0.581 \times 10^6$ cells/mL; $p < 0.05$).

To further investigate the effect of EP54 on immune cells, we used the 4T1 model to analyze tumor infiltrating leukocyte populations by flow cytometry. As shown in Figure 3, there was a slight (but not significant) increase in total ($CD45^+$) leukocytes infiltrating 4T1 tumors from EP54-treated mice. Although there were no differences in myeloid cell populations (myeloid derived suppressor cells (MDSC) or macrophages) between EP54- and control (vehicle)-treatment groups, the percentage of total ($CD3^+$) T lymphocytes was significantly higher following EP54 treatment ($8.3\% \pm 5.6\%$) compared with the control group ($5.3\% \pm 2.6\%$; $p < 0.05$), as was the percentage of $CD4^+$ T cells ($3.6\% \pm 1.5\%$ compared with $2.6\% \pm 0.9\%$; $p < 0.05$). Moreover, the proportions of CD4+ T cell subsets, Th1 and Th17, were increased within EP54-treated tumors. There was also a slight increase in the proportion of $CD8^+$ T cells and reduction in Tregs, although these were not significant. Taken together, these results suggest that EP54 may inhibit mammary tumor growth by promoting an effective T cell-mediated response.

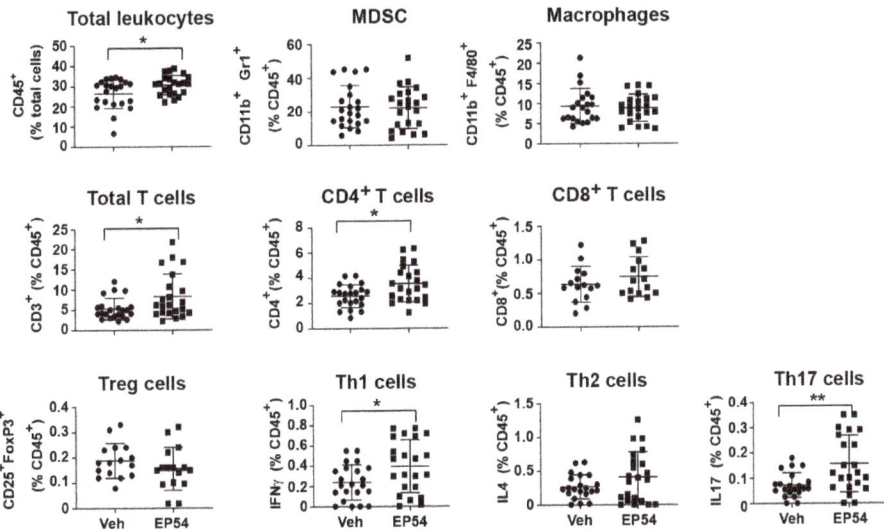

Figure 3. Effect of EP54-treatment on leukocyte sub-populations in mice with established 4T1 mammary tumors. Flow cytometric analysis of leukocyte sub-populations in tumor tissue from BALB/c mice treated with vehicle (control) ● or EP54 ■: total leukocytes ($CD45^+$), myeloid derived suppressor cells (MDSC; $CD11b^+Gr-1^+$), macrophages ($F4/80^+$), total ($CD3^+$), $CD4^+$ and $CD8^+$ T lymphocytes; $CD4^+$ T lymphocyte subsets: Treg ($CD4^+CD25^+FoxP3^+$), Th1 ($CD4^+IFN\gamma^+$), Th2 ($CD4^+IL4^+$) and Th17 ($CD4^+IL17^+$). Results of three independent experiments (n = 6–8/group). Data expressed as % positive cells (mean ± SD); ** $p < 0.01$; * $p < 0.05$, Student's t-test.

4. Discussion

Chronic inflammation plays a critical role in the development and progression of cancer [47]. As key mediators of inflammation [48], the complement proteins C3a and

C5a have been implicated for roles in tumorigenesis. Our laboratory and others have demonstrated that C3a and C5a promote tumor growth in a number of murine cancer models, including cervical [24], lung [25,30], ovarian [26], colon and melanoma [27,28]. However, the few studies investigating the role of these proteins in breast cancer models have produced conflicting results. Thus, the current study sought to clarify the role of complement proteins in murine syngeneic breast cancer models, EMT6 and 4T1.

In accordance with the previous study by Vadrevu and co-workers, we found no effect of PMX53 on primary EMT6 mammary tumor growth [23]. However, treatment with a dual C3aR/C5aR1 agonist (EP54) inhibited development and growth of both EMT6 and 4T1 mammary tumors. These results are in agreement with the work of Kim et al., who demonstrated a protective role for C5a in the EMT6 mammary cancer model [21]. They are also in accordance with those of Bandini et al. [22], who showed that C3-deficiency (in which both C3a and C5a are lacking) accelerated tumor growth in a transgenic mouse model of mammary adenocarcinoma. This raises the question of whether the anti-tumor effects are mediated solely by C5a or whether C3a may also play a role. Our previous demonstration that C3aR signaling promotes 4T1 tumor growth, along with the evidence from Kim and co-workers that C5a alone has a protective role in EMT6 tumors, suggest that C5a is primarily responsible for the observed protective effects.

Another question still to be resolved is the mechanism by which EP54 exerts its anti-tumor effects. Kim and co-workers showed that C5a-expressing EMT6 tumors had high rates of apoptosis and cell cycle progression was blocked. Although this group demonstrated C5aR1 expression by EMT6 cells, we found that both C3aR and C5aR1 were undetectable on EMT6 and 4T1 cells at the protein level, suggesting that the anti-tumor effects of EP54 are indirect. Indeed, Kim and co-workers also showed that mice whose tumors regressed were immune to subsequent challenge with unmodified tumors (i.e., not expressing C5a), suggesting that at least some of the effects of C5a were indirect, via enhancement of the anti-tumor immune response. Moreover, Bandini et al. showed that mammary tumors from C3-deficient mice have a more immunosuppressive microenvironment [22]. The present study supports the premise that the tumor inhibitory effects of EP54 are due to immunoregulatory mechanisms, with EP54-treated mice showing increased tumor infiltration by T lymphocytes, in particular CD4+ T cell subsets, Th1 and Th17. While the presence of Th1 cells is linked to favorable prognoses in many cancers, the role of Th17 remains controversial [49]. However, Th17 cells have recently been identified as the most favorable prognostic indicator for triple-negative breast cancers with low T cell infiltrate [50]. Thus, the increased Th1–Th17 response in EP54-treated tumors suggests that these cells contribute to the anti-tumor response. Our results are in contrast to previous reports demonstrating that inhibition of C5aR1 signaling in MDSC favors Th1 and Th17 responses [23,51]. Although we found no significant difference in the proportions of tumor-infiltrating myeloid cells, qualitative differences are possible. For example, Markiewski and co-workers showed in the TC-1 cervical cancer model that C5a regulates the production of reactive oxygen and nitrogen species by MDSC [24]. In addition to immunoregulation, other effects are possible. For example, Nunez-Cruz and co-workers [26] demonstrated a primary role for C5a in neovascularization of ovarian cancers. Although beyond the scope of the present study, future studies could determine more precisely the mechanisms by which C3aR/C5aR1 agonism influences breast cancer growth, including potential effects on the function of myeloid and lymphocyte cell populations, and the ability to regulate tumor angiogenesis.

The few studies investigating the role of complement proteins in mammary tumor models have yielded results that are in contrast to the majority of studies in other murine cancer models which show that pharmacological blockade of C5aR1 or C3aR inhibits tumor progression by limiting recruitment of immunosuppressive myeloid cells and Tregs into the tumor and promoting effective T cell responses [24,25,27,28,30]. The reasons for differing effects of complement proteins on different tumor types are yet to be determined, but likely include intrinsic differences in tumor mutational load, immunogenicity of tumor lines and immune profiles of the host mice [52]. One possible reason for differing responses between tumors is the variability in expression of complement receptors. Although we found no evidence of C3aR or C5aR1 expression by EMT6 or 4T1 mammary tumor cells, expression of these receptors has been reported for a range of human and mouse tumor cells, including melanoma [27], lung [53] and ovarian [31] cancers—all of which are inhibited by C3aR or C5aR1 receptor antagonism. While the lack of C3aR or C5aR1 expression by EMT6 and 4T1 tumor cells precludes direct effects of complement proteins on tumor growth, direct effects are possible for other (receptor-expressing) tumor models.

Compared with other common tumor models, 4T1 and EMT6 tumors are relatively immunogenic, with high levels of immune infiltration [54,55]. Our own experience shows that 4T1 mammary tumors have higher percentages of tumor-infiltrating leukocyte populations than poorly immunogenic B16.F0 melanoma tumors [28]. The site of tumor cell injection may also influence the response, due to tissue-specific variation in resident immune cells, differences in vascularization and the ability of immune cells to infiltrate the site [56]. The nature of the immune infiltrate is also likely to depend on the immune profile of the host strain. Most previous studies showing tumor-promoting effects of complement C3a and/or C5a have utilized tumor models syngeneic in C57Bl/6 mice whose immune system is skewed towards a Th1-M1 response [24–28,57]. Conversely, mammary tumor (EMT6 and 4T1 and the spontaneous neuT transgenic) models are on a BALB/c background in which Th2-M2 responses are dominant [58].

Differences in levels of complement proteins within the tumor microenvironment are also possible. Although C57Bl/6 and BALB/c mice have normal complement function [59], complement activation levels may differ, and tumor intrinsic complement production may also vary. As demonstrated in this study, both EMT6 and 4T1 cells express C3 mRNA, and at levels that are relatively higher than other murine cell lines, such as B16 melanoma, MC38 colon carcinoma and Lewis lung carcinoma (LLC) [55]. As suggested by Gunn and co-workers [57], differing levels of tumor-derived complement proteins could contribute to observed differences in immune responses to the tumor, with low C5a levels inhibiting tumor growth by promoting Th1 cell differentiation, and high levels promoting Treg differentiation and stimulating tumor growth. Clearly, further work is required to clarify the roles of complement receptors in different tumor types, and how this is influenced by factors such as tumor immunogenicity, tumor site and the immune status of the host.

5. Conclusions

The present study demonstrated a protective role for C3aR/C5aR1 agonism in murine models of mammary carcinoma and suggests that this may be due to an enhanced T cell response. The results provide further evidence that complement proteins can exert distinct responses depending on the cancer type, possibly due to differences in the host's immune response to the tumor. They also suggest that in the mammary tumor environment, exogenous C3a/C5a stimulation is required to trigger tumor inhibitory mechanisms. As proposed by Pio et al. [60], the immune system establishes a balance between tumor-promoting and tumor-inhibitory elements. By modulating the levels of complement activation, the balance may be altered towards a more (or less) favorable outcome. Thus, before complement-regulating drugs can be developed for clinical application, it is important to understand the mechanisms by which they exert their effects, and how this varies with cancer type.

Supplementary Materials: The following are available online at https://www.mdpi.com/article/10.3390/10.3390/antib10010002/s1, Figure S1: Gating strategies for flow cytometric analysis of the tumor inflammatory infiltrate.

Author Contributions: Conceptualization, H.D.M., I.A.S., P.C.M., T.M.W. and B.E.R.; Formal analysis, J.A.N. and H.D.M.; Funding acquisition, T.M.W. and B.E.R.; Investigation, F.N.M.A., K.W.K.L., J.A.N., S.E.S., J.N.T.F. and C.E.M.; Methodology, M.H.M.N., H.D.M., T.M.W. and B.E.R.; Resources, T.M.W. and B.E.R.; Supervision, H.D.M., P.C.M., T.M.W. and B.E.R.; Writing—original draft, F.N.M.A.,

M.H.M.N. and K.W.K.L.; Writing—review and editing, H.D.M., T.M.W. and B.E.R. All authors have read and agreed to the published version of the manuscript.

Funding: This research was funded by Australian National Health and Medical Research Council (NHMRC; APP1103951), Cancer Council Queensland (CCQ) and The University of Queensland Collaboration and Industry Fund (CIEF). F.A. was supported by Skim Latihan Akademik Bumiputera (SLAB), Ministry of Higher Education Malaysia, M.H. by the Malaysian Government Public Universities Academic Training Scholarship Scheme and J.N. by a University of Queensland Post-Graduate Research Scholarship.

Acknowledgments: We thank Darryl Whitehead for histological advice and Geoff Osborne for advice on flow cytometry.

Conflicts of Interest: The authors declare no conflict of interest.

References

1. Bray, F.; Ferlay, J.; Soerjomataram, I.; Siegel, R.L.; Torre, L.A.; Jemal, A. Global cancer statistics 2018: GLOBOCAN estimates of incidence and mortality worldwide for 36 cancers in 185 countries. *CA Cancer J. Clin.* **2018**, *68*, 394–424. [CrossRef] [PubMed]
2. Garrido-Castro, A.C.; Lin, N.U.; Polyak, K. Insights into Molecular Classifications of Triple-Negative Breast Cancer: Improving Patient Selection for Treatment. *Cancer Discov.* **2019**, *9*, 176–198. [CrossRef] [PubMed]
3. Coussens, L.M.; Werb, Z. Inflammation and cancer. *Nature* **2002**, *420*, 860–867. [CrossRef] [PubMed]
4. Qu, X.; Tang, Y.; Hua, S. Immunological Approaches towards Cancer and Inflammation: A Cross Talk. *Front. Immunol.* **2018**, *9*, 563. [CrossRef]
5. Reis, E.S.; Mastellos, D.C.; Ricklin, D.; Mantovani, A.; Lambris, J.D. Complement in cancer: Untangling an intricate relationship. *Nat. Rev. Immunol.* **2018**, *18*, 5–18. [CrossRef]
6. Niculescu, F.; Rus, H.G.; Retegan, M.; Vlaicu, R. Persistent complement activation on tumor cells in breast cancer. *Am. J. Pathol.* **1992**, *140*, 1039–1043.
7. Chung, L.; Moore, K.; Phillips, L.; Boyle, F.M.; Marsh, D.J.; Baxter, R.C. Novel serum protein biomarker panel revealed by mass spectrometry and its prognostic value in breast cancer. *Breast Cancer Res.* **2014**, *16*, R63. [CrossRef]
8. Imamura, T.; Yamamoto-Ibusuki, M.; Sueta, A.; Kubo, T.; Irie, A.; Kikuchi, K.; Kariu, T.; Iwase, H. Influence of the C5a-C5a receptor system on breast cancer progression and patient prognosis. *Breast Cancer* **2016**, *23*, 876–885. [CrossRef]
9. Ricklin, D.; Hajishengallis, G.; Yang, K.; Lambris, J.D. Complement: A key system for immune surveillance and homeostasis. *Nat. Immunol.* **2010**, *11*, 785–797. [CrossRef]
10. Ostrand-Rosenberg, S. Cancer and complement. *Nat. Biotechnol.* **2008**, *26*, 1348–1349. [CrossRef]
11. Gelderman, K.A.; Tomlinson, S.; Ross, G.D.; Gorter, A. Complement function in mAb-mediated cancer immunotherapy. *Trends Immunol.* **2004**, *25*, 158–164. [CrossRef] [PubMed]
12. Geller, A.; Yan, J. The Role of Membrane Bound Complement Regulatory Proteins in Tumor Development and Cancer Immunotherapy. *Front. Immunol.* **2019**, *10*, 1074. [CrossRef]
13. Ouyang, Q.; Zhang, L.; Jiang, Y.; Ni, X.; Chen, S.; Ye, F.; Du, Y.; Huang, L.; Ding, P.; Wang, N.; et al. The membrane complement regulatory protein CD59 promotes tumor growth and predicts poor prognosis in breast cancer. *Int. J. Oncol.* **2016**, *48*, 2015–2024. [CrossRef] [PubMed]
14. Maciejczyk, A.; Szelachowska, J.; Szynglarewicz, B.; Szulc, R.; Szulc, A.; Wysocka, T.; Jagoda, E.; Lage, H.; Surowiak, P. CD46 Expression is an unfavorable prognostic factor in breast cancer cases. *Appl. Immunohistochem. Mol. Morphol.* **2011**, *19*, 540–546. [CrossRef] [PubMed]
15. Klos, A.; Wende, E.; Wareham, K.J.; Monk, P.N. International Union of Pharmacology. LXXXVII. Complement peptide C5a, C4a, and C3a receptors. *Pharmacol. Rev.* **2013**, *65*, 500–543. [CrossRef]
16. Lo, M.W.; Woodruff, T.M. Complement: Bridging the innate and adaptive immune systems in sterile inflammation. *J. Leukoc. Biol.* **2020**, *108*, 339–351. [CrossRef] [PubMed]
17. Li, X.X.; Lee, J.D.; Kemper, C.; Woodruff, T.M. The complement receptor C5aR2: A powerful modulator of innate and adaptive immunity. *J. Immunol.* **2019**, *202*, 3339–3348. [CrossRef]
18. Pandey, S.; Maharana, J.; Li, X.X.; Woodruff, T.M.; Shukla, A.K. Emerging Insights into the Structure and Function of Complement C5a Receptors. *Trends Biochem. Sci.* **2020**, *45*, 693–705. [CrossRef]
19. Wu, M.C.; Brennan, F.H.; Lynch, J.P.; Mantovani, S.; Phipps, S.; Wetsel, R.A.; Ruitenberg, M.J.; Taylor, S.M.; Woodruff, T.M. The receptor for complement component C3a mediates protection from intestinal ischemia-reperfusion injuries by inhibiting neutrophil mobilization. *Proc. Natl. Acad. Sci. USA* **2013**, *110*, 9439–9444. [CrossRef]
20. Coulthard, L.G.; Woodruff, T.M. Is the complement activation product C3a a proinflammatory molecule? Re-evaluating the evidence and the myth. *J. Immunol.* **2015**, *194*, 3542–3548. [CrossRef]
21. Kim, D.Y.; Martin, C.B.; Lee, S.N.; Martin, B.K. Expression of complement protein C5a in a murine mammary cancer model: Tumor regression by interference with the cell cycle. *Cancer Immunol. Immunother.* **2005**, *54*, 1026–1037. [CrossRef] [PubMed]

22. Bandini, S.; Curcio, C.; Macagno, M.; Quaglino, E.; Arigoni, M.; Lanzardo, S.; Hysi, A.; Barutello, G.; Consolino, L.; Longo, D.L.; et al. Early onset and enhanced growth of autochthonous mammary carcinomas in C3-deficient Her2/neu transgenic mice. *Oncoimmunology* **2013**, *2*, e26137. [CrossRef] [PubMed]
23. Vadrevu, S.K.; Chintala, N.K.; Sharma, S.K.; Sharma, P.; Cleveland, C.; Riediger, L.; Manne, S.; Fairlie, D.P.; Gorczyca, W.; Almanza, O.; et al. Complement c5a receptor facilitates cancer metastasis by altering T-cell responses in the metastatic niche. *Cancer Res.* **2014**, *74*, 3454–3465. [CrossRef]
24. Markiewski, M.M.; DeAngelis, R.A.; Benencia, F.; Ricklin-Lichtsteiner, S.K.; Koutoulaki, A.; Gerard, C.; Coukos, G.; Lambris, J.D. Modulation of the antitumor immune response by complement. *Nat. Immunol.* **2008**, *9*, 1225–1235. [CrossRef]
25. Corrales, L.; Ajona, D.; Rafail, S.; Lasarte, J.J.; Riezu-Boj, J.I.; Lambris, J.D.; Rouzaut, A.; Pajares, M.J.; Montuenga, L.M.; Pio, R. Anaphylatoxin C5a creates a favorable microenvironment for lung cancer progression. *J. Immunol.* **2012**, *189*, 4674–4683. [CrossRef]
26. Nunez-Cruz, S.; Gimotty, P.A.; Guerra, M.W.; Connolly, D.C.; Wu, Y.Q.; DeAngelis, R.A.; Lambris, J.D.; Coukos, G.; Scholler, N. Genetic and pharmacologic inhibition of complement impairs endothelial cell function and ablates ovarian cancer neovascularization. *Neoplasia* **2012**, *14*, 994–1004. [CrossRef] [PubMed]
27. Nabizadeh, J.A.; Manthey, H.D.; Panagides, N.; Steyn, F.J.; Lee, J.D.; Li, X.X.; Akhir, F.N.M.; Chen, W.; Boyle, G.M.; Taylor, S.M.; et al. C5a receptors C5aR1 and C5aR2 mediate opposing pathologies in a mouse model of melanoma. *FASEB J.* **2019**, *33*, 11060–11071. [CrossRef] [PubMed]
28. Nabizadeh, J.A.; Manthey, H.D.; Steyn, F.J.; Chen, W.; Widiapradja, A.; Md Akhir, F.N.; Boyle, G.M.; Taylor, S.M.; Woodruff, T.M.; Rolfe, B.E. The Complement C3a Receptor Contributes to Melanoma Tumorigenesis by Inhibiting Neutrophil and CD4+ T Cell Responses. *J. Immunol.* **2016**, *196*, 4783–4792. [CrossRef] [PubMed]
29. Guglietta, S.; Chiavelli, A.; Zagato, E.; Krieg, C.; Gandini, S.; Ravenda, P.S.; Bazolli, B.; Lu, B.; Penna, G.; Rescigno, M. Coagulation induced by C3aR-dependent NETosis drives protumorigenic neutrophils during small intestinal tumorigenesis. *Nat. Commun.* **2016**, *7*, 11037. [CrossRef] [PubMed]
30. Kwak, J.W.; Laskowski, J.; Li, H.Y.; McSharry, M.V.; Sippel, T.R.; Bullock, B.L.; Johnson, A.M.; Poczobutt, J.M.; Neuwelt, A.J.; Malkoski, S.P.; et al. Complement Activation via a C3a Receptor Pathway Alters CD4(+) T Lymphocytes and Mediates Lung Cancer Progression. *Cancer Res.* **2018**, *78*, 143–156. [CrossRef]
31. Cho, M.S.; Vasquez, H.G.; Rupaimoole, R.; Pradeep, S.; Wu, S.; Zand, B.; Han, H.D.; Rodriguez-Aguayo, C.; Bottsford-Miller, J.; Huang, J.; et al. Autocrine effects of tumor-derived complement. *Cell Rep.* **2014**, *6*, 1085–1095. [CrossRef] [PubMed]
32. Boire, A.; Zou, Y.; Shieh, J.; Macalinao, D.G.; Pentsova, E.; Massague, J. Complement Component 3 Adapts the Cerebrospinal Fluid for Leptomeningeal Metastasis. *Cell* **2017**, *168*, 1101–1113.e1113. [CrossRef] [PubMed]
33. Rockwell, S.C.; Kallman, R.F.; Fajardo, L.F. Characteristics of a serially transplanted mouse mammary tumor and its tissue-culture-adapted derivative. *J. Natl. Cancer Inst.* **1972**, *49*, 735–749. [PubMed]
34. Pulaski, B.A.; Ostrand Rosenberg, S. Mouse 4T1 Breast Tumor Model. *Curr. Protoc. Immunol.* **2001**, *20*, 20.2.1–20.2.16. [CrossRef] [PubMed]
35. Finch, A.M.; Wong, A.K.; Paczkowski, N.J.; Wadi, S.K.; Craik, D.J.; Fairlie, D.P.; Taylor, S.M. Low-molecular-weight peptidic and cyclic antagonists of the receptor for the complement factor C5a. *J. Med. Chem.* **1999**, *42*, 1965–1974. [CrossRef] [PubMed]
36. Wu, M.C.L.; Lee, J.D.; Ruitenberg, M.J.; Woodruff, T.M. Absence of the C5a Receptor C5aR2 Worsens Ischemic Tissue Injury by Increasing C5aR1-Mediated Neutrophil Infiltration. *J. Immunol.* **2020**, *205*, 2834–2839. [CrossRef]
37. Proctor, L.M.; Arumugam, T.V.; Shiels, I.; Reid, R.C.; Fairlie, D.P.; Taylor, S.M. Comparative anti-inflammatory activities of antagonists to C3a and C5a receptors in a rat model of intestinal ischaemia/reperfusion injury. *Br. J. Pharm.* **2004**, *142*, 756–764. [CrossRef]
38. Manthey, H.D.; Thomas, A.C.; Shiels, I.A.; Zernecke, A.; Woodruff, T.M.; Rolfe, B.; Taylor, S.M. Complement C5a inhibition reduces atherosclerosis in ApoE-/- mice. *FASEB J.* **2011**, *25*, 2447–2455. [CrossRef]
39. Campbell, W.D.; Lazoura, E.; Okada, N.; Okada, H. Inactivation of C3a and C5a octapeptides by carboxypeptidase R and carboxypeptidase N. *Microbiol. Immunol.* **2002**, *46*, 131–134. [CrossRef]
40. Woodruff, T.M.; Strachan, A.J.; Sanderson, S.D.; Monk, P.N.; Wong, A.K.; Fairlie, D.P.; Taylor, S.M. Species dependence for binding of small molecule agonist and antagonists to the C5a receptor on polymorphonuclear leukocytes. *Inflammation* **2001**, *25*, 171–177. [CrossRef]
41. Finch, A.M.; Vogen, S.M.; Sherman, S.A.; Kirnarsky, L.; Taylor, S.M.; Sanderson, S.D. Biologically active conformer of the effector region of human C5a and modulatory effects of N-terminal receptor binding determinants on activity. *J. Med. Chem.* **1997**, *40*, 877–884. [CrossRef] [PubMed]
42. Li, X.X.; Lee, J.D.; Massey, N.L.; Guan, C.; Robertson, A.A.B.; Clark, R.J.; Woodruff, T.M. Pharmacological characterisation of small molecule C5aR1 inhibitors in human cells reveals biased activities for signalling and function. *Biochem. Pharm.* **2020**, *180*, 114156. [CrossRef] [PubMed]
43. Kumar, V.; Lee, J.D.; Clark, R.J.; Noakes, P.G.; Taylor, S.M.; Woodruff, T.M. Preclinical Pharmacokinetics of Complement C5a Receptor Antagonists PMX53 and PMX205 in Mice. *ACS Omega* **2020**, *5*, 2345–2354. [CrossRef] [PubMed]
44. Hegde, G.V.; Meyers-Clark, E.; Joshi, S.S.; Sanderson, S.D. A conformationally-biased, response-selective agonist of C5a acts as a molecular adjuvant by modulating antigen processing and presentation activities of human dendritic cells. *Int. Immunopharmacol.* **2008**, *8*, 819–827. [CrossRef]

45. Tomayko, M.M.; Reynolds, C.P. Determination of subcutaneous tumor size in athymic (nude) mice. *Cancer Chemother. Pharm.* **1989**, *24*, 148–154. [CrossRef]
46. Spang-Thomsen, M.; Nielsen, A.; Visfeldt, J. Growth curves of three human malignant tumors transplanted to nude mice. *Exp. Cell Biol.* **1980**, *48*, 138–154. [CrossRef]
47. Greten, F.R.; Grivennikov, S.I. Inflammation and Cancer: Triggers, Mechanisms, and Consequences. *Immunity* **2019**, *51*, 27–41. [CrossRef]
48. Klos, A.; Tenner, A.J.; Johswich, K.O.; Ager, R.R.; Reis, E.S.; Kohl, J. The role of the anaphylatoxins in health and disease. *Mol. Immunol.* **2009**, *46*, 2753–2766. [CrossRef]
49. Bailey, S.R.; Nelson, M.H.; Himes, R.A.; Li, Z.; Mehrotra, S.; Paulos, C.M. Th17 cells in cancer: The ultimate identity crisis. *Front. Immunol.* **2014**, *5*, 276. [CrossRef]
50. Faucheux, L.; Grandclaudon, M.; Perrot-Dockes, M.; Sirven, P.; Berger, F.; Hamy, A.S.; Fourchotte, V.; Vincent-Salomon, A.; Mechta-Grigoriou, F.; Reyal, F.; et al. A multivariate Th17 metagene for prognostic stratification in T cell non-inflamed triple negative breast cancer. *Oncoimmunology* **2019**, *8*, e1624130. [CrossRef]
51. Markiewski, M.M.; Vadrevu, S.K.; Sharma, S.K.; Chintala, N.K.; Ghouse, S.; Cho, J.H.; Fairlie, D.P.; Paterson, Y.; Astrinidis, A.; Karbowniczek, M. The Ribosomal Protein S19 Suppresses Antitumor Immune Responses via the Complement C5a Receptor 1. *J. Immunol.* **2017**, *198*, 2989–2999. [CrossRef] [PubMed]
52. Yu, J.W.; Bhattacharya, S.; Yanamandra, N.; Kilian, D.; Shi, H.; Yadavilli, S.; Katlinskaya, Y.; Kaczynski, H.; Conner, M.; Benson, W.; et al. Tumor-immune profiling of murine syngeneic tumor models as a framework to guide mechanistic studies and predict therapy response in distinct tumor microenvironments. *PLoS ONE* **2018**, *13*, e0206223. [CrossRef] [PubMed]
53. Ajona, D.; Zandueta, C.; Corrales, L.; Moreno, H.; Pajares, M.J.; Ortiz-Espinosa, S.; Martinez-Terroba, E.; Perurena, N.; de Miguel, F.J.; Jantus-Lewintre, E.; et al. Blockade of the Complement C5a/C5aR1 Axis Impairs Lung Cancer Bone Metastasis by CXCL16-mediated Effects. *Am. J. Respir. Crit. Care Med.* **2018**, *197*, 1164–1176. [CrossRef] [PubMed]
54. Mosely, S.I.; Prime, J.E.; Sainson, R.C.; Koopmann, J.O.; Wang, D.Y.; Greenawalt, D.M.; Ahdesmaki, M.J.; Leyland, R.; Mullins, S.; Pacelli, L.; et al. Rational Selection of Syngeneic Preclinical Tumor Models for Immunotherapeutic Drug Discovery. *Cancer Immunol. Res.* **2017**, *5*, 29–41. [CrossRef] [PubMed]
55. Zhong, W.; Myers, J.S.; Wang, F.; Wang, K.; Lucas, J.; Rosfjord, E.; Lucas, J.; Hooper, A.T.; Yang, S.; Lemon, L.A.; et al. Comparison of the molecular and cellular phenotypes of common mouse syngeneic models with human tumors. *BMC Genom.* **2020**, *21*, 2. [CrossRef]
56. Devaud, C.; Westwood, J.A.; John, L.B.; Flynn, J.K.; Paquet-Fifield, S.; Duong, C.P.; Yong, C.S.; Pegram, H.J.; Stacker, S.A.; Achen, M.G.; et al. Tissues in different anatomical sites can sculpt and vary the tumor microenvironment to affect responses to therapy. *Mol. Ther. J. Am. Soc. Gene Ther.* **2014**, *22*, 18–27. [CrossRef]
57. Gunn, L.; Ding, C.; Liu, M.; Ma, Y.; Qi, C.; Cai, Y.; Hu, X.; Aggarwal, D.; Zhang, H.G.; Yan, J. Opposing roles for complement component C5a in tumor progression and the tumor microenvironment. *J. Immunol.* **2012**, *189*, 2985–2994. [CrossRef]
58. Mills, C.D.; Kincaid, K.; Alt, J.M.; Heilman, M.J.; Hill, A.M. M-1/M-2 macrophages and the Th1/Th2 paradigm. *J. Immunol.* **2000**, *164*, 6166–6173. [CrossRef]
59. Sellers, R.S.; Clifford, C.B.; Treuting, P.M.; Brayton, C. Immunological variation between inbred laboratory mouse strains: Points to consider in phenotyping genetically immunomodified mice. *Vet. Pathol.* **2012**, *49*, 32–43. [CrossRef]
60. Pio, R.; Ajona, D.; Lambris, J.D. Complement inhibition in cancer therapy. *Semin. Immunol.* **2013**, *25*, 54–64. [CrossRef]

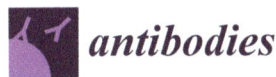

Article

Anti gC1qR/p32/HABP1 Antibody Therapy Decreases Tumor Growth in an Orthotopic Murine Xenotransplant Model of Triple Negative Breast Cancer

Ellinor I. Peerschke [1,*], Elisa de Stanchina [2], Qing Chang [2], Katia Manova-Todorova [2], Afsar Barlas [2], Anne G. Savitt [3], Brian V. Geisbrecht [4] and Berhane Ghebrehiwet [5]

1. Department of Laboratory Medicine, Memorial Sloan Kettering Cancer Center, New York, NY 10065, USA
2. Sloan Kettering Institute, Memorial Sloan Kettering Cancer Center, New York, NY 10065, USA; destance@mskcc.org (E.d.S.); changq@mskcc.org (Q.C.); manovak@mskcc.org (K.M.-T.); barlasa@mskcc.org (A.B.)
3. Department of Microbiology and Immunology, Renaissance School of Medicine, Stony Brook University, Stony Brook, NY 11794, USA; anne.savitt@stonybrook.edu
4. Department of Biochemistry and Molecular Biophysics, Kansas State University, Manhattan, KS 66506, USA; geisbrechtb@ksu.edu
5. Departments of Medicine and Pathology, Renaissance School of Medicine, Stony Brook University, Stony Brook, NY 11794, USA; Berhane.ghebrehiwet@stonybrookmedicine.edu
* Correspondence: peersche@mskcc.org; Tel.: +1-646-608-1357

Received: 6 August 2020; Accepted: 8 September 2020; Published: 6 October 2020

Abstract: gC1qR is highly expressed in breast cancer and plays a role in cancer cell proliferation. This study explored therapy with gC1qR monoclonal antibody 60.11, directed against the C1q binding domain of gC1qR, in a murine orthotopic xenotransplant model of triple negative breast cancer. MDA231 breast cancer cells were injected into the mammary fat pad of athymic nu/nu female mice. Mice were segregated into three groups (n = 5, each) and treated with the vehicle (group 1) or gC1qR antibody 60.11 (100 mg/kg) twice weekly, starting at day 3 post-implantation (group 2) or when the tumor volume reached 100 mm^3 (group 3). At study termination (d = 35), the average tumor volume in the control group measured 895 ± 143 mm^3, compared to 401 ± 48 mm^3 and 701 ± 100 mm^3 in groups 2 and 3, respectively ($p < 0.05$). Immunohistochemical staining of excised tumors revealed increased apoptosis (caspase 3 and TUNEL staining) in 60.11-treated mice compared to controls, and decreased angiogenesis (CD31 staining). Slightly decreased white blood cell counts were noted in 60.11-treated mice. Otherwise, no overt toxicities were observed. These data are the first to demonstrate an in vivo anti-tumor effect of 60.11 therapy in a mouse model of triple negative breast cancer.

Keywords: gC1qR; breast cancer; xenotransplant model

1. Introduction

Triple negative breast cancer is characterized by the absence of estrogen and progesterone receptors, as well as human epidermal growth factor receptor 2 [1–3]. Due to the absence of hormone receptors, chemotherapy represents the major therapeutic modality for triple negative breast cancer. The median survival, especially for patients with advanced disease [2,3], remains poor. For this reason, the development of additional therapies directed against novel cellular targets is an important goal to deepen disease response and improve patient outcomes [4,5].

The complement system is emerging as a novel target in cancer therapy. Complement is involved not only in shaping the inflammatory tumor microenvironment, but also in tumor growth and spread [6–10]. In this regard, the complement component C1q is increasingly recognized as a tumor promoting factor, enhancing cancer cell adhesion, migration, proliferation, and angiogenesis [11,12].

We have identified gC1qR (also known as/p32/HABP1) as the major cellular binding site for C1q [13]. Marked upregulation of gC1qR expression has been observed in proliferating cells, particularly in cancers of epithelial cell origin including breast, colon, and lung cancers [14,15]. Moreover, overexpression of gC1qR has been associated with poor prognosis in patients with breast cancer [16,17], prostate cancer [18], serous ovarian adenocarcinoma [19], and endometrial cell cancer [20]. In addition, gC1qR has been identified as a potential molecular target for delivery of cytotoxic agents [21,22].

The present study used a mouse xenograft model to investigate the C1q-gC1qR axis in triple negative breast cancer with the 60.11 murine monoclonal antibody, 60.11, which is directed specifically against the C1q binding domain of gC1qR [23]. Human tumor xenograft models provide important insights into tumor progression and metastasis. We selected the MDA-MB-231 (MDA231) human breast cancer cell line, as it represents a triple negative breast cancer cell line that has been widely studied in xenotransplantation [24]. Moreover, MDA231 cells bind the 60.11 antibody [21], and the role of gC1qR in MDA231 cell proliferation has been described [25,26].

2. Materials and Methods

2.1. Antibody Production

The therapeutic murine monoclonal antibody (60.11) (IgG) is directed against N-terminal amino acids 76–93 of human gC1qR, and specifically inhibits C1q binding [27,28]. Surface plasmon resonance studies estimate the binding affinity of 60.11 for gC1qR at 67 nM (Appendix A). The antibody recognizes human, mouse, and rat gC1qR [27,28]. Human and rodent (rat/mouse) gC1qR (C1qBP) cDNA sequences are 89.9% identical [29,30].

The study antibody was prepared using in vitro ascites (IVA), as described [31]. Hybridoma 60.11 was cultured in DMEM (Gibco/Thermo Fisher Scientific, Waltham, MA, USA supplemented with 10% Fetal Clone I serum (HyClone, Logan, UT, USA), penicillin and streptomycin (Gibco), and non-essential amino acids (NEAA, Gibco), and subcloned by limiting dilution to identify a high-producing subclone. Hybridoma supernatants were tested by ELISA against recombinant gC1qR antigen. The selected subclone was then adapted into an animal-derived component-free medium (ADCF, HyClone) supplemented with NEAA and inoculated into a CELLine CL1000 flask (Wheaton) according to the manufacturer's instructions. Antibody-containing supernatants (IVA) were harvested under sterile conditions according to manufacturer's instructions. Collected supernatants were transferred to sterile tubes (Falcon/Corning Life Sciences, Teterboro, NJ, USA) and stored at −20 °C until used. Antibody quantitation was accomplished by quantitative Western blot. Low-endotoxin, azide-free (LEAF) IgG$_1$ kappa (BioLegend, Dedham, MA, USA) was used to generate a standard curve. Antibody was detected in the blot using Alexa Fluor 680-labeled anti mouse IgG (Thermo Fisher, Waltham, MA, USA). Visualization and densitometry were performed on a Licor Odyssey Infrared Imager.

2.2. Murine Xenotransplantation Model

An orthotopic xenograft model was used to test the in vivo efficacy of 60.11 antibody therapy, in collaboration with the MSK Antitumor Assessment Core, according to established protocols [32–34]. All procedures were performed under approved Institutional Animal Care and Use Committee protocols (04–03–009). Briefly, 5 million MDA231 breast cancer cells (ATCC) were injected into the 4th left mammary fat pad of athymic nu/nu female mice (5–6 weeks old). Animals were treated with gC1qR antibody 60.11 (100mg/kg) starting either 3 days post-MDA231 cell implantation (group 2) before tumors were measurable, or on day 13, after tumor volume reached approximately 100 mm^3 (groups 1 and 3). Control mice (group 1) were treated with the vehicle, starting 3 days after MDA231 cell implantation. Each treatment group consisted of 5 mice, exposed to twice-weekly intraperitoneal antibody or vehicle injection. Over the course of the experiment, animals in group 2 received 16 doses of 60.11 antibody, whereas animals in group 3 received 11 doses. Animal weights and tumor volumes were recorded twice weekly. Tumor volumes were calculated using the following equation, $((\text{width}^2 \times \text{length} \times 3.14)/6)$. In addition, clinical assessments of animal distress (weight loss, disruption of locomotor coordination, hunching, lack of grooming, lethargy) were made and recorded daily to assess toxicity. At time of sacrifice (35 days after MDA231 cell implantation), automated blood cell counts (Element HT5 veterinary hematology analyzer, Heska, Loveland, CO, USA) were obtained and tumors were removed, fixed, and processed for histologic (hematoxylin and eosin staining) and immunohistochemical evaluation. In addition, vital organs were harvested for histologic examination. Serum 60.11 antibody levels were quantified using a solid-phase ELISA assay using immobilized recombinant gC1qR and 60.11 antibody standards [35].

2.3. Immunohistochemical Analysis

Tissue processing and immunohistochemical analysis was performed by the Molecular Cytology Core Facility of Memorial Sloan Kettering Cancer Center as previously described [36,37]. In brief, tissues were fixed in 4% formaldehyde and processed by paraffin embedding, using a tissue processor (Leica ASP6025). Next, 5 μm sections were obtained and applied to superfrost plus slides. Immunohistochemical detection of Ki 67, Cleaved Caspase 3, TUNEL (Terminal deoxynucleotidyl dUTP nick end labeling), and CD31 was performed using a Discovery XT processor (Ventana Medical Systems, Oro Valley, AZ, USA). Slides were counterstained with hematoxylin and cover-slipped with Permount (Fisher Scientific).

2.3.1. Ki 67 Immunostaining

The Discovery XT autostainer was programmed to incubate slides with primary rabbit polyclonal Ki 67 antibody (Abcam, Cambridge, MA, USA) at 1 μg/mL for 4 h, followed by incubation with secondary antibody (biotinylated goat anti-rabbit IgG; Vector Labs, San Diego, CA, USA) at a concentration of 5.75 μg/mL for 30 min. Blocker D, Streptavidin—HRP, and DAB detection kit (Ventana Medical Systems) were used according to the manufacturer's instructions.

2.3.2. Cleaved Caspase 3 Immunostaining

A rabbit polyclonal Cleaved Caspase 3 antibody (Cell Signaling) was used at 0.1 μg/mL concentration. Slides were incubated in the Discovery XT autostainer for 3 h. Incubation with secondary antibody (biotinylated goat anti-rabbit IgG; Vector labs) at a concentration of 5.75 μg/mL occurred for 20 min. Blocker D, Streptavidin—HRP, and DAB detection kit (Ventana Medical Systems, Oro Valley, AZ, USA) were used according to the manufacturer's instructions.

2.3.3. TUNEL Immunostaining

TUNEL analysis was performed as follows. Slides were manually de-paraffinized in xylene, rehydrated in a series of alcohol dilutions (100%, 95%, and 70%) and tap water, and placed into the autostainer. Tissue sections were treated with Proteinase K (20 μg/mL in PBS) for 8 min, incubated with endogenous biotin blocking kit (Roche Diagnostics, Florham Park, NJ, USA) for 12 min, and incubated with labeling mix: TdT (Roche, 1000 U/mL) and biotin-dUTP (Roche, 4.5 nmol/mL) for 2 h. Detection was performed with Streptavidin—HRP and DAB detection kit (Ventana Medical Systems) according to the manufacturer's instruction.

2.3.4. CD31 Immunostaining

Primary antibody, a rat anti-mouse CD31 antibody (Dianova, Pine Bush, NY, USA), was used at 2 μg/mL. Slides were incubated in the autostainer for 6 h, followed by exposure to biotinylated rabbit anti-rat IgG (Vector Laboratories, Inc., Burlingame, CA, USA, 1:200 dilution) for 60 min. Blocker D,

Streptavidin—HRP, and DAB detection kit (Ventana Medical Systems) were used according to the manufacturer's instructions.

2.4. Quantitative Analysis of Target Staining

Quantitative analysis of immunohistochemical staining was performed using a scanning microscope (Panoramic Flash 250, 3DHisttech, Budapest, Hungary) with image processing analytical software. Findings were confirmed by microscopic evaluation.

3. Results

Previous studies have shown that gC1qR is upregulated in a variety of breast cancer cell lines including MDA231 triple negative cells [12,25,26], and human breast cancer tumors [14,15]. In the present study, we used the 60.11 monoclonal antibody directed against the C1q binding domain of gC1qR to assess tumor development in mice transplanted with MDA-231 cells. Compared to control mice, animals treated with 60.11 antibody developed smaller tumors (Figure 1, Table 1). A statistically significant difference in tumor volume was noted after 9 doses of 60.11 therapy (day 20) when treatment was initiated 3 days after tumor implantation (group 2), and after 10 doses of 60.11 therapy (day 35) when treatment was initiated after tumors had reached 100 mm^3 (group 3). Antibody treatment had no effect on mouse weight or physical and behavioral characteristics. Serum 60.11 concentrations, measured at study termination, were variable, with an average of 50 µg/mL (Table 1).

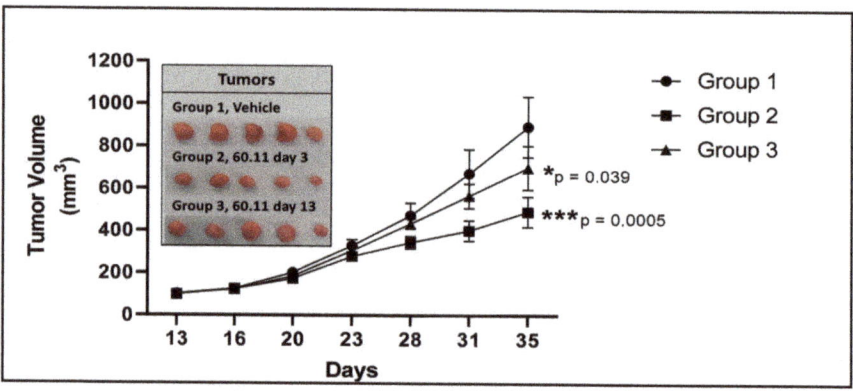

Figure 1. Tumor development in vehicle control and 60.11-treated mice. Figure 1. gC1qR therapy with 60.11 antibody inhibits MDA231 cell proliferation. Tumor volumes of vehicle-treated control mice (group 1) and mice treated with 60.11 antibody are presented over time (35 days). 60.11 therapy was initiated either three days after MDA231 cell implantation (group 2) or on day 13, when tumor volume had reached approximately 100 mm^3 (group 3). Mean and standard deviation (SD) of tumor volume is shown for each treatment group (n = 5 animals per group). P values were determined by Student t-test. (*) designates statistically significant differences in tumor volume between control and treatment groups (p < 0.05). Images of individual tumors resected at study termination are shown in the inset.

Table 1. 60.11 therapy reduces MDA231 tumor volume.

	Vehicle	60.11 Treatment (Group 2)	60.11 Treatment (Group 3)
Tumor Volume (mm^3)	894 ± 143	401 ± 48 ($p = 8.34 \times 10^{-5}$)	700 ± 104 ($p = 0.040$)
Mouse Weight (g)	24.80 ± 2.16	25.00 ± 2.00 ($p = 0.883$)	23.60 ± 1.67 ($p = 0.356$)
Serum 60.11 (µg/mL)	undetectable	52 ± 40 (median 34; range 31–124)	49 ± 25 (median 47; range 28–89)

Results obtained at study termination (day 35) represent mean ± S.D., $n = 5$. Mice in group 2 were treated with 60.11 antibody, 3 days after MDA 231 cell implantation before tumors were measurable, and received a total of 16 doses of antibody by study termination. Mice in group 3 began 60.11 treatment when tumors were measurable (100mm^3), and received a total of 11 treatment doses by study termination.

Immunohistochemical studies of excised tumors were performed to gain insight into the mechanism of action of 60.11 therapy. Results were compared between controls and treatment group 2. The data demonstrate an increase in early and late apoptosis markers, cleaved caspase 3, and TUNEL, respectively, in the treatment group (Figure 2). No difference in cell proliferation index (Ki 67) was noted.

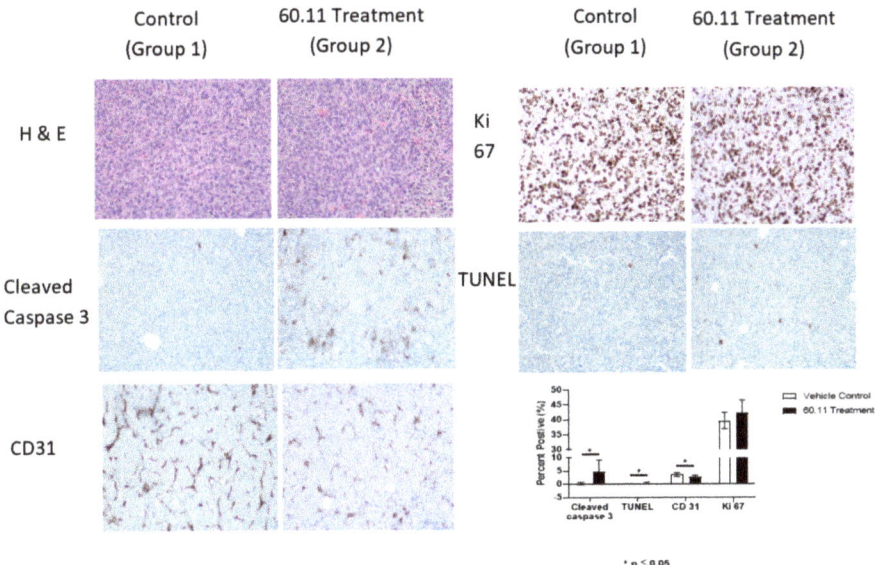

Figure 2. Histologic and immunohistochemical evaluation of MDA231 breast tumors. Figure 2 Representative histologic images (20 × original magnification) of MDA231 tumors obtained from control (group 1) and 60.11-treated (group 2) mice. Sections were stained with hematoxylin and eosin (H&E), cleaved caspase 3, CD31, Ki 76, and TUNEL. Positive immunohistochemical reactivity is represented by brown stain. Quantitative immunohistochemical evaluation is shown in the bar graph. Results represent mean ± S.D. ($n = 5$) of proportional (%) surface area staining positively for the indicated markers. (*) designates statistical significance, $p < 0.05$.

Interestingly, 60.11 therapy was associated also with decreased CD31 staining. CD31 is a murine endothelial cell marker that is widely used to assess angiogenesis in tumor models. Since gC1qR has been implicated in angiogenesis [8,25], tumors were stained with CD31 to quantify vascular structures in the developing MDA231 tumors. Fewer CD31-positive structures (brown staining) were observed in tumors from treated mice, and the CD31-positive structures appeared small, as compared to their control counterparts.

Since gC1qR is expressed not only by malignant cells but also by blood cells (B lymphocytes [13], platelets [38], neutrophils [39], eosinophils [40], and macrophages and dendritic cells [41,42]) as well as by proliferating normal cells [15], blood cell counts and vital organs were examined at study termination for on target/off tumor effects. Table 2 compares blood cell counts of control mice and mice with the greatest 60.11 exposure (group 2). Small but statistically significant differences in WBC counts, reflected by decreases in granulocytes (neutrophils, eosinophils, basophils) and lymphocytes, were noted. Reference values are influenced by differences in laboratory instrumentation, methods, collection sites, mouse age, and sex, as well as by environmental factors. Therefore, group comparisons, as shown here (control vs. treatment groups), may be more appropriate than comparisons to reference ranges alone [43].

Table 2. Comparison of peripheral blood cell counts in vehicle control and 60.11-treated mice.

Cell Count	Treatment Groups		Reference Values *
	Vehicle Control (Group 1)	60.11 Treatment (Group 2)	
RBC (10^{12}/L)	9.77 ± 0.05	9.68 ± 0.41 ($p = 0.779$)	7.4–10.1
Hgb (g/dL)	15.95 ± 0.81	15.58 ± 0.54 ($p = 0.441$)	13.2–18.0
Platelets (10^9/L)	769 ± 133	778 ± 137 ($p = 0.923$)	659–1372
WBC (10^9/L)	7.38 ± 3.50	5.09 ± 1.40 ($p = 0.005$)	2.1–11.3
Neutrophils (10^9/L)	2.10 ± 0.93	1.42 ± 0.44 ($p = 0.064$)	0.4–2.1
Lymphocytes (10^9/L)	4.98 ± 2.54	3.46 ± 1.07 ($p = 0.002$)	0.7–9.3
Monocytes (10^9/L)	0.20 ± 0.10	0.106 ± 0.052 ($p = 0.42$)	0.01–0.43
Eosinophils (10^9/L)	0.090 ± 0.24	0.094 ± 0.017 ($p = 7 \times 10^{-5}$)	0–0.4
Basophils (10^9/L)	0.010 ± 0.005	0.006 ± 0.005 ($p = 2 \times 10^{-5}$)	0–0.03

Results represent mean ± S.D., $n = 5$. * Reference values reflect locally established ranges for athymic nude mice. Blood was obtained from the retro-orbital plexus before sacrifice.

No evidence of tissue damage was observed by histologic examination of vital organs (Appendix B). In particular, lining cells of the gastrointestinal tract, previously reported to express higher levels of gC1qR than other normal tissue [15], were closely examined and showed no differences between treatment and control groups.

4. Discussion

The present study represents the first in vivo proof-of-concept study to evaluate the efficacy of 60.11 monoclonal gC1qR antibody therapy in a murine orthotopic xenotransplant model of triple negative breast cancer. Human gC1qR is a multiligand multicompartmental cellular protein, which is found in the cytosol, plasma membrane, and mitochondria. In addition, soluble forms are released into the surrounding milieu by proliferating cells [21,44,45]. Indeed, in vitro studies by Kandov et al. [12] suggested not only that gC1qR blockade inhibits breast cancer cell proliferation, but also that extracellular, soluble gC1qR enhances cancer cell proliferation via interaction with cell surface-associated C1q. C1q has been detected on breast cancer cells in vitro by flow cytometry [12], and in human tumors by immunohistochemistry [7].

Based on this information, we tested the therapeutic potential of a gC1qR antibody (60.11), which is directed against the C1q binding site of gC1qR (aa 74–282) [23], in an orthotopic xenotransplant mouse model using the MDA231 cell line, which was previously shown to bind the 60.11 antibody [21]. In the absence of formal pharmacokinetic studies, the 60.11 dosing strategy was based on our previous experience in rats [35] and the desire to achieve plasma concentrations in excess of 10 µg/mL, which are required to demonstrate antiproliferative effects in vitro [12]. Serum 60.11 levels at study termination averaged 50 µg/mL, ranging from 28 to 124 µg/mL.

The results demonstrate that 60.11 therapy inhibits MDA231 breast cancer cell proliferation in vivo. When treatment was begun three days after MDA231 cell implantation (group 2), a statistically significant antibody effect was observed after nine doses of antibody therapy (day 20). Differences in tumor volume between controls and treatment group 2 continued to increase for the remainder of the treatment period (15 days). At the time of study termination, day 35, the average tumor size of treated mice in group 2 was 50% smaller compared to controls. Significant reductions in tumor size were also achieved when the 60.11 treatment was begun after visible tumors had formed (group 3). A statistically significant difference in tumor volume was noted after 10 doses of 60.11 therapy (day 35). Treatment with the 60.11 antibody was associated with increased MDA231 tumor cell apoptosis and decreased angiogenesis.

Previous studies have documented that MDA231 breast cancer tumors in mice retain gC1qR expression, and that the intratumoral distribution of gC1qR, when assessed by immunohistochemical staining, is consistent with a cell surface gC1qR expression pattern [46]. Despite the ubiquitous expression of gC1qR by normal cells and tissues, previous studies showed highly selective anti-gC1qR antibody uptake by MDA231 tumors in vivo [46]. These observations are consistent with our finding that 60.11 therapy is not associated with overt toxicities in vital organs.

Animal weights remained constant, and histologic examination of vital organs, showed no pathologic, inflammatory, or degenerative lesions. However, a small decrease in blood leukocyte counts (granulocytes, lymphocytes) was observed in the 60.11 treatment group. Formal toxicity studies are required to further evaluate the on target/off tumor effects of 60.11 antibody therapy. It is important to note that any observations of toxicity may be limited in an immunocompromised mouse model. Therefore, our limited studies explored potential toxicities related to the antiproliferative effect of 60.11 antibody therapy.

gC1qR is involved in a variety of cellular processes [11]. Although this pilot study was performed with a single breast cancer cell line, the results support the concept that gC1qR may play a broader role in breast cancer cell proliferation. The observed 60.11 treatment-induced inhibition of MDA231 cell proliferation via increased apoptosis suggests a direct effect on cell proliferation. These findings are consistent with previous observations demonstrating reduced proliferation of MDA231 breast cancer cells following gC1qR knock-down [26]. Additionally, the present study provides evidence that modulation of MDA231 tumor development by 60.11 treatment may also occur via impaired angiogenesis.

Angiogenesis is essential for tumor growth in vivo. Tumor angiogenesis requires endothelial cell migration into the tumor, followed by endothelial cell organization into hollow tubes that develop into functional blood vessels [47]. C1q is an important factor in endothelial cell tube formation [8]. In the present study, immunohistochemical staining of tumors from 60.11 antibody-treated mice was remarkable, not only for decreased staining with the endothelial cell marker CD31 compared to controls, but also for the presence of much smaller CD31 staining vascular structures.

Results from this pilot study generate several important questions. Pharmacokinetic and pharmacodynamic studies are needed to better understand the therapeutic potential and toxicologic profile of 60.11 therapy. At a mechanistic level, the contribution of antibody inhibition of the cell surface and extracellular gC1qR warrants further exploration. Further, the role of antibody-dependent cytotoxicity in any observed antitumor effect must be considered but cannot be assessed in the present study with immunodeficient mice.

The expanding non-traditional roles of complement have been identified in recent years, including the participation of C1q in cancer [48]. C1q, a constituent of the first component of complement, has been identified in the microenvironment of breast cancer, as well as colon, lung, and pancreatic cancers, in addition to melanoma [7]. Interestingly, C1q localization in the tumor microenvironment appears concentrated on tumor microvascular endothelial cells and stroma, and is independent of peripheral blood C1q levels, suggesting local synthesis. Indeed, the genes for C1q A, B, and C chains are highly expressed in the stroma of human breast cancers, and high expression levels are associated with poor prognosis [49]. Moreover, C1q deficiency has been associated with decreased tumor growth and enhanced survival in a mouse melanoma model [7]. Results from the present study support the concept that blocking C1q–gC1qR interactions may represent a novel treatment approach in breast cancer, and potentially other malignancies associated with increased gC1qR expression.

5. Patents

EP and BG hold a licensed patent for the use of gC1qR antibodies in angioedema and cancer.

Author Contributions: Conceptualization, E.I.P. and B.G.; methodology, E.I.P., B.G., E.d.S., K.M.-T., Q.C., A.B., A.G.S., B.V.G.; formal analysis, E.I.P.,Q.C.; investigation, E.d.S., Q.C., K.M.-T., A.B., A.G.S., B.G., B.V.G.; writing—original draft preparation, E.I.P., B.G.; writing—review and editing, all authors. All authors have read and agreed to the published version of the manuscript.

Funding: This research was funded by in part by grants from the National Institutes of Allergy and Infectious Diseases R01 AI 060866 and R01 AI-084178 (to BG),the NIH/NCI Cancer Center Support grant P30 CA008748 (to MSKCC), and a grant from the Terry Johnson Cancer Research Center (to BVG).

Conflicts of Interest: EIP and BG have licensed the 60.11 antibody for commercial distribution through Stony Brook Research Foundation and receive royalties.

Appendix A

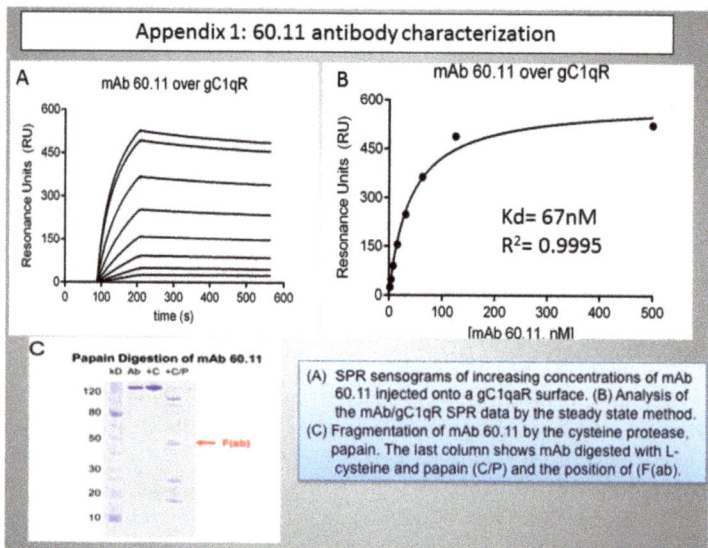

Figure A1. 60.11 antibody characterization.

Appendix B

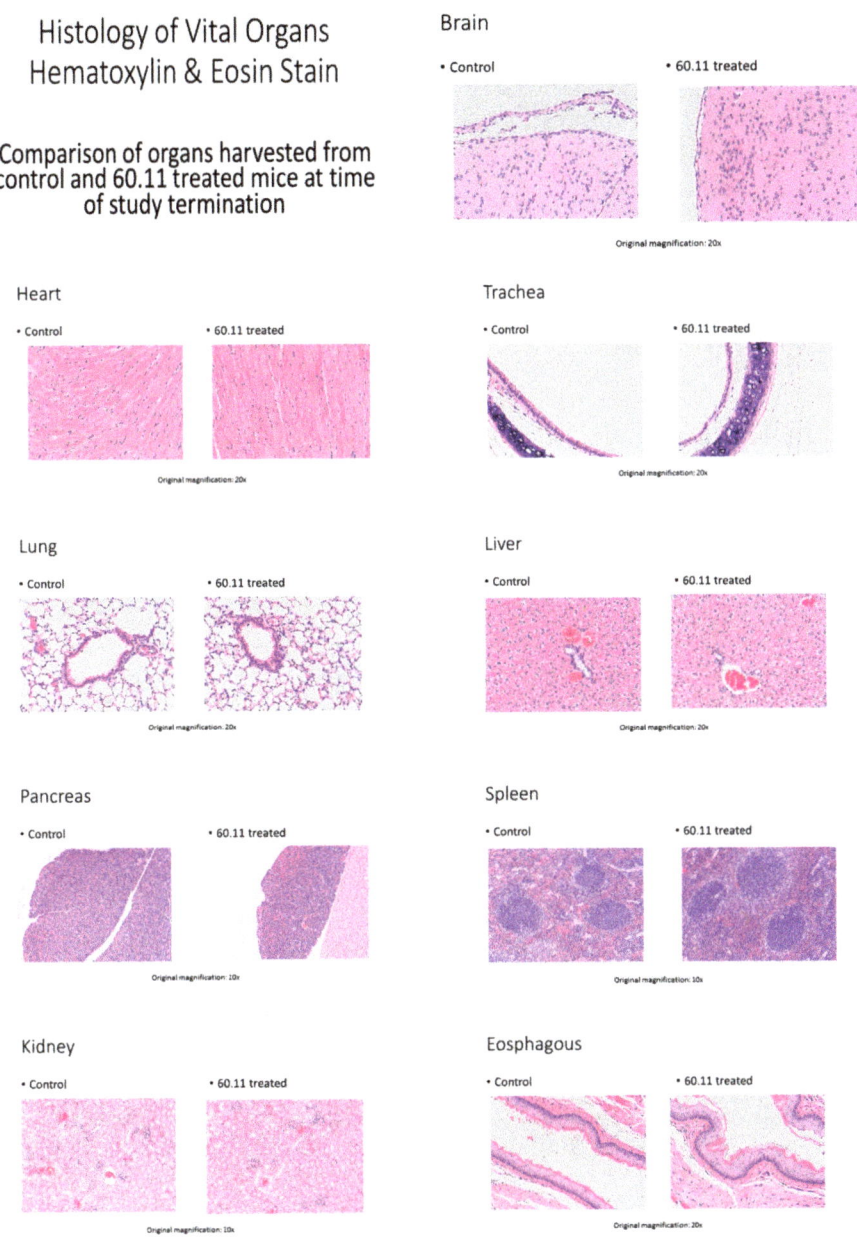

Figure A2. *Cont.*

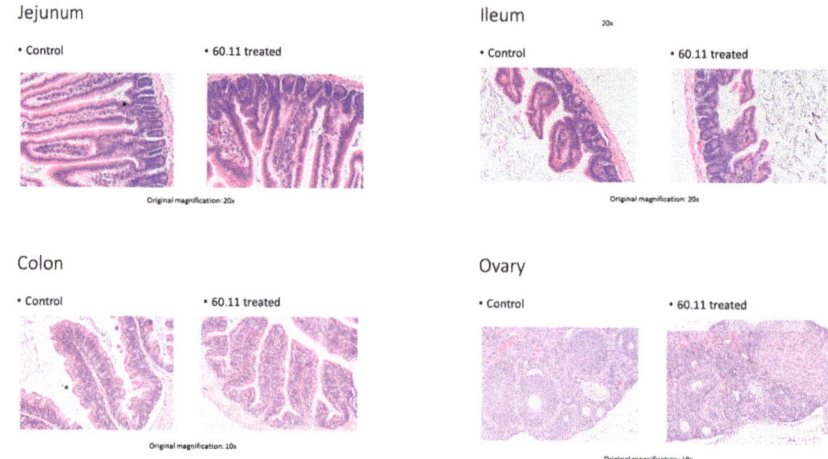

Figure A2. Representative histology of vital organs from control and 60.11 treated animals.

References

1. Shah, S.P.; Roth, A.; Goya, R.; Oloumi, A.; Ha, G.; Zhao, Y.; Turashvili, G.; Ding, J.; Tse, K.; Haffari, G. The clonal and mutational evolution spectrum of primary triple-negative breast cancers. *Nature* **2012**, *486*, 395–399. [CrossRef] [PubMed]
2. Dawood, S.; Broglio, K.; Esteva, F.J.; Yang, W.; Kau, S.W.; Islam, R.; Albarracin, C.; Yu, T.K.; Green, M.; Hortobagyi, G.N.; et al. Survival among women with triple receptor-negative breast cancer and brain metastases. *Ann. Oncol.* **2009**, *20*, 621–628. [CrossRef] [PubMed]
3. Haffty, B.G.; Yang, Q.; Reiss, M.; Kearney, T.; Higgins, S.A.; Weidhaas, J.; Harris, L.; Hait, W.; Toppmeyer, D. Locoregional relapse and distant metastasis in conservatively managed triple negative early-stage breast cancer. *J. Clin. Oncol.* **2006**, *24*, 5652–5657. [CrossRef] [PubMed]
4. Dianan, A.; Franzese, E.; Centonze, S.; Carlino, F.; Della Corte, C.M.; Ventriglia, J.; Petrillo, A.; De Vita, F.; Alfano, R.; Ciardiello, F.; et al. Triple-negative breast cancers: Systematic review of the literature on molecular and clinical features with a focus on treatment with innovative drugs. *Curr. Oncol. Rep.* **2018**, *20*, 76. [CrossRef]
5. Tray, N.; Adams, S.; Esteva, F.J. Antibody-drug conjugates in triple negative breast cancer. *Future Oncol.* **2018**, *14*, 2651–2661. [CrossRef]
6. Kourtzelis, I.; Rafail, S. The dual role of complement in cancer and its implication in anti-tumor therapy. *Ann. Transl. Med.* **2016**, *4*, 265. [CrossRef]
7. Bulla, R.; Tripodo, C.; Rami, D.; Ling, G.S.; Agostinis, C.; Guarnotta, C.; Zorzet, S.; Durigutto, P.; Botto, M.; Tedesco, F. C1q acts in the tumor microenvironment as a cancer-promoting factor independently of complement activation. *Nature Commun.* **2016**, *7*, 10346. [CrossRef]
8. Bossi, F.; Tripodo, C.; Rizzi, L.; Bulla, R.; Agostinis, C.; Guarnotta, C.; Munaut, C.; Baldassarre, G.; Papa, G.; Zorzet, S.; et al. C1q as a unique player in angiogenesis with therapeutic implication in wound healing. *Proc. Natl. Acad. Sci. USA* **2014**, *111*, 4209–4214. [CrossRef]
9. Ghebrehiwet, B.; Hosszu, K.K.; Valentino, A.; Peerschke, E.I.B. The C1q family of proteins: Insights into the emerging non-traditional functions. *Front. Immunol.* **2012**, *3*, 52. [CrossRef]
10. Peerschke, E.I.B.; Ghebrehiwet, B. cC1qR/CR and gC1qR/p33: Observations in cancer. *Mol. Immunol.* **2014**, *61*, 100–109. [CrossRef]
11. Saha, P.; Datta, K. Multifunction, multicompartmental hyaluronan-binding protein 1 (HABP1/p32/gC1qR: Implication in cancer progression and metastasis. *Oncotarget* **2018**, *9*, 10784–10807. [CrossRef] [PubMed]
12. Kandov, E.; Kaur, A.; Kishore, U.; Ji, P.; Williams, J.; Peerschke, E.I.B.; Ghebrehiwet, B. C1q and C1q receptors (gC1qR and cC1qR) as potential novel targets for therapy against breast cancer. *Cur. Trends Immunol.* **2018**, *19*, 59–76.

13. Ghebrehiwet, B.; Lim, B.L.; Peerschke, E.I.; Willis, A.C.; Reid, K.B. Isolation, cDNA cloning, and overexpression of a 33-kDa cell surface glycoprotein that binds to the globular "heads" of C1q. *J. Exp. Med.* **1994**, *179*, 1809–1821. [CrossRef] [PubMed]
14. Rubinstein, D.B.; Stortchevoi, A.; Boosalis, M.; Ashfaq, R.; Ghebrehiwet, B.; Peerschke, E.I.; Calvo, F.; Guillaume, T. Receptor for the globular heads of C1q (gC1q-R, p33, hyaluronan binding protein) is preferentially expressed by adenocarcinoma cells. *Int. J. Cancer* **2004**, *110*, 741–750. [CrossRef] [PubMed]
15. Dembitzer, F.R.; Kinoshita, Y.; Burstein, D.; Phelps, R.G.; Beasley, M.B.; Garcia, R.; Harpaz, N.; Jaffer, S.; Thung, S.N.; Unger, P.D.; et al. gC1qR expression in normal and pathologic human tissues: Differential expression in tissues of epithelial and mesenchymal origin. *J. Histochem. Cytochem.* **2012**, *60*, 467–474. [CrossRef]
16. Chen, Y.B.; Jiang, C.T.; Zhang, G.Q.; Wang, J.S.; Pang, D. Increased expression of hyaluronic acid binding protein 1 is correlated with poor prognosis in patients with breast cancer. *J. Surg. Oncol.* **2009**, *100*, 382–386. [CrossRef]
17. Jiang, Y.; Wu, H.; Liu, J.; Chen, Y.; Xie, J.; Zhao, Y.; Pang, D. Increased breast cancer risk with HABP1/p32/gC1qR genetic polymorphism rs2285747 and its upregulation in northern Chinese women. *Oncotarget* **2017**, *8*, 13932–13941. [CrossRef]
18. Amamoto, R.; Yagi, M.; Song, Y.; Oda, Y.; Tsuneyoshi, M.; Naito, S.; Yokomizo, A.; Kuroiwa, K.; Tokunaga, S.; Kato, S.; et al. Mitochondrial p32/C1QBP is highly expressed in prostate cancer and is associated with shorter prostate-specific antigen relapse time after radical prostatectomy. *Cancer Sci.* **2011**, *102*, 639–647. [CrossRef]
19. Yu, G.; Wang, J. Significance of hyaluronan binding protein [HABP1/P32/gC1qR] expression in advanced serous ovarian cancer patients. *Exp. Mol. Pathol.* **2013**, *94*, 210–215. [CrossRef]
20. Zhao, J.; Liu, T.; Yu, G.; Wang, J. Overexpression of HABP1 correlated with clinicopathological characteristics and unfavorable prognosis in endometrial cancer. *Tumour Biol.* **2015**, *36*, 1299–1306. [CrossRef]
21. Fogal, V.; Zhang, L.; Krajewski, S.; Ruoslahti, E. Mitochondria/cell surface protein p32/gC1qR as a molecular target in tumor cells and tumor stroma. *Cancer Res.* **2008**, *68*, 7210–7218. [CrossRef] [PubMed]
22. Paasonen, L.; Sharma, S.; Braun, G.B.; Katamraju, V.R.; Chung, T.D.Y.; She, Z.; Sugahara, K.N.; Yliperttula, M.; Wu, B.; Pellecchia, M.; et al. New p32/gC1qR ligands for targeted drug delivery. *Chembiochemistry* **2016**, *17*, 570–575. [CrossRef]
23. Ghebrehiwet, B.; Jesty, J.; Peerschke, E.I.B. gC1qR/p33: Structure-function predictions from the crystal structure. *Immunobiology* **2002**, *205*, 421–432. [CrossRef] [PubMed]
24. Park, M.K.; Lee, C.H.; Lee, H. Mouse models of breast cancer in preclinical research. *Lab. Anim. Res.* **2018**, *34*, 160–165. [CrossRef] [PubMed]
25. Kim, B.-C.; Hwang, H.-J.; An, H.-T.; Lee, H.; Partk, J.-S.; Hong, J.; Ko, J.; Kim, C.; Lee, J.-S.; Ko, Y.-G. Antibody neutralization of cell-surface gC1qR/HABP1/SF2-p32 prevents lamellipodia formation and tumorigenesis. *Oncotarget* **2016**, *7*, 49972–49985. [CrossRef]
26. McGee, A.M.; Douglas, D.L.; Liang, Y.; Hyder, S.M.; Baines, C.P. The mitochondrial protein C1qbp promotes cell proliferation, migration and resistance to cell death. *Cell Cycle* **2011**, *10*, 4119–4127. [CrossRef]
27. Ghebrehiwet, B.; Lu, P.D.; Zhang, W.; Lim, B.-L.; Eggleton, P.; Leigh, L.E.A.; Reid, K.B.M.; Peerschke, E.I.B. Identification of functional domins on gC1q-R, a cell surface protein, which binds to the globular heads of C1q, using monoclonal antibodies and synthetic peptides. *Hybridoma* **1996**, *15*, 333–344. [CrossRef]
28. Ghebrehiwet, B.; Geisbrecht, B.V.; Xu, X.; Savitt, A.G.; Peerschke, E.I.B. The C1q receptors: Focus on gC1qR [C1qBP, p32, HABP-1]. *Semin. Immunol.* **2019**, *45*, 101338. [CrossRef]
29. Lim, B.L.; White, R.A.; Hummel, G.S.; Mak, S.C.; Schwaeble, W.J.; Reid, K.B.M.; Peerschke, E.I.B.; Ghebrehiwet, B. Characterization of the murine gene for gC1q-BP [gC1q-R], a novel cell protein that binds the globular heads of C1q, vitronectin, high molecular weight kinogen and factor XII. *Gene* **1998**, *209*, 229–237. [CrossRef]
30. Lynch, N.J.; Reid, K.B.M.; van den Berg, R.H.; Daha, M.R.; Leigh, L.E.A.; Lim, B.L.; Ghebrehiwet, B.; Schwaeble, W.J. The murine homologues of gC1qBP, a 33kDa protein that binds to the globular 'heads' of C1q. *FEBS Lett.* **1997**, *418*, 111–114. [CrossRef]
31. Savitt, A.G.; Mena-Taboada, P.; Monsalve, G.; Benach, J.L. Francisella tularensis infection-derived monoclonal antibodies provide detection, protection and therapy. *Clin. Vacc. Immunol.* **2009**, *16*, 414–422. [CrossRef]

32. Chang, Q.; Bournazou, E.; Sansone, P.; Berishaj, M.; Gao, S.P.; Daly, L.; Wels, J.; Theilen, T.; Granitto, S.; Zhang, X.; et al. The IL-6/JAK/STAT3 feed-forward loop drives tumorigenesis and metastasis. *Neoplasia* **2013**, *15*, 848–862. [CrossRef] [PubMed]
33. Gao, S.P.; Chang, Q.; Mao, N.; Daly, L.A.; Vogel, R.; Chan, T.; Liu, S.H.; Bournazou, E.; Schori, E.; Zhang, H.; et al. JAK2 inhibition sensitizes resistant EGFR-mutant lung adenocarcinoma to tyrosine kinase inhibitors. *Cancer* **2016**, *9*, 421–445. [CrossRef] [PubMed]
34. Moroz, M.A.; Kochetkov, T.; Cai, S.; Wu, J.; Shamis, M.; Nair, J.; de Stanchina, E.; Serganova, I.; Schwartz, G.K.; Banerjee, D.; et al. Imaging colon cancer response following treatment with AZD1152: A preclinical analysis of [^{18}F]Fluoro-2-deoxuglucose and 3′-deoxy-3′-[^{18}F]Fluorothymidine imaging. *Clin. Cancer Res.* **2011**, *17*, 1099–1110. [CrossRef] [PubMed]
35. Peerschke, E.I.B.; Bayer, A.S.; Ghebrehiwet, B.; Xiong, Y.Q. gC1qR/p33 blockade reduces *Staphylococcus aureus* colonization of target tissues in an animal model of infective endocarditis. *Infect. Immun.* **2006**, *74*, 4418–4423. [CrossRef]
36. Rodrik-Outmezguine, V.S.; Okaniwa, M.; Yao, Z.; Novotny, C.J.; McWhirter, C.; Banaji, A.; Won, H.; Wong, W.; Berger, M.; de Stanchina, E.; et al. Overcoming mTOR resistance mutations with a new-generation mTOR inhibitor. *Nature* **2016**, *534*, 272–276. [CrossRef]
37. Shaffer, D.R.; Viale, A.; Ishiwata, R.; Leversha, M.; Olgac, S.; Manova, K.; Satagopan, J.; Scher, H.; Koff, A. Evidence for a p27 tumor suppressive function independent of its role regulating cell proliferation in the prostate. *Proc. Natl. Acad. Sci. USA* **2005**, *102*, 210–215. [CrossRef]
38. Peerschke, E.I.B.; Reid, K.B.M.; Ghebrehiwet, B. Identification of a novel 33-kDa C1q binding site on human blood platelets. *J. Immunol.* **1994**, *152*, 5896–5901.
39. Eggleton, P.; Ghebrehiwet, B.; Sastry, K.N.; Coburn, J.P.; Zaner, K.S.; Reid, K.B.M.; Tauber, A.I. Identification of a gC1q-bindin protein [gC1q-R] on the surface of human neutrophils. Subcellular localization and binding properties in comparison with cC1q-R. *J. Clin. Investig.* **1995**, *95*, 1569–1578. [CrossRef]
40. Kuna, P.; Iyer, M.; Peerschke, E.I.; Kaplan, A.P.; Reid, K.B.; Ghebrehiwet, B. Human C1q induces eosinophil migration. *Clin. Immunol. Immunopathol.* **1996**, *81*, 48–54. [CrossRef]
41. Steinberger, P.; Szekeres, A.; Wille, S.; Stockl, J.; Selenko, N.; Prager, E.; Staffler, G.; Madic, O.; Stockinger, H.; Knapp, W. Identification of human CD93 as the phagocytic C1q receptor [C1qRP] by expression cloning. *J. Leukoc. Biol.* **2002**, *71*, 33–140.
42. Vegh, Z.; Goyarts, E.C.; Rozengarten, K.; Mazumder, A.; Ghebrehiwet, B. Maturation-dependent expression of C1q-binding proteins on the cell surface of human monocyte-derived dendritic cells. *Int. Immunopharmacol.* **2003**, *3*, 345–357. [CrossRef]
43. O'Connell, D.E.; Mikkola, A.M.; Stepanek, A.M.; Vernet, A.; Hall, C.D.; Sun, C.C.; Yildririm, E.; Starpoli, J.F.; Lee, J.T.; Brown, D.E. Practical murine hematopathology: A comparative review and implications for research. *Comp. Med.* **2015**, *65*, 96–113.
44. Ghebrehiwet, B.; Peerschke, E.I.B. Structure and function of gC1qR: A multiligand binding cellular protein. *Immunobiology* **1998**, *199*, 225–238. [CrossRef]
45. Peterson, K.L.; Zhang, W.; Lu, P.D.; Keilbaugh, S.A.; Peerschke, E.I.; Ghebrehiwet, B. The C1q-binding cell membrane proteins cC1qR and gC1qR are released from activated cells: Subcellular distribution and immunochemical characterization. *Clin. Immunol. Immunopathol.* **1997**, *84*, 17–26. [CrossRef]
46. Sanchez-Martin, D.; Cuesta, A.M.; Fogal, V.; Ruoslahti, E.; Alvarez-Vallin, L. The multicompartmental p32/gC1qR as a new target for antibody-based tumor targeting strategies. *J. Biol. Chem.* **2011**, *286*, 5197–5203. [CrossRef]
47. Nishida, N.; Yano, H.; Nishida, T.; Kamura, T.; Kojiro, M. Angiogenesis in Cancer. *Vasc. Health Risk Manag.* **2006**, *2*, 213–219. [CrossRef]
48. Loveland, B.E.; Cebon, J. Cancer exploiting complement: A clue or an exception? *Nat. Immunol.* **2008**, *9*, 1205–1206. [CrossRef]
49. Winslow, S.; Leandersson, K.; Edsjo, A.; Larssen, C. Prognostic stromal gene signatures in breast cancer. *Breast Cancer Res.* **2015**, *17*, 23. [CrossRef]

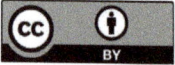

© 2020 by the authors. Licensee MDPI, Basel, Switzerland. This article is an open access article distributed under the terms and conditions of the Creative Commons Attribution (CC BY) license (http://creativecommons.org/licenses/by/4.0/).

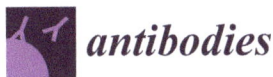

Article

Enhancing CDC and ADCC of CD19 Antibodies by Combining Fc Protein-Engineering with Fc Glyco-Engineering

Sophia Roßkopf [1], Klara Marie Eichholz [1], Dorothee Winterberg [2], Katarina Julia Diemer [1], Sebastian Lutz [3], Ira Alexandra Münnich [3], Katja Klausz [1], Thies Rösner [1], Thomas Valerius [1], Denis Martin Schewe [2], Andreas Humpe [3], Martin Gramatzki [1], Matthias Peipp [1,*,†] and Christian Kellner [3,†]

[1] Division of Stem Cell Transplantation and Immunotherapy, Department of Medicine II Christian-Albrechts-University Kiel and University Hospital Schleswig-Holstein, Campus Kiel, 24105 Kiel, Germany; sophia.rosskopf@onlinehome.de (S.R.); klara.eichholz@gmx.de (K.M.E.); katarina_julia@icloud.com (K.J.D.); k.klausz@med2.uni-kiel.de (K.K.); t.roesner@med2.uni-kiel.de (T.R.); t.valerius@med2.uni-kiel.de (T.V.); m.gramatzki@med2.uni-kiel.de (M.G.)
[2] Pediatric Hematology/Oncology, Christian-Albrechts-University Kiel and University Hospital Schleswig-Holstein, Campus Kiel, 24105 Kiel, Germany; Dorothee.Winterberg@uksh.de (D.W.); Denis.Schewe@uksh.de (D.M.S.)
[3] Department of Transfusion Medicine, Cell Therapeutics and Hemostaseology, University Hospital, LMU Munich, 81377 Munich, Germany; Sebastian.Lutz@med.uni-muenchen.de (S.L.); Ira.Muennich@med.uni-muenchen.de (I.A.M.); Andreas.Humpe@med.uni-muenchen.de (A.H.); Christian.Kellner@med.uni-muenchen.de (C.K.)
* Correspondence: m.peipp@med2.uni-kiel.de; Tel.: +49-431-500-22701
† These authors contributed equally to this work.

Received: 16 September 2020; Accepted: 9 November 2020; Published: 17 November 2020

Abstract: Background: Native cluster of differentiation (CD) 19 targeting antibodies are poorly effective in triggering antibody-dependent cell-mediated cytotoxicity (ADCC) and complement-dependent cytotoxicity (CDC), which are crucial effector functions of therapeutic antibodies in cancer immunotherapy. Both functions can be enhanced by engineering the antibody's Fc region by altering the amino acid sequence (Fc protein-engineering) or the Fc-linked glycan (Fc glyco-engineering). We hypothesized that combining Fc glyco-engineering with Fc protein-engineering will rescue ADCC and CDC in CD19 antibodies. Results: Four versions of a CD19 antibody based on tafasitamab's V-regions were generated: a native IgG1, an Fc protein-engineered version with amino acid exchanges S267E/H268F/S324T/G236A/I332E (EFTAE modification) to enhance CDC, and afucosylated, Fc glyco-engineered versions of both to promote ADCC. Irrespective of fucosylation, antibodies carrying the EFTAE modification had enhanced C1q binding and were superior in inducing CDC. In contrast, afucosylated versions exerted an enhanced affinity to Fcγ receptor IIIA and had increased ADCC activity. Of note, the double-engineered antibody harboring the EFTAE modification and lacking fucose triggered both CDC and ADCC more efficiently. Conclusions: Fc glyco-engineering and protein-engineering could be combined to enhance ADCC and CDC in CD19 antibodies and may allow the generation of antibodies with higher therapeutic efficacy by promoting two key functions simultaneously.

Keywords: antibody therapy; cluster of differentiation 19 (CD19); CD19; Fc fragment crystallizable (Fc); Fc engineering; complement-dependent cytotoxicity (CDC); antibody-dependent cell-mediated cytotoxicity (ADCC)

1. Introduction

Therapeutic antibodies have considerably improved treatment outcomes both in solid tumors and in hematological malignancies [1]. In the treatment of lymphomas, antibody therapy is well established and both native antibodies such as rituximab and immunoconjugates have been approved for clinical use. Besides cluster of differentiation (CD) 20, the CD19 antigen represents an attractive target for antibody-based immunotherapy of B-lineage lymphomas and leukemias [2,3]. CD19 shows a favorable expression pattern, since its expression is restricted to the B-cell lineage, where it is displayed from very early to mature stages of B cell differentiation. However, the clinical development of CD19 antibodies was hampered by a lack of efficacy of native IgG1 antibodies. Thus, in contrast to CD20 antibodies, native CD19 antibodies are unable to elicit antibody key effector functions, since they do not induce growth arrest or programmed cell death and are only poorly effective in triggering complement-dependent cytotoxicity (CDC), antibody-dependent cell-mediated cytotoxicity (ADCC) or antibody-dependent cellular phagocytosis (ADCP). Strategies to target CD19 mainly focused on T cell recruitment [4], which led to clinical approval of the [CD19 × CD3] bispecific T cell engager (BiTE) molecule blinatumomab and two chimeric antigen receptor (CAR) T cell products, tisagenlecleucel and axicabtagen–ciloleucel [5,6]. However, most recently, the CD19 antibody tafasitamab (formerly MOR208 or Xmab®5574), which was optimized by engineering its fragment crystalizable (Fc) domain to overcome limitations of native CD19 antibodies, has demonstrated clinical efficacy and has received approval by the FDA for combination treatment with the immunomodulatory drug lenalidomide in diffuse large B cell lymphoma (DLBCL) patients [7,8].

Key observations underlining the importance of antibody functions that depend on the Fc domain such as CDC or the recruitment of effector cells for ADCC by engagement of Fcγ receptors (FcγR) on various effector cells have provided a rational basis for the development of Fc engineering strategies for the generation of tailor-made antibodies with enhanced efficacy [9]. The importance of CDC has been demonstrated in selected murine xenograft models [10] and clinical observations have suggested a role for CDC in CD20 antibody therapy. Thus, the consumption of complement proteins following rituximab injection has been observed in lymphoma patients and individual patients benefited from the administration of plasma as a complement source [11,12]. In addition, augmented expression of the inhibitory membrane-bound complement regulatory protein (mCRP) CD59 has been related to rituximab resistance in chronic lymphocytic leukemia (CLL) patients [13]. Besides its potential contribution to the therapeutic activity of monoclonal antibodies, complement activation has also been associated with first infusion reactions.

The importance of effector cell recruitment was demonstrated in murine xenograft models [14,15]. Moreover, clinical observations suggest the importance of effective FcγR engagement also in patients. Thus, lymphoma patients homozygous for the FcγRIIIA-158V allelic version, which is bound by the antibody's Fc region with higher affinity, showed better responses to rituximab therapy than did patients carrying the low-affinity FcγRIIIA-158F allele, suggesting functions as ADCC or ADCP as important mechanisms by which the antibody depletes lymphoma cells [16–18]. However, a consistent effect of FcγR genotype on the clinical anti-tumour activity of therapeutic IgG1 antibodies has not been observed in all published clinical studies [19,20].

Currently, two main Fc engineering technologies exist, which either rely on modifying the Fc-associated glycan linked to amino acid N297 or on altering the amino acid sequence in the C1q and FcγR binding sites within the antibody constant heavy chain 2 (CH2) domain [9]. For example, the fucose content in antibody preparations was reduced and afucosylated antibodies or antibodies with significantly reduced fucose content exerted a higher affinity to FcγRIII (CD16), whose activating isoform (FcγRIIIA) is expressed by natural killer (NK) cells, macrophages and certain γδ-T cell subsets in humans, while binding to other FcγR was not affected. Alternatively, Fc protein-engineering was shown to be a valid approach to improve Fc mediated antibody functions. Amino acid substitutions were identified that greatly improved binding to activating FcγR and enhanced the antibody's ability to trigger NK cell ADCC or ADCP by macrophages. Other substitutions were demonstrated to enhance

CDC by improving binding to C1q [21,22]. However, maintenance of ADCC function was difficult in such engineered antibodies optimized for C1q binding, because certain modifications that on the one side enhanced CDC diminished on the other side FcγR binding and ADCC. Therefore, additional amino acid substitutions were necessary. For example, a gain in CDC was achieved by the introduction of amino acid exchanges S267E/H268F/S324T in the CH2 domain, but the two additional substitutions G236A/I332E were also necessary to preserve ADCC activity ("EFTAE modification") [21]. Moreover, mixed isotype IgG1/IgG3 antibodies exerted improved CDC activity, and also the introduction of certain amino acid exchanges that promote assembly of antibody hexamers augmented CDC [23]. CDC was further improved by combinations of such antibodies recognizing different antigens such as CD20 and CD37 that are co-expressed on certain lymphomas [24]. Yet, simultaneous enhancement of both ADCC and CDC functions to increase the potency of native IgG1 molecules by amino acid alteration was difficult, presumably because the binding sites for FcγR and C1q overlap [25–27].

Fc engineering technologies are particularly important for improving CD19 antibodies that in general exert poor effector functions [4]. Thus, Fc engineering has been applied for CD19 antibodies to favor effector cell recruitment and resulted in CD19 antibodies now being capable of triggering ADCC and ADCP effectively. Thus, CD19 antibodies carrying amino acid substitutions S239D/I332E ("DE modification") such as antibody tafasitamab (formerly MOR208 or Xmab®5574) were found to be more effective in inducing NK-cell-mediated ADCC and ADCP by macrophages [7,28,29]. Importantly, the comparison of tafasitamab with its native counterpart revealed that in non-human primates Fc engineering was essential for B cell depletion [30]. Clinically, promising results were obtained with tafasitamab single-agent therapy in B cell Non-Hodgkin lymphoma [31], and therapeutic efficacy has been demonstrated for this antibody in combination with lenalidomide in DLBCL not eligible for autologous stem-cell transplantation [8]. Recently, tafasitamab in combination with lenalidomide has received approval by the FDA for the treatment of adult patients with relapsed or refractory DLBCL, making the antibody the fourth clinically approved Fc engineered antibody optimized for enhanced FcγR binding in oncology next to mogamulizumab, obinutuzumab and Belantamab–Mafodotin, which bind the CC chemokine receptor 4, CD20 and B cell maturation antigen (BCMA), respectively [32]. Besides, Fc glyco-engineered, afucosylated CD19 antibodies demonstrated enhanced efficacy in triggering ADCC or ADCP and exerted therapeutic efficacy in pre-clinical models [33,34]. Clinically, promising results were obtained for monotherapy with the CD19 antibody inebilizumab, which is approved for treatment of the autoimmune disease neuromyelitis optica spectrum disorder, in a phase I study in relapsed or refractory lymphoma patients [35,36]. Finally, the feasibility to enhance CDC activity of CD19 antibodies by Fc engineering has been demonstrated by introducing the EFTAE amino acid modifications to optimize C1q binding, resulting in a CD19 antibody with potent CDC function [21]. However, Fc engineered CD19 antibodies with established CDC and ADCC activity have not been described yet.

Recently, we have shown that ADCC and CDC by CD20 antibodies can be enhanced simultaneously by concomitant Fc glyco- and Fc protein-engineering [37]. Thus, an Fc double-engineered version of rituximab was generated, in which CDC was enhanced by introducing the EFTAE modification, while ADCC was improved by expression of the antibody as an afucosylated variant in Lec13 cells. Here, we investigated whether Fc double engineering was applicable to CD19 antibody using differentially engineered versions based on V-regions of tafasitamab, of which a native IgG1 derivative is ineffective in ADCC and CDC reactions.

2. Materials and Methods

2.1. Cell Culture

Raji, Ramos, SK-BR-3 (DSMZ—German Collection of Microorganisms and Cell Cultures, Braunschweig, Germany) and baby hamster kidney (BHK)-21 cells (American Type Culture Collection, ATCC, Manassas, VA, USA) were kept in RPMI 1640 Glutamax-I medium (Thermo Fisher Scientific,

Waltham, MA, USA) containing 10% fetal calf serum (FCS; Thermo Fisher Scientific, Waltham, MA, USA), 100 U/mL penicillin and 100 µg/mL streptomycin (Thermo Fisher Scientific; R10+ medium). BHK-21 cells that were co-transfected with plasmids encoding the FcɛRI γ chain and either human FcγRIIIA 158F (BHK-CD16-158F) or FcγRIIIA 158V (BHK-CD16-158V) were cultured as described [38]. CHO glycosylation mutant Lec13 cells [39,40] were maintained in MEM alpha medium with nucleosides (Thermo Fisher Scientific, Waltham, MA, USA) supplemented with 10% dialyzed FCS (Thermo Fisher Scientific, Waltham, MA, USA) and penicillin (100 U/mL)/streptomycin (100 µg/mL). For culturing CHO-K1 and Lec13 cells transfected with antibody expression vectors, hygromycin B (Thermo Fisher Scientific, Waltham, MA, USA) was added to a concentration of 500 µg/mL. CHO cells stably transfected with a plasmid coding for the cDNA of human CD19 (Origene Technologies Inc., Rockville, MD, USA) were generated using standard procedures (Peipp, unpublished).

2.2. Antibodies

For generation of a CD19 antibody variant carrying the EFTAE amino acid modification the variable heavy chain region (VH) of a CD19 antibody (tafasitamab) was excised from vector pSectag2-CD19-HC-DE [28] and cloned as NheI/PpuMI cassette into vector pSectag2-HC-EFTAE [37] encoding a modified human IgG1 Fc region with amino acid modification, harboring the exchanges S267E/H268F/S324T/G236A/I332E [21]. The generation of expression vectors encoding tafasitamab light chain (LC) and a native CD19 IgG1 heavy chain (HC) has been described previously [28]. Fucosylated or non-fucosylated CD19 antibodies were expressed in stably transfected CHO-K1 or Lec13 cells, respectively, and purified by affinity chromatography as described previously [37]. Corresponding control antibodies against HER2 as well as the Fc engineered variant of rituximab CD20-EFTAE-CHO were produced as described earlier [37]. Trastuzumab and rituximab were obtained from Roche (Penzberg, Bavaria, Germany).

2.3. Sodium Dodecyl Sulfate Polyacrylamide Gel Electrophoresis (SDS-PAGE), Lectin Blot Analysis, WESTERN Transfer Experiments and Size Exclusion Chromatography (SEC)

Antibody integrity and concentration were determined by reducing or non-reducing SDS-PAGE following published procedures [41]. Lectin blots with biotinylated A. aurantia lectin (Vector Laboratories, Burlingame, CA, USA) and Western Transfer experiments employing goat-anti-human-IgG-HRP conjugates (Sigma Aldrich, St. Louis, MO, USA) for detection of human IgG heavy chains were performed as described [41]. SEC was performed according to standard procedures using an Äkta Pure chromatography system.

2.4. Flow Cytometry

Antibody binding to antigen-positive cells was analyzed using secondary Fluorescein isothiocyanate (FITC) or Phycoerythrin (PE) conjugates of anti-human IgG Fc F(ab')2 fragments of polyclonal goat antibodies (Dianova) and flow cytometry as described [37]. Deposition of C1q was analyzed by incubating 3×10^5 Raji cells with antibodies (25 µg/mL) in 50 µL R10+ medium on ice for 20 min. In parallel, human serum (final concentration of 2%) and antibody eculizumab (200 µg/mL) (Alexion Pharma GmbH; Munich, Germany) were incubated in R10+ medium at room temperature for 20 min to neutralize C5, before 50 µL were reacted with antibody-treated cells. After three washing steps, cell-associated C1q was detected with FITC-conjugated rabbit anti-C1q antibody (DAKO, Glostrup, Denmark) by flow cytometry.

2.5. Cytotoxicity Assay

CDC and ADCC were analyzed in 51Cr release assays following published procedures [41]. Mononuclear cells (MNC) and plasma were prepared from citrate-anticoagulated blood from healthy volunteers by density gradient centrifugation employing Easycoll (Biochrom, Berlin, Germany). In CDC experiments, plasma was added to the reactions (25%) as a source of complement and Refludan®

(Bayer HealthCare Pharmaceuticals, Wayne, NJ, USA) was used as anticoagulant at concentration of 10 µg/mL. In ADCC experiments, antibodies were analyzed at an effector-to-target cell ratio of 40:1.

2.6. Statistical Analysis

Statistical and graphical analyses were performed using software GraphPad Prism 8.0 (GraphPad Software, San Diego, CA, USA). *p*-values were calculated using repeated measures ANOVA and Bonferroni post-tests. Differences between treatment groups were regarded as statistically significant for $p < 0.05$.

3. Results

In an effort to equip CD19 antibodies with both CDC and ADCC functions, an Fc double-engineered antibody version of the CD19 antibody tafasitamab was generated by applying Fc protein-engineering and Fc glyco-engineering technologies (Figure 1A). First, the amino acid substitutions S267E/H268F/S324T/G236A/I332E (EFTAE) were introduced to establish CDC activity [21]. Second, the antibody was produced as an afucosylated variant by expression in Lec13 cells to also enhance its ability to trigger ADCC in parallel. In addition to this double-engineered CD19 antibody referred to as CD19-EFTAE-Lec13, also a native IgG1 version (CD19-wt-CHO) and corresponding mono-engineered variants, i.e., the fucosylated variant with the EFTAE modification (CD19-EFTAE-CHO) and the afucosylated antibody with native IgG1 Fc (CD19-wt-Lec13) were produced using CHO-K1 or Lec13 cells as expression hosts, respectively (Figure 1B). The antibodies were purified from cell culture supernatant by affinity chromatography of established monoclonal production lines, and the integrity of purified antibodies was verified by SDS-PAGE under reducing or non-reducing conditions and Coomassie Blue staining (Figure 1C). Selected variants were analyzed by SEC to investigate the content of multimers/aggregates (Supplementary Figure S1) Analysis of fucosylation status by lectin blot employing A. aurantia lectin revealed that antibodies produced in CHO-K1 cells were fucosylated, while fucose was almost absent in the Fc domain of antibody versions expressed in Lec13 cells (Figure 1D). Binding studies using flow cytometry indicated that all CD19 antibody variants bound to CD19-positive Ramos cells (Figure 2A) and did not react with CD19-negative SK-BR-3 breast cancer cells used as control (Figure 2B). Importantly, the four antibodies showed similar binding to CD19-transfected CHO-K1 cells and exerted almost equal affinity to the target antigen (Figure 2C). EC50 values for binding were between 2 µg/mL (13 nM) and 3 µg/mL (20 nM) for the different CD19 antibodies, in agreement with results obtained for the CD19 antibody variant with DE modification [28].

To analyze the impact of fucosylation on FcγRIIIA engagement, dose-dependent binding of the CD19 antibody variants to BHK cells transfected with expression vectors encoding either FcγRIIIA-158V or FcγRIIIA-158F expression constructs was analyzed (Figure 3A). Here, antibody variants differed considerably in their binding affinity. Of note, afucosylated antibodies bound both FcγRIIIA allelic variants with a significantly higher affinity. Thus, Fc glyco-engineering improved binding of both the antibody variant with native amino acid sequence and the version carrying the EFTAE modification. A comparison between the two afucosylated antibodies revealed that whereas they had equal binding to the high-affinity FcγRIIIA-158V allele (EC50 = 50 nM), the double-engineered antibody CD19-EFTAE-Lec13 was superior to CD19-wt-Lec13 in binding to the low-affinity FcγRIIIA-158F allele. Thus, FcγRIIIA-158V transfected cells were bound by CD19-EFTAE-Lec13 as effectively as FcγRIIIA-158F transfected cells (EC50 = 50 nM), whereas CD19-wt-Lec13 bound with lower affinity to FcγRIIIA-158F (EC50 = 180 nM). A benefit of the EFTAE modification was also observed for the fucosylated antibodies, since also CD19-EFTAE-CHO showed better binding than CD19-wt-CHO when FcγRIIIA-158F transfected cells were analyzed (Figure 3A).

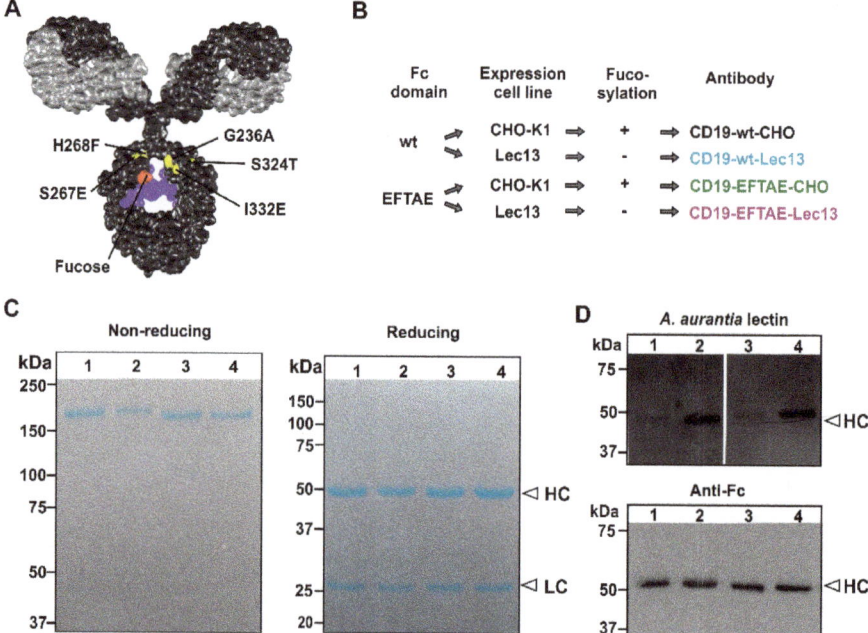

Figure 1. Generation of Fc engineered CD19 antibodies. (**A**) Structural model of an IgG molecule and illustration of amino acid exchanges S267E/H268F/S324T/G236A/I332E (EFTAE modification; in yellow) in the antibody CH2 domain, and the critical fucose residue in red. The light and heavy chains are depicted in light grey and dark grey, respectively. The N297-associated carbohydrate is colored in blue. The model is based on the pdb-file provided by Dr. Mike Clark [42] and was edited employing Discovery Studio Visualizer software (Biovia, San Diego, CA, USA). (**B**) Expression constructs for CD19 heavy chains with native (wt) or with EFTAE modified Fc domain sequences were generated and transfected into CHO-K1 and Lec13 cells for production of fucosylated antibodies (CD19-wt-CHO and CD19-EFTAE-CHO) as well as their afucosylated counterparts (CD19-wt-Lec13 and CD19-EFTAE-Lec13), respectively. (**C**) After purification by affinity chromatography antibodies were analyzed by SDS-PAGE and Coomassie blue staining under non-reducing (left gel) or reducing (right gel) conditions. Amounts of 1–2 µg protein were loaded on 6% and 12% polyacrylamide gels, respectively (Lanes: (1) CD19-EFTAE-Lec13, (2) CD19-EFTAE-CHO, (3) CD19-wt-Lec13, (4) CD19-wt-CHO). Results from one representative experiment are shown ($n = 3$). HC, heavy chain; LC, light chain. (**D**) The fucosylation status of the different antibody versions was determined by lectin blot experiments employing biotinylated A. aurantia lectin and HRP-conjugated neutrAvidin protein (upper panel), indicating that fucose was almost absent in antibodies produced in Lec13 cells. As a control, antibody heavy chains (HC) were detected in Western Transfer experiments with an HRP-coupled anti-human IgG Fc antibody (lower panel). Results from one representative experiment are shown ($n = 3$). Lanes: (1) CD19-EFTAE-Lec13 (2) CD19-EFTAE-CHO (3) CD19-wt-Lec13 (4) CD19-wt-CHO).

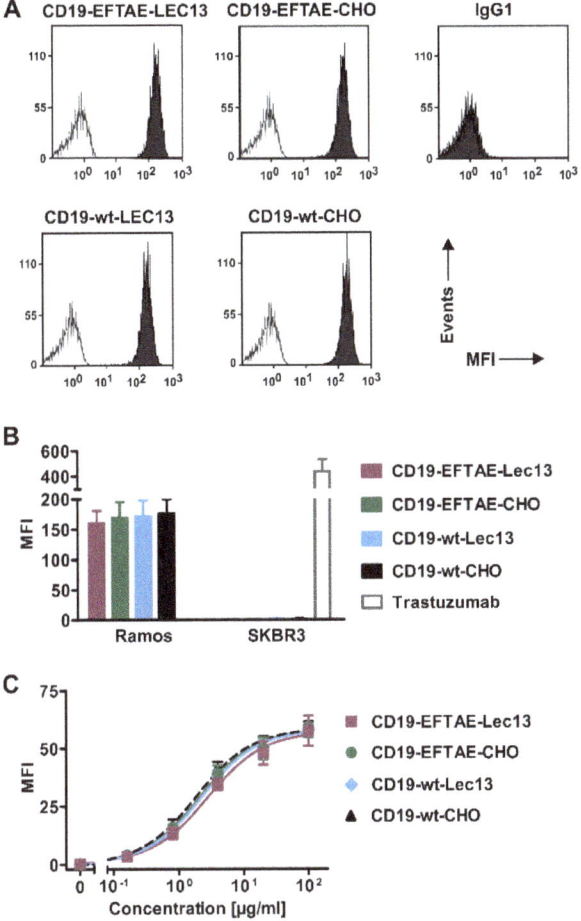

Figure 2. CD19 binding analysis. (**A**) CD19-positive Ramos cells were incubated with antibodies as indicated (concentration: 50 µg/mL; grey peaks) or in PBA buffer alone (white peaks), stained with FITC-coupled anti-human IgG Fc F(ab′)2 and then analyzed by flow cytometry. As a control, trastuzumab was added (IgG1). (**B**) CD19-wt-CHO, CD19-EFTAE-CHO, CD19-wt-Lec13 and CD19-EFTAE-Lec13 (concentration: 50 µg/mL) bound to CD19-expressing Ramos cells but did not react with CD19-negative SK-BR-3 cells. Bars indicate mean values ± SEM ($n = 3$) of mean fluorescence intensity (MFI). PE-labeled anti-human IgG Fc F(ab′)2 fragments were used as secondary antibodies. Trastuzumab was employed as a control antibody and bound to HER2-positive SK-BR-3 cells. (**C**) Binding of antibody versions to CHO-K1-CD19 cells was analyzed at varying concentrations employing FITC-coupled anti-human IgG Fc F(ab′)2 fragments as detection reagents and MFI values were determined by flow cytometry. Mean values ± SEM are shown ($n = 4$).

To determine the abilities of the antibodies to trigger ADCC, 51Cr release experiments with MNC effector cells and Raji lymphoma target cells were performed (Figure 3B). At saturating conditions, CD19-wt-Lec13 and CD19-EFTAE-Lec13 showed an enhanced potency relative to fucosylated antibodies CD19-EFTAE-CHO and CD19-wt-CHO, which both induced only moderate ADCC. None of the corresponding control antibodies against HER2, which is not expressed by Raji cells, induced ADCC, showing the antigen-specific mode of action even when the antibodies had been Fc engineered. Analysis of dose-dependent ADCC induction using MNC and either Raji or Ramos target cells revealed that CD19-EFTAE-Lec13 and CD19-wt-Lec13 had similar efficacy, although the double-engineered antibody was slightly more effective (Figure 3C). In experiments with Raji cells, EC50 values were 0.4 nM and 1.3 nM for CD19-EFTAE-Lec13 and CD19-wt-Lec13, respectively. However, these differences did not reach statistical significance. A comparison between rituximab and CD19-EFTAE-Lec13 revealed that this antibody now almost reached the potency of rituximab, although rituximab was slightly more effective in terms of maximum lysis at saturating concentrations (Figure 3D). Thus, Fc glyco-engineering by the generation of afucosylated antibodies improved the ADCC of CD19 antibodies, and the inclusion of the EFTAE modification in the afucosylated CD19 antibody even improved ADCC slightly further.

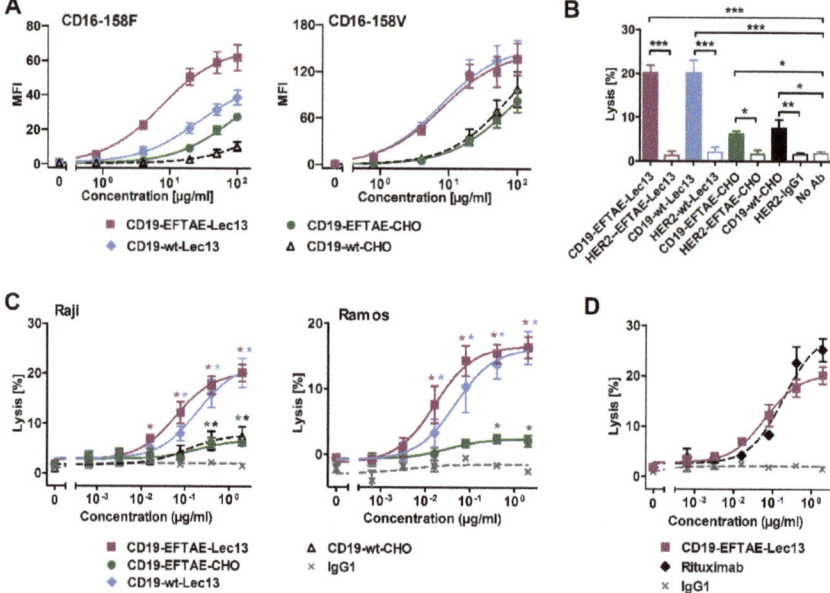

Figure 3. FcγRIIIA binding and induction of ADCC by differentially engineered CD19 antibodies. (**A**) Binding of antibodies CD19-wt-CHO, CD19-EFTAE-CHO, CD19-wt-Lec13 and CD19-EFTAE-Lec13 to transfected BHK cells stably expressing human FcγRIIIA-158V (BHK-CD16-158V) or FcγRIIIA-158F (BHK-CD16-158F) alleles was analyzed by flow cytometry. Secondary FITC-coupled anti-human IgG Fc F(ab')2 fragments were employed for detection. MFI, mean fluorescence intensity. (**B**) Induction of ADCC by antibody versions (concentration: 2 μg/mL) was investigated in 51Cr release experiments using Raji as target cells and human MNC as effector cells. Similarly designed variants of trastuzumab were used as controls. Bars represent mean values of specific lysis ± SEM. Significant differences between CD19 antibodies and HER2-specific control antibodies or the control reaction performed in the absence of any added antibody (no Ab) are indicated (*, $p \leq 0.05$; **, $p \leq 0.01$; ***, $p \leq 0.001$ $n = 3$). (**C**) Dose-dependent induction of ADCC by CD19 variants was analyzed using Raji ($n = 3$) or Ramos cells as targets and MNC as effector cells. Data points indicate mean values of specific lysis ± SEM. Statistically significant differences in ADCC between CD19 antibodies and the control antibody trastuzumab (IgG1) are indicated (*, $p \leq 0.05$; **, $p \leq 0.01$; $n = 3$). (**D**) Comparison of ADCC by the Fc double-engineered antibody CD19-EFTAE-Lec13 (purple) and by the CD20 antibody rituximab (black). Trastuzumab served as an additional negative control (IgG1). Raji cells were used as target cells and MNC served as effector cells. Mean values of specific lysis ± SEM are shown ($n = 3$).

Since the induction of CDC along the classical pathway requires efficient C1q deposition, we investigated whether the EFTAE amino acid substitutions in engineered CD19 antibodies promoted C1q fixation on lymphoma cells and whether this was affected by the antibody fucosylation status

(Figure 4A). To test this, CD19-expressing Raji cells were first incubated in the presence of antibodies CD19-wt-CHO, CD19-EFTAE-CHO, CD19-wt-Lec13 or CD19-EFTAE-Lec13. Then cells were reacted with human serum as a source of C1q, which finally was detected using an antibody specific for human C1q. Analysis by flow cytometry demonstrated that cell-bound C1q was only detectable when Raji cells were pre-incubated with CD19 antibody variants carrying the EFTAE modification. Of note, CD19-EFTAE-CHO and CD19-EFTAE-Lec13 were similarly effective in binding C1q, but none of them reached the efficacy of rituximab (Figure 4A).

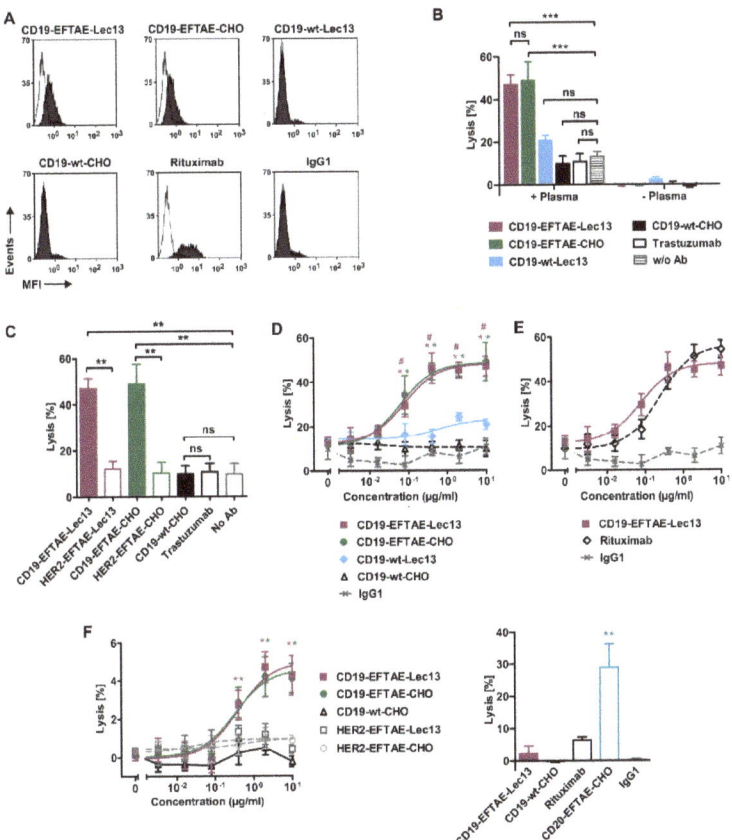

Figure 4. C1q binding capacities and induction of CDC by CD19 antibody versions. (**A**) Raji cells were left untreated (white peaks) or coated with antibodies CD19-wt-CHO, CD19-EFTAE-CHO, CD19-wt-Lec13 or CD19-EFTAE-Lec13 (grey peaks) at a concentration of 50 μg/mL. Then cells were incubated with human serum (1%) as a source of C1q and C1q binding to antibody coated cells was determined using a FITC-conjugated mouse anti-human C1q antibody and flow cytometry. Rituximab, which binds C1q efficiently, and trastuzumab, which does not react with HER2-negative Raji cells, were included as control reagents. MFI, mean fluorescence intensity. (**B**) CDC by CD19 antibodies was determined by 51Cr release experiments with Ramos cells as target cells in the presence or in the absence of 25% human plasma. Antibodies were analyzed at a concentration of 10 μg/mL. Bars represent mean values of specific lysis ± SEM. Significant differences between antibody-treated groups and the control group without any added antibody (w/o Ab) are indicated (***, $p \leq 0.001$; ns, not significant; $n = 3$). (**C**) CDC against Ramos by antibodies CD19-EFTAE-Lec13, CD19-EFTAE-CHO and CD19-wt-CHO compared to corresponding engineered control antibodies against HER2 and the native anti-HER2 IgG1

antibody trastuzumab. Antibodies were analyzed at a concentration of 10 µg/mL. Bars show mean values of specific lysis ± SEM. Significant differences between CD19 antibodies and the corresponding versions of the HER2-specific antibody trastuzumab or between antibody treatment and the control reaction without any added antibody (no Ab) are indicated (**, $p \leq 0.01$; $n = 3$). (**D**) Dose-dependent induction of CDC against Ramos cells ($n = 3$). Human plasma (25%) was added as a source of complement. *, statistically significant differences ($p \leq 0.05$) in CDC between CD19 antibodies and the native CD19-wt-CHO IgG1 molecule; #, statistically significant differences ($p \leq 0.05$) between CD19-EFTAE-Lec13 and CD19-wt-Lec13. Trastuzumab served as an additional negative control (IgG1). (**E**) Comparison of CDC induced by the Fc double-engineered antibody CD19-EFTAE-Lec13 and by the CD20 antibody rituximab. Trastuzumab served as an additional negative control (IgG1). Ramos cells were employed as target cells and serum was added to 25% as a source for complement. Mean values of specific lysis ± SEM are shown ($n = 3$). (**F**) Left graph: CD19 antibody variants were analyzed at varying concentrations for their ability to induce CDC against Raji cells, which in comparison to Ramos cells are rather resistant to CDC. Mean values of specific lysis ± SEM are shown ($n = 3$). Right graph: CD19 antibody variants were compared with rituximab and an Fc engineered version of rituximab-containing the EFTAE modification (CD20-EFTAE-CHO). Trastuzumab served as an additional negative control (IgG1). Mean values of specific lysis ± SEM are shown and statistically significant differences are indicated (**, $p < 0.01$).

To investigate CDC induction by CD19 antibodies, 51Cr release assays were performed employing human plasma and CDC-sensitive Ramos cells (Figure 4B). As a result, only antibodies CD19-EFTAE-CHO and CD19-EFTAE-Lec13 were able to trigger efficient CDC, while antibodies CD19-wt-CHO and CD19-wt-Lec13 were not effective. No lysis occurred in the absence of plasma, indicating that under these experimental conditions no direct induction of cell death was induced. Additionally, no CDC was found when HER2-specific control antibodies were applied, revealing that the observed CDC was induced in a target antigen-dependent manner (Figure 4C). Importantly, the analysis of dose-dependent induction of CDC indicated that CD19-EFTAE-Lec13 was as effective as CD19-EFTAE-CHO (Figure 4D). Both antibodies triggered CDC at nanomolar concentrations with EC50 values of 0.5 nM and 0.4 nM for CD19-EFTAE-Lec13 and CD19-EFTAE-CHO, respectively. The Fc double-engineered antibody CD19-EFTAE-Lec13 almost reached the potency of rituximab (Figure 4E). Finally, CDC was analyzed with Raji cells that are rather resistant to CDC (Figure 4F). Both CD19-EFTAE-Lec13 and CD19-EFTAE-CHO were able to trigger CDC against Raji cells in a dose-dependent manner. However, lysis of Raji cells was quite low. Reduced CDC induction was also observed for rituximab, which was employed for comparison (Figure 4F). However, an Fc-engineered variant of rituximab carrying the EFTAE modification (CD20-EFTAE-CHO) [37] was able to trigger substantial CDC, showing that although Fc engineering improves CDC of CD19 antibodies leading to a considerable efficacy, limitations associated with unfavorable antigen characteristics or specific antibody features are not fully overcome, when CDC insensitive target cells are analyzed.

4. Discussion

The CD19 antigen has attractive features for antibody therapy of B-cell lineage leukemias and lymphomas, but native CD19 IgG1 isotype antibodies only poorly mediate CDC and ADCC. In an effort to enhance both functions concomitantly, Fc protein-engineering was combined with Fc glyco-engineering to generate a double-engineered version of a CD19 antibody based on the v-regions of the clinically approved antibody tafasitamab. We found that the double-engineered afucosylated CD19 antibody harboring the EFTAE modifications was more efficacious in triggering both ADCC and CDC than the native IgG1 molecule, which had only weak effects in ADCC and which was unable to induce CDC. These findings demonstrate that CDC and ADCC functions can be established in CD19 antibodies by combined glyco-engineering and protein-engineering technologies and show that these technologies are applicable to the same antibody molecule.

The underlying reasons why native CD19 antibodies are not efficacious as for example CD20 antibodies are not fully understood and presumably are not due to antigen expression levels. Potential reasons may be specific antigen characteristics such as antigen membrane fluidity, size and structure or the antigen's plasma membrane microdomain localization, as well as antibody characteristics such as the epitope specificity and its location [43]. However, even when native antibodies elicit weak effects, they can be turned into effective agents by applying Fc engineering technologies, which allow fine-tuning of individual antibody effector functions and the generation of tailor-made antibodies [9,32].

Regarding CD19, the clinically approved Fc protein engineered antibody tafasitamab with amino acid substitutions S239D/I332E has demonstrated promising results in clinical studies. However, the antibody is optimized for FcγR binding and still lacks CDC activity [29]. Several observations suggest that CDC activity is an important antibody function and establishing CDC activity in CD19 antibodies may be beneficial in certain situations. Thus, in murine tumor models, variation in the relative contribution of CDC and FcγR-mediated functions were observed and an impact of tumor burden and anatomic localization has been suggested [44]. Additionally, the immune status of the patient and the tumor microenvironment may play a role [45]. Moreover, different phenotypes of tumor cells may impact the susceptibility of tumor cells to different antibody functions differentially, and cell phenotypes of individual tumor cells may differ even in the same patient. Thus, susceptibility to ADCC may be hampered by strong expression of inhibitory human leukocyte antigen (HLA) molecules or promoted by increased expression of NK cell-activating danger signals such as NKG2D ligands [46]. In contrast, tumor cells may be protected from CDC by expression of mCRP [47]. Interestingly, studies with CD20 transgenic cell clones revealed that individual CDC resistant cell clones were eliminated by ADCC and vice versa [48]. Thus, CDC as well as effector cell-mediated killing may be required for effective eradication of tumor cells in certain situations, and Fc double-engineered CD19 antibodies optimized for ADCC and CDC activity may be advantageous. Whether the double engineering strategy demonstrated here can be applied also to other CD19 antibodies remains to be investigated.

Of note, Fc glyco-engineering by lowering fucose content enhances only FcγRIIIA affinity, while Fc protein-engineering often leads to improved affinity for different activating FcγR [9]. Therefore, Fc protein-engineered antibodies carrying for example the DE modification may have advantages in engaging macrophages that express FcγRI and FcγRIIA next to FcγRIIIA. In addition, the comparison of Fc protein-engineered and Fc glyco-engineered antibody derivatives revealed that antibodies harboring the DE modification had a significantly higher affinity to FcγRIIIA than afucosylated antibodies [41]. However, afucosylated antibodies had an almost equal potency to trigger ADCC by NK cells, suggesting that the gain in affinity achieved by Fc glyco-engineering is sufficient for potent effector cell recruitment and ADCC. However, whether also the Fc double-engineered antibody CD19-EFTAE-Lec13 is as effective in mediating ADCC as a corresponding CD19 antibody with the DE modification needs to be investigated.

In previous studies, we have demonstrated that neutrophil-mediated ADCC is diminished when antibodies engineered for improved FcγRIIIA binding were compared to wildtype IgG [49,50]. This may be less relevant for CD19 antibodies, since CD19 antibodies do not trigger neutrophil-mediated ADCC (unpublished observation). When applied in vivo, the situation might even be more complex, since FcR-positive cells and complement proteins may compete for Fc binding. For example, Wang and colleagues demonstrated that complement binding to the Fc domain of wildtype antibodies diminishes NK cell activation [51]. Addressing this aspect in vivo in preclinical mouse models is challenging since FcR binding and complement activation of the described engineered Fc domains in commonly used xenograft models may not reflect the human situation. While certain protein-engineered Fc variants demonstrate enhanced binding to all mouse FcγR, glyco-engineering of human IgG1 results in a very minor improvement in mouse FcγR binding [7,52]. Even in complex transgenic mouse models engineered to express all human FcγR on the respective murine effector populations the contribution of the complement system might not be adequately reflected and tumor location and tumor burden may have a significant impact on which effector mechanisms contribute to the therapeutic activity in a given situation [15,53,54]. Therefore, the impact of double-engineering could probably ultimately only be tested in non-human primates or clinical trials.

In conclusion, the combination of Fc glyco-engineering and Fc protein-engineering technologies promotes both CDC and ADCC activity in CD19 antibodies simultaneously and allows the generation of CD19 antibodies with appreciable efficacy. Thus, Fc double-engineering may represent an attractive strategy, which may be in particular advantageous for antibodies directed against antigens as CD19, which are not that well-suited as target antigens for antibody therapy as CD20 or CD38. Thus, the Fc double-engineering approach may offer an opportunity to enhance the efficacy of CD19 antibody therapy and deserves further evaluation.

Supplementary Materials: The following are available online at http://www.mdpi.com/2073-4468/9/4/63/s1, Figure S1: Size exclusion chromatography (SEC) of CD19 antibody variants.

Author Contributions: Conceptualization, M.G., M.P. and C.K.; Methodology, S.R., T.R., T.V., M.P. and C.K.; Formal Analysis, S.R., M.P. and C.K.; Investigation, S.R., K.M.E., D.W., K.J.D., S.L., I.A.M. and K.K.; Writing—Original Draft Preparation, M.P. and C.K.; Writing—Review and Editing, A.H., T.V., M.G. and D.M.S.; Visualization, R.S. and C.K.; Project Administration, M.P. and C.K. All authors have read and agreed to the published version of the manuscript.

Funding: This study was supported by research grants from the José Carreras Leukämie-Stiftung (to D.M.S., C.K. and M.P.), Wilhelm Sander-Stiftung (to M.P. and C.K.) and from the Deutsche Krebshilfe (to D.M.S. and C.K.). M.P. is supported by the Deutsche Krebshilfe Mildred-Scheel professorship program.

Acknowledgments: We kindly thank Pamela Stanley (Albert Einstein College of Medicine of Yeshiva University, New York, NY, USA) for providing us Lec13 cells. Anja Muskulus and Britta von Below are kindly acknowledged for expert technical assistance.

Conflicts of Interest: The authors declare no conflict of interest.

References

1. Carter, P.J.; Lazar, G.A. Next generation antibody drugs: Pursuit of the 'high-hanging fruit'. *Nat. Rev. Drug Discov.* **2018**, *17*, 197–223. [CrossRef] [PubMed]
2. Hammer, O. CD19 as an attractive target for antibody-based therapy. *mAbs* **2012**, *4*, 571–577. [CrossRef] [PubMed]
3. Yazawa, N.; Hamaguchi, Y.; Poe, J.C.; Tedder, T.F. Immunotherapy using unconjugated CD19 monoclonal antibodies in animal models for B lymphocyte malignancies and autoimmune disease. *Proc. Natl. Acad. Sci. USA* **2005**, *102*, 15178–15183. [CrossRef] [PubMed]
4. Kellner, C.; Peipp, M.; Gramatzki, M.; Schrappe, M.; Schewe, D.M. Perspectives of Fc engineered antibodies in CD19 targeting immunotherapies in pediatric B-cell precursor acute lymphoblastic leukemia. *Oncoimmunology* **2018**, *7*, e1448331. [CrossRef] [PubMed]
5. Frigault, M.J.; Maus, M.V. State of the art in CAR T cell therapy for CD19+ B cell malignancies. *J. Clin. Investig.* **2020**, *130*, 1586–1594. [CrossRef] [PubMed]
6. Kantarjian, H.; Stein, A.; Gokbuget, N.; Fielding, A.K.; Schuh, A.C.; Ribera, J.M.; Wei, A.; Dombret, H.; Foa, R.; Bassan, R.; et al. Blinatumomab versus Chemotherapy for Advanced Acute Lymphoblastic Leukemia. *N. Engl. J. Med.* **2017**, *376*, 836–847. [CrossRef] [PubMed]
7. Horton, H.M.; Bernett, M.J.; Pong, E.; Peipp, M.; Karki, S.; Chu, S.Y.; Richards, J.O.; Vostiar, I.; Joyce, P.F.; Repp, R.; et al. Potent in vitro and in vivo activity of an Fc-engineered anti-CD19 monoclonal antibody against lymphoma and leukemia. *Cancer Res.* **2008**, *68*, 8049–8057. [CrossRef]
8. Salles, G.; Duell, J.; Gonzalez Barca, E.; Tournilhac, O.; Jurczak, W.; Liberati, A.M.; Nagy, Z.; Obr, A.; Gaidano, G.; Andre, M.; et al. Tafasitamab plus lenalidomide in relapsed or refractory diffuse large B-cell lymphoma (L-MIND): A multicentre, prospective, single-arm, phase 2 study. *Lancet Oncol.* **2020**, *21*, 978–988. [CrossRef]
9. Kellner, C.; Otte, A.; Cappuzzello, E.; Klausz, K.; Peipp, M. Modulating Cytotoxic Effector Functions by Fc Engineering to Improve Cancer Therapy. *Transfus. Med. Hemother.* **2017**, *44*, 327–336. [CrossRef]
10. Di Gaetano, N.; Cittera, E.; Nota, R.; Vecchi, A.; Grieco, V.; Scanziani, E.; Botto, M.; Introna, M.; Golay, J. Complement activation determines the therapeutic activity of rituximab in vivo. *J. Immunol.* **2003**, *171*, 1581–1587. [CrossRef]

11. Kennedy, A.D.; Beum, P.V.; Solga, M.D.; DiLillo, D.J.; Lindorfer, M.A.; Hess, C.E.; Densmore, J.J.; Williams, M.E.; Taylor, R.P. Rituximab infusion promotes rapid complement depletion and acute CD20 loss in chronic lymphocytic leukemia. *J. Immunol.* **2004**, *172*, 3280–3288. [CrossRef] [PubMed]
12. Klepfish, A.; Schattner, A.; Ghoti, H.; Rachmilewitz, E.A. Addition of fresh frozen plasma as a source of complement to rituximab in advanced chronic lymphocytic leukaemia. *Lancet Oncol.* **2007**, *8*, 361–362. [CrossRef]
13. Bannerji, R.; Kitada, S.; Flinn, I.W.; Pearson, M.; Young, D.; Reed, J.C.; Byrd, J.C. Apoptotic-regulatory and complement-protecting protein expression in chronic lymphocytic leukemia: Relationship to in vivo rituximab resistance. *J. Clin. Oncol.* **2003**, *21*, 1466–1471. [CrossRef] [PubMed]
14. Clynes, R.A.; Towers, T.L.; Presta, L.G.; Ravetch, J.V. Inhibitory Fc receptors modulate in vivo cytotoxicity against tumor targets. *Nat. Med.* **2000**, *6*, 443–446. [CrossRef]
15. De Haij, S.; Jansen, J.H.; Boross, P.; Beurskens, F.J.; Bakema, J.E.; Bos, D.L.; Martens, A.; Verbeek, J.S.; Parren, P.W.; van de Winkel, J.G.; et al. In vivo cytotoxicity of type I CD20 antibodies critically depends on Fc receptor ITAM signaling. *Cancer Res.* **2010**, *70*, 3209–3217. [CrossRef]
16. Cartron, G.; Dacheux, L.; Salles, G.; Solal-Celigny, P.; Bardos, P.; Colombat, P.; Watier, H. Therapeutic activity of humanized anti-CD20 monoclonal antibody and polymorphism in IgG Fc receptor FcgammaRIIIa gene. *Blood* **2002**, *99*, 754–758. [CrossRef]
17. Weng, W.K.; Levy, R. Two immunoglobulin G fragment C receptor polymorphisms independently predict response to rituximab in patients with follicular lymphoma. *J. Clin. Oncol.* **2003**, *21*, 3940–3947. [CrossRef]
18. Persky, D.O.; Dornan, D.; Goldman, B.H.; Braziel, R.M.; Fisher, R.I.; Leblanc, M.; Maloney, D.G.; Press, O.W.; Miller, T.P.; Rimsza, L.M. Fc gamma receptor 3a genotype predicts overall survival in follicular lymphoma patients treated on SWOG trials with combined monoclonal antibody plus chemotherapy but not chemotherapy alone. *Haematologica* **2012**, *97*, 937–942. [CrossRef]
19. Dahal, L.N.; Roghanian, A.; Beers, S.A.; Cragg, M.S. FcgammaR requirements leading to successful immunotherapy. *Immunol. Rev.* **2015**, *268*, 104–122. [CrossRef]
20. Cartron, G.; Houot, R.; Kohrt, H.E. Scientific Significance of Clinically Insignificant FcgammaRIIIa-V158F Polymorphism. *Clin. Cancer Res.* **2016**, *22*, 787–789. [CrossRef]
21. Moore, G.L.; Chen, H.; Karki, S.; Lazar, G.A. Engineered Fc variant antibodies with enhanced ability to recruit complement and mediate effector functions. *mAbs* **2010**, *2*, 181–189. [CrossRef] [PubMed]
22. Idusogie, E.E.; Wong, P.Y.; Presta, L.G.; Gazzano-Santoro, H.; Totpal, K.; Ultsch, M.; Mulkerrin, M.G. Engineered antibodies with increased activity to recruit complement. *J. Immunol.* **2001**, *166*, 2571–2575. [CrossRef] [PubMed]
23. Diebolder, C.A.; Beurskens, F.J.; de Jong, R.N.; Koning, R.I.; Strumane, K.; Lindorfer, M.A.; Voorhorst, M.; Ugurlar, D.; Rosati, S.; Heck, A.J.; et al. Complement is activated by IgG hexamers assembled at the cell surface. *Science* **2014**, *343*, 1260–1263. [CrossRef] [PubMed]
24. Oostindie, S.C.; van der Horst, H.J.; Lindorfer, M.A.; Cook, E.M.; Tupitza, J.C.; Zent, C.S.; Burack, R.; VanDerMeid, K.R.; Strumane, K.; Chamuleau, M.E.D.; et al. CD20 and CD37 antibodies synergize to activate complement by Fc-mediated clustering. *Haematologica* **2019**, *104*, 1841–1852. [CrossRef] [PubMed]
25. Schneider, S.; Zacharias, M. Atomic resolution model of the antibody Fc interaction with the complement C1q component. *Mol. Immunol.* **2012**, *51*, 66–72. [CrossRef]
26. Radaev, S.; Motyka, S.; Fridman, W.H.; Sautes-Fridman, C.; Sun, P.D. The structure of a human type III Fcgamma receptor in complex with Fc. *J. Biol. Chem.* **2001**, *276*, 16469–16477. [CrossRef]
27. Sondermann, P.; Huber, R.; Oosthuizen, V.; Jacob, U. The 3.2-A crystal structure of the human IgG1 Fc fragment-Fc gammaRIII complex. *Nature* **2000**, *406*, 267–273. [CrossRef]
28. Schewe, D.M.; Alsadeq, A.; Sattler, C.; Lenk, L.; Vogiatzi, F.; Cario, G.; Vieth, S.; Valerius, T.; Rosskopf, S.; Meyersieck, F.; et al. An Fc-engineered CD19 antibody eradicates MRD in patient-derived MLL-rearranged acute lymphoblastic leukemia xenografts. *Blood* **2017**, *130*, 1543–1552. [CrossRef]
29. Kellner, C.; Zhukovsky, E.A.; Potzke, A.; Bruggemann, M.; Schrauder, A.; Schrappe, M.; Kneba, M.; Repp, R.; Humpe, A.; Gramatzki, M.; et al. The Fc-engineered CD19 antibody MOR208 (XmAb5574) induces natural killer cell-mediated lysis of acute lymphoblastic leukemia cells from pediatric and adult patients. *Leukemia* **2013**, *27*, 1595–1598. [CrossRef]

30. Zalevsky, J.; Leung, I.W.; Karki, S.; Chu, S.Y.; Zhukovsky, E.A.; Desjarlais, J.R.; Carmichael, D.F.; Lawrence, C.E. The impact of Fc engineering on an anti-CD19 antibody: Increased Fcgamma receptor affinity enhances B-cell clearing in nonhuman primates. *Blood* **2009**, *113*, 3735–3743. [CrossRef]
31. Jurczak, W.; Zinzani, P.L.; Gaidano, G.; Goy, A.; Provencio, M.; Nagy, Z.; Robak, T.; Maddocks, K.; Buske, C.; Ambarkhane, S.; et al. Phase IIa study of the CD19 antibody MOR208 in patients with relapsed or refractory B-cell non-Hodgkin's lymphoma. *Ann. Oncol.* **2018**, *29*, 1266–1272. [CrossRef]
32. Dalziel, M.; Beers, S.A.; Cragg, M.S.; Crispin, M. Through the barricades: Overcoming the barriers to effective antibody-based cancer therapeutics. *Glycobiology* **2018**, *28*, 697–712. [CrossRef] [PubMed]
33. Matlawska-Wasowska, K.; Ward, E.; Stevens, S.; Wang, Y.; Herbst, R.; Winter, S.S.; Wilson, B.S. Macrophage and NK-mediated killing of precursor-B acute lymphoblastic leukemia cells targeted with a-fucosylated anti-CD19 humanized antibodies. *Leukemia* **2013**, *27*, 1263–1274. [CrossRef] [PubMed]
34. Lang, P.; Barbin, K.; Feuchtinger, T.; Greil, J.; Peipp, M.; Zunino, S.J.; Pfeiffer, M.; Handgretinger, R.; Niethammer, D.; Fey, G.H. Chimeric CD19 antibody mediates cytotoxic activity against leukemic blasts with effector cells from pediatric patients who received T-cell-depleted allografts. *Blood* **2004**, *103*, 3982–3985. [CrossRef] [PubMed]
35. Ohmachi, K.; Ogura, M.; Suehiro, Y.; Ando, K.; Uchida, T.; Choi, I.; Ogawa, Y.; Kobayashi, M.; Fukino, K.; Yokoi, Y.; et al. A multicenter phase I study of inebilizumab, a humanized anti-CD19 monoclonal antibody, in Japanese patients with relapsed or refractory B-cell lymphoma and multiple myeloma. *Int. J. Hematol.* **2019**, *109*, 657–664. [CrossRef]
36. Cree, B.A.C.; Bennett, J.L.; Kim, H.J.; Weinshenker, B.G.; Pittock, S.J.; Wingerchuk, D.M.; Fujihara, K.; Paul, F.; Cutter, G.R.; Marignier, R.; et al. Inebilizumab for the treatment of neuromyelitis optica spectrum disorder (N-MOmentum): A double-blind, randomised placebo-controlled phase 2/3 trial. *Lancet* **2019**, *394*, 1352–1363. [CrossRef]
37. Wirt, T.; Rosskopf, S.; Rosner, T.; Eichholz, K.M.; Kahrs, A.; Lutz, S.; Kretschmer, A.; Valerius, T.; Klausz, K.; Otte, A.; et al. An Fc Double-Engineered CD20 Antibody with Enhanced Ability to Trigger Complement-Dependent Cytotoxicity and Antibody-Dependent Cell-Mediated Cytotoxicity. *Transfus. Med. Hemother.* **2017**, *44*, 292–300. [CrossRef]
38. Glorius, P.; Baerenwaldt, A.; Kellner, C.; Staudinger, M.; Dechant, M.; Stauch, M.; Beurskens, F.J.; Parren, P.W.; Winkel, J.G.; Valerius, T.; et al. The novel tribody [(CD20)(2)xCD16] efficiently triggers effector cell-mediated lysis of malignant B cells. *Leukemia* **2013**, *27*, 190–201. [CrossRef]
39. Ripka, J.; Adamany, A.; Stanley, P. Two Chinese hamster ovary glycosylation mutants affected in the conversion of GDP-mannose to GDP-fucose. *Arch. Biochem. Biophys.* **1986**, *249*, 533–545. [CrossRef]
40. Patnaik, S.K.; Stanley, P. Lectin-resistant CHO glycosylation mutants. *Methods Enzymol.* **2006**, *416*, 159–182. [CrossRef]
41. Repp, R.; Kellner, C.; Muskulus, A.; Staudinger, M.; Nodehi, S.M.; Glorius, P.; Akramiene, D.; Dechant, M.; Fey, G.H.; van Berkel, P.H.; et al. Combined Fc-protein- and Fc-glyco-engineering of scFv-Fc fusion proteins synergistically enhances CD16a binding but does not further enhance NK-cell mediated ADCC. *J. Immunol. Methods* **2011**, *373*, 67–78. [CrossRef] [PubMed]
42. Clark, M.R. IgG effector mechanisms. *Chem. Immunol.* **1997**, *65*, 88–110. [PubMed]
43. Cleary, K.L.S.; Chan, H.T.C.; James, S.; Glennie, M.J.; Cragg, M.S. Antibody Distance from the Cell Membrane Regulates Antibody Effector Mechanisms. *J. Immunol.* **2017**, *198*, 3999–4011. [CrossRef] [PubMed]
44. Boross, P.; Jansen, J.H.; de Haij, S.; Beurskens, F.J.; van der Poel, C.E.; Bevaart, L.; Nederend, M.; Golay, J.; van de Winkel, J.G.; Parren, P.W.; et al. The in vivo mechanism of action of CD20 monoclonal antibodies depends on local tumor burden. *Haematologica* **2011**, *96*, 1822–1830. [CrossRef]
45. Gong, Q.; Ou, Q.; Ye, S.; Lee, W.P.; Cornelius, J.; Diehl, L.; Lin, W.Y.; Hu, Z.; Lu, Y.; Chen, Y.; et al. Importance of cellular microenvironment and circulatory dynamics in B cell immunotherapy. *J. Immunol.* **2005**, *174*, 817–826. [CrossRef]
46. Inagaki, A.; Ishida, T.; Yano, H.; Ishii, T.; Kusumoto, S.; Ito, A.; Ri, M.; Mori, F.; Ding, J.; Komatsu, H.; et al. Expression of the ULBP ligands for NKG2D by B-NHL cells plays an important role in determining their susceptibility to rituximab-induced ADCC. *Int. J. Cancer* **2009**, *125*, 212–221. [CrossRef]
47. Meyer, S.; Leusen, J.H.; Boross, P. Regulation of complement and modulation of its activity in monoclonal antibody therapy of cancer. *mAbs* **2014**, *6*, 1133–1144. [CrossRef]

48. Van Meerten, T.; van Rijn, R.S.; Hol, S.; Hagenbeek, A.; Ebeling, S.B. Complement-induced cell death by rituximab depends on CD20 expression level and acts complementary to antibody-dependent cellular cytotoxicity. *Clin. Cancer Res.* **2006**, *12*, 4027–4035. [CrossRef]
49. Derer, S.; Glorius, P.; Schlaeth, M.; Lohse, S.; Klausz, K.; Muchhal, U.; Desjarlais, J.R.; Humpe, A.; Valerius, T.; Peipp, M. Increasing FcgammaRIIa affinity of an FcgammaRIII-optimized anti-EGFR antibody restores neutrophil-mediated cytotoxicity. *mAbs* **2014**, *6*, 409–421. [CrossRef]
50. Peipp, M.; Lammerts van Bueren, J.J.; Schneider-Merck, T.; Bleeker, W.W.; Dechant, M.; Beyer, T.; Repp, R.; van Berkel, P.H.; Vink, T.; van de Winkel, J.G.; et al. Antibody fucosylation differentially impacts cytotoxicity mediated by NK and PMN effector cells. *Blood* **2008**, *112*, 2390–2399. [CrossRef]
51. Wang, S.Y.; Veeramani, S.; Racila, E.; Cagley, J.; Fritzinger, D.C.; Vogel, C.W.; St John, W.; Weiner, G.J. Depletion of the C3 component of complement enhances the ability of rituximab-coated target cells to activate human NK cells and improves the efficacy of monoclonal antibody therapy in an in vivo model. *Blood* **2009**, *114*, 5322–5330. [CrossRef] [PubMed]
52. Junttila, T.T.; Parsons, K.; Olsson, C.; Lu, Y.; Xin, Y.; Theriault, J.; Crocker, L.; Pabonan, O.; Baginski, T.; Meng, G.; et al. Superior in vivo efficacy of afucosylated trastuzumab in the treatment of HER2-amplified breast cancer. *Cancer Res.* **2010**, *70*, 4481–4489. [CrossRef] [PubMed]
53. Nimmerjahn, F.; Ravetch, J.V. Antibodies, Fc receptors and cancer. *Curr. Opin. Immunol.* **2007**, *19*, 239–245. [CrossRef] [PubMed]
54. Casey, E.; Bournazos, S.; Mo, G.; Mondello, P.; Tan, K.S.; Ravetch, J.V.; Scheinberg, D.A. A new mouse expressing human Fcgamma receptors to better predict therapeutic efficacy of human anti-cancer antibodies. *Leukemia* **2018**, *32*, 547–549. [CrossRef] [PubMed]

Publisher's Note: MDPI stays neutral with regard to jurisdictional claims in published maps and institutional affiliations.

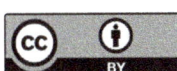

© 2020 by the authors. Licensee MDPI, Basel, Switzerland. This article is an open access article distributed under the terms and conditions of the Creative Commons Attribution (CC BY) license (http://creativecommons.org/licenses/by/4.0/).

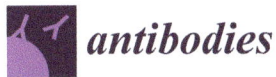

Review

CD46 and Oncologic Interactions: Friendly Fire against Cancer

Michelle Elvington [1,†], **M. Kathryn Liszewski** [2,†] **and John P. Atkinson** [2,*]

1. Kypha, Inc., Saint Louis, MO 63110, USA; melvington@kypha.net
2. Division of Rheumatology, Department of Medicine, Washington University School of Medicine, Saint Louis, MO 63110, USA; kliszews@wustl.edu
* Correspondence: j.p.atkinson@wustl.edu; Tel.: +1-314-362-8391
† These authors contributed equally to this work.

Received: 1 September 2020; Accepted: 25 October 2020; Published: 2 November 2020

Abstract: One of the most challenging aspects of cancer therapeutics is target selection. Recently, CD46 (membrane cofactor protein; MCP) has emerged as a key player in both malignant transformation as well as in cancer treatments. Normally a regulator of complement activation, CD46 is co-expressed as four predominant isoforms on almost all cell types. CD46 is highly overexpressed on a variety of human tumor cells. Clinical and experimental data support an association between increased CD46 expression and malignant transformation and metastasizing potential. Further, CD46 is a newly discovered driver of metabolic processes and plays a role in the intracellular complement system (complosome). CD46 is also known as a pathogen magnet due to its role as a receptor for numerous microbes, including several species of measles virus and adenoviruses. Strains of these two viruses have been exploited as vectors for the therapeutic development of oncolytic agents targeting CD46. In addition, monoclonal antibody-drug conjugates against CD46 also are being clinically evaluated. As a result, there are multiple early-phase clinical trials targeting CD46 to treat a variety of cancers. Here, we review CD46 relative to these oncologic connections.

Keywords: CD46; membrane cofactor protein (MCP); complement; cancer therapeutics; measles virus; adenovirus; antibody-drug conjugates

---

1. Introduction to CD46

CD46 is a ubiquitously expressed membrane protein in humans that regulates C3b/C4b that deposits on host cells and serves as a receptor for multiple pathogens. CD46 was originally discovered as a C3b-interacting protein based on its ability in surface-labeled, solubilized cell preparations to bind to C3b and C3(H_2O) affinity columns [1]. Subsequently, it was demonstrated to be a cofactor protein for the plasma serine protease factor I (FI) to mediate cleavage of C3b to iC3b and C4b to C4c and C4d [2,3]. Further, CD46 performs its function intrinsically; that is, this inhibitor binds its two ligands, C3b and C4b, only if they are deposited on the same cell on which CD46 is expressed. As a membrane protein, CD46 does not bind to C3b or C4b free in blood, attached to immune complexes or bound to other cells. CD46 has a wide tissue distribution, being expressed by almost all human cell populations except erythrocytes [3,4]. Thus, CD46 protects healthy human cells from complement attack.

CD46 is rather unique among complement proteins, receptors and regulators in that most cell types co-express four primary isoforms (Figure 1). These arise from alternative splicing of a single gene (Figure 2) located within the regulators of complement activation (RCA) cluster on the long arm of chromosome 1 at position q3.2 [5]. The N-terminus of CD46 consists of four contiguous complement control protein (CCP) repeats. Following this is an alternatively spliced segment enriched in serines, threonines and prolines (i.e., the STP domain) that is variably *O*-glycosylated. The STP domain of the regularly expressed proteins consists of B+C or C alone, although rarer isoforms exist.

Following the STP domain and common to all isoforms is a juxtamembraneous segment of 12 amino acids of undefined function and a hydrophobic transmembrane domain. CD46 also contains one of two cytoplasmic tails (termed CYT-1 or CYT-2), each of which has distinct signaling motifs (reviewed in [3]). Much remains to be learned about the biological reasons for CD46 isoform variation among cell types.

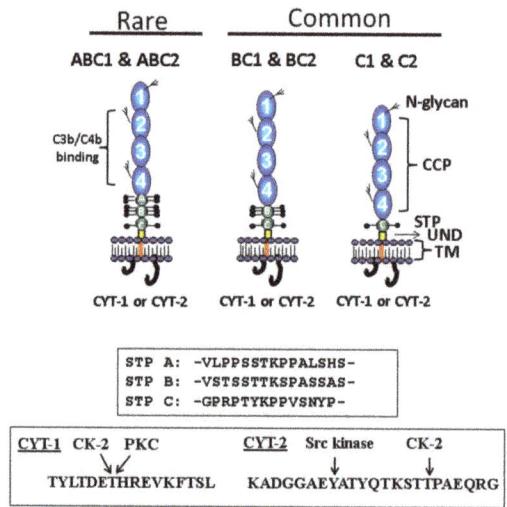

Figure 1. CD46 (membrane cofactor protein; MCP) is a widely expressed, alternatively spliced complement regulatory protein whose structure is dominated by four complement control protein modules (CCPs). CCPs 2–4 house the main sites for C3b and C4b interactions. CCPs 1, 2 and 4 feature N-glycans. Alternative splicing of the STP region (enriched in serines, threonines and prolines, and a site of variable levels for O-glycosylation) and of the cytoplasmic tails (CYT-1 or CYT-2, which have distinct signaling motifs) generates four common isoforms co-expressed to variable levels on most cells. These are called BC1, BC2, C1 and C2. Rarer isoforms also exist. UND, undefined juxtamembraneous segment; TM, transmembrane domain; CK-2, casein kinase 2; PKC, protein kinase C.

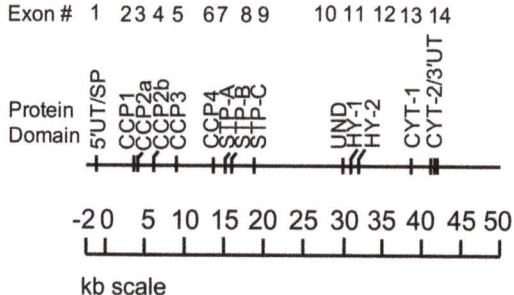

Figure 2. The gene for CD46. The alternatively spliced *MCP* gene lies at 1q3.2 and consists of 14 exons and 13 introns for a minimum length of 43 Kb. The exon number and corresponding domain are indicated. Note that CCP2 and the hydrophobic domain (HY) are encoded by two exons. Abbreviations per Figure 1: 5′UT/SP (5′ untranslated area and signal peptide); CYT-2/3′UT (cytoplasmic tail 2 and 3′ untranslated region).

Since its original discovery in 1987, CD46 is now known to play a broader role in human biology (reviewed in [6,7]). This includes modulation of immune cell function through its intracellular signaling capabilities; namely, CD46 is an important modulator of adaptive immunity and a central participant in human infectious and Th1 biology [8,9]. Individuals with a homozygous CD46 deficiency are hampered in mounting Th1 responses and suffer from recurrent severe infections [10] and, more commonly, atypical hemolytic uremic syndrome at a young age [11]. CD46 engagement on CD4$^+$ T cells results in a Th1 response; however, as IL-2 accumulates, a switch occurs to a T regulatory phenotype characterized by production of IL-10 that is mediated by the CYT-1 tail of CD46 [12,13]. In this manner, CD46 also contributes to the contraction phase of a Th1 response. CD46 cytoplasmic tail switching links Th1 cell activation (CYT-1) and then contraction (CYT-2) to a pathway for metabolic reprogramming [14]. The bulk of the work on this subject has been performed by the Kemper laboratory employing human CD4$^+$ T cells and is reviewed extensively elsewhere [6,8,15].

Four additional key observations relevant to this review are CD46's: (1) enhanced expression by many types of malignant cell populations; (2) "abuse" by ten human-specific pathogens that use CD46 as a receptor, including species of measles virus and adenovirus; (3) modulation of immune cell function via its intracellular signaling capabilities; (4) role as a driver of cellular metabolism [16]. Point #3 is briefly noted in the preceding paragraph while the other three points will be further highlighted in this review because of their oncologic implications.

2. CD46 as Tumor Target

CD46 is emerging as an important player in both malignant transformation as well as in cancer immunotherapy. Complement expression is often dysregulated in tumors [17] (reviewed in [18]). Although heterogeneous relative to tumor type, complement proteins expressed by malignant cells are variable; in general, tumor cells express low C8 and C9 but highly express C3 and the regulators factor H, factor I and especially the membrane regulators CD46, CD55 and CD59 [19]. Notably, CD46 expression is increased up to 14-fold in relapsed multiple myeloma (MM) patients who have the region on chromosome 1q carrying CD46 genomically amplified (mean antigen density 313,190 for MM vs. 22,475 for healthy donor plasma cells) [20]. The overexpression of CD46 occurs in many, although not all, other common tumor types but usually to a lesser magnitude. For example, in hepatocellular carcinoma cells, the relative density of CD46 is increased approximately 6-fold [21]. Complement deposition also is frequently noted in tumor tissue and soluble activation fragments are identified in patients' sera [22,23], including increased levels of soluble CD46 [24]. Further, clinical and experimental data in ovarian and breast cancer as well as multiple myeloma support an association between increased CD46 expression and malignant transformation and metastasizing potential [25–27]. Indeed, increased CD46 expression is a prognostic indicator in multiple common malignancies, including ovarian cancer, breast cancer and hepatocellular carcinoma [25,26,28].

In the context of cancer, the view of the complement system has traditionally been that of an anti-tumor effector, particularly to enhance the efficacy of anti-cancer monoclonal antibodies (mAb) [29,30]. Complement engagement following Ab binding to a tumor Ag has several potential mechanisms to enhance cell killing [31]. These include direct complement-mediated lysis or complement-dependent cytotoxicity (CDC) and enhancing antibody-dependent cellular cytotoxicity (ADCC). Additionally, C3a and C5a can recruit immune cells that then may modulate the adaptive immune response. The upregulation of complement inhibitors, including CD46, has historically been considered an evasion mechanism against Ab therapy that may also prevent the generation of an acquired immune response (reviewed in [17]). The interference of membrane complement regulators with the efficacy of anti-cancer mAb therapy has been demonstrated in animal models ([32] and reviewed in [33,34]). Several strategies have been employed to target the overexpression of complement regulators and thereby improve the therapeutic outcome [34]. These include small interfering RNAs [35–37], neutralizing (blocking) mAbs to complement inhibitors [38,39], bispecific antibodies [40–43] and a targeted complement activator (CR2-Fc) [30,44].

Targeted downregulation of the in vivo expression of a complement inhibitor, such as CD46, is technically challenging due to its ubiquitous presence on normal cells. However, the feasibility of this approach has been demonstrated both in vitro and in animal models where tumor cells can be manipulated ex vivo. For example, siRNA-mediated downregulation of CD46, CD55 and/or CD59 on several primary tumors and tumor cell lines sensitizes them to CDC [35,36]. Furthermore, the downregulation of the complement inhibitor Crry (the murine counterpart of CD46) on tumor cells in a mouse model of metastatic bladder cancer induced a protective anti-tumor CD8$^+$ T cell response [37]. In another model, complement inhibitor neutralization on tumor cells prior to vaccination elicited protective immunity [38]. Proof of principle also has been demonstrated in murine models for the efficacy of neutralizing mAbs [39] and bispecific antibodies [40–43]. Another study determined that in primary myeloma cells derived from bone marrow aspirates, a macropinocytosing CD46-antibody drug conjugate induced apoptosis and cell death but did not affect the viability of nontumor mononuclear cells [20]. In a slightly different approach, a strategy to utilize the targeting specificity of a mAb to amplify complement activation on tumor cells (CR2-Fc) demonstrated efficacy in murine models [30,44].

Unfortunately, complement activation does not always act to the host's benefit [45,46]. The protumor roles of complement were discussed recently in an excellent review [19]. C5a, in particular, has been shown to be protumor by recruitment of myeloid-derived suppressor cells and T regulatory cells that suppress anti-tumor T cell responses [47,48]. Complement may also promote tumorigenesis by triggering tumor cell proliferation, invasiveness and metastasis, as well as by enhancing angiogenesis [49]. Therefore, although increased CD46 on tumor cells is generally considered an immune evasion mechanism, in certain situations, preventing complement activation may also benefit the host. For example, suppressing complement activation at the level of C3 will also inhibit downstream C5 cleavage and generation of C5a, which has been shown to have protumor effects [45,47]. Another possibility is that the role of complement in promoting the clearance of apoptotic cells, which is a generally tolerogenic process, supports tumor growth. Indeed, apoptotic cells have been shown to directly activate complement [50–52]. This possibility was demonstrated in a murine model of lymphoma in which delivering a targeted complement inhibitor enhanced the outcome of radiation therapy by inhibiting apoptotic cell clearance, thereby promoting inflammation within the tumor and driving a systemic antitumor immune response [53].

Notably, a body of literature, as well as online resources such as The Cancer Genome Atlas (TCGA) Program reveal that the involvement of CD46 in cancer varies. CD46 expression in malignancies may: (1) correlate with a poorer prognosis (e.g., breast, colorectal, prostate and cervical cancers); (2) correlate with a positive outcome (e.g., renal or stomach cancers); (3) have no apparent impact. Further, there can be variability in expression even among specific tumor cell types. For example, one study reported that 35% of patients with colon or prostate carcinoma overexpressed CD46, while in other cancers (such as brain, lymphoma and lung), ~11% of tissue samples overexpressed CD46 [54]. Such variability suggests differences in the potential mode of action of CD46 in different contexts. Dissecting the role CD46 plays in multiple settings will support which patient cohorts would benefit from specific CD46-targeted therapeutics.

3. CD46 as a Receptor for Anti-Tumor Therapeutic Vectors

Interestingly, CD46 is known as a "pathogen magnet" because it is a target for ten (and counting) human pathogens [55–58], including the Edmonston vaccine strain of the measles virus [59] and some species of adenovirus (see below). Moreover, bovine and swine CD46 are receptors for the bovine viral diarrhea virus and the classical swine fever virus, respectively [60,61]. CD46 is utilized as a receptor for pathogens to gain entry into the cell. The exact reason why so many microbes target CD46 is unclear. However, several issues likely drive this phenomenon, including its high level of and ubiquitous expression across human cell types. In addition, because pathogens bind to different sites on the protein (see Figure 3) and utilize distinct methods for cellular entry, CD46 is likely targeted not simply due to its wide distribution and high level of expression but also because of its immune-modulatory signaling functions including immune suppression [56]. For example, *Neisseria gonorrhoeae* dysregulates the CD46-CYT-1 autophagic pathway to disturb lysosome homeostasis and promote its survival [62]. Furthermore, measles virus downregulates IL-12 production by monocytes through its binding to CD46 [63,64].

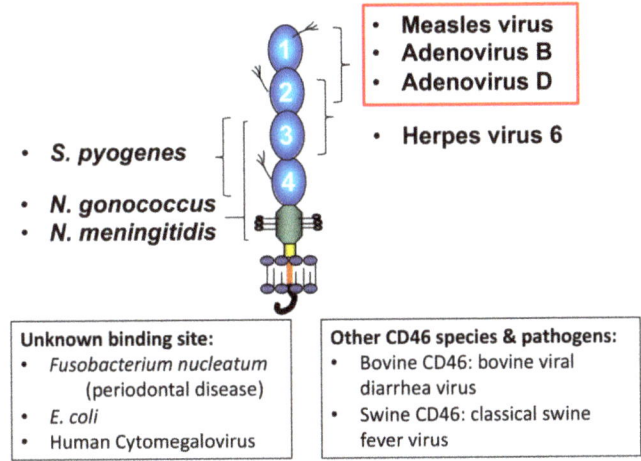

Figure 3. CD46 is a receptor for 10 human-specific pathogens; bovine and swine CD46 are also pathogen receptors. For seven of the human pathogens, the binding site has been identified (indicated above), including strains of measles virus and adenovirus. Two features make CD46 an attractive target for oncology applications: (1) it is overexpressed on many cancer cell types and (2) measles and adenoviral vectors can be constructed to target CD46 for cancer treatment. More than 20 CD46-targeted cancer treatments trials are currently being conducted.

One of the most challenging aspects of cancer therapy development is target selection. In this regard, two features make CD46 an attractive candidate. First, as noted in the preceding paragraph, it is a receptor for some strains of measles- and adenoviruses. Second, as outlined above, CD46 is commonly overexpressed on a variety of tumor cells [27,33]. Thus, a number of therapeutic agents, including more than 20 now in clinical trials (Table 1), employ CD46-targeted oncolytic adenoviral- or measles virus-based vectors [20,54,65–68]. More than 500 gene therapy trials have been conducted, most with human adenoviral vectors. Many have been conducted using Adenovirus type C that binds to the coxsackie-adenovirus receptor (CAR) (reviewed by [69]). However, the low expression level of CAR by cancer cells has limited the efficiency of such targeted oncolytic therapies. Alternatively, some species B adenoviruses target CD46, thus presenting an improved approach to increase the effectiveness of cancer targeting. As an example, comparisons between CD46 and CAR-targeted adenoviral therapy have demonstrated superior outcomes with CD46 targeting in bladder cancer [69] and ovarian cancer [70], despite comparable receptor expression by the tumor cells.

Table 1. Clinical trials of CD46-based cancer therapeutics.

Name	Category	Target	Phase	Clinicaltrials.gov#	Sponsor
Enadenotucirev [1]	Oncolytic adenovirus	Epithelial tumors; colorectal cancer; bladder cancer	Phase 1/2	NCT02028442	PsiOxus Therapeutics
Enadenotucirev	Oncolytic adenovirus + chemotherapy	Platinum-resistant epithelial ovarian cancer	Phase 1	NCT02028117	PsiOxus Therapeutics
Enadenotucirev	Oncolytic adenovirus + immunotherapy	Metastatic or advanced epithelial tumors	Phase 1	NCT02636036	PsiOxus Therapeutics
Enadenotucirev	Oncolytic adenovirus + chemoradiotherapy	Advanced rectal cancer	Phase 1	NCT03916510	University of Oxford
NG-350A [2]	Oncolytic adenovirus	Advanced or metastatic epithelial tumors	Phase 1	NCT03852511	PsiOxus Therapeutics
NG-641 [2]	Oncolytic adenovirus	Advanced or metastatic epithelial tumors	Phase 1	NCT04053283	PsiOxus Therapeutics
LOAd703 [3]	Oncolytic adenovirus + chemotherapy or immunotherapy	Pancreatic cancer	Phase 1/2	NCT02705196	Lokon Pharma AB
LOAd703	Oncolytic adenovirus + immunotherapy	Malignant melanoma	Phase 1/2	NCT04123470	Lokon Pharma AB
LOAd703	Oncolytic adenovirus + chemotherapy or immune conditioning	Pancreatic adenocarcinoma; ovarian cancer; biliary cancer; colorectal cancer	Phase 1/2	NCT03225989	Lokon Pharma AB
MV-NIS [4]	Oncolytic measles virus + chemotherapy	Cancer of ovaries, fallopian tubes or peritoneal cancer	Phase 2	NCT02364713	Mayo Clinic
MV-NIS	Oncolytic measles virus	Squamous cell carcinoma neck/head or breast cancer	Phase 1	NCT01846091	Mayo Clinic
MV-NIS	Oncolytic measles virus	Ovarian epithelial cancer; peritoneal cancer	Phase 1	NCT00408590	Mayo Clinic
MV-NIS	Oncolytic measles virus	Malignant pleural mesothelioma	Phase 1	NCT01503177	Mayo Clinic
MV-NIS	Oncolytic measles virus	Recurrent or refractory multiple myeloma	Phase 1/2	NCT00450814	Mayo Clinic
MV-NIS	Oncolytic measles virus	Peripheral nerve sheath tumor; neurofibromatosis type 1	Phase 1	NCT02700230	Mayo Clinic

Table 1. *Cont.*

Name	Category	Target	Phase	Clinicaltrials.gov#	Sponsor
MV-NIS	Oncolytic measles virus	Multiple myeloma	Phase 2	NCT02192775	University of Arkansas
MV-NIS	Oncolytic measlesvirus-infected mesenchymal stem cells	Recurrent ovarian cancer	Phase 1/2	NCT02068794	Mayo Clinic
MV-CEA [5]	Oncolytic measles virus	Recurrent glioblastoma multiforme	Phase 1	NCT00390299	Mayo Clinic
MV-CEA	Oncolytic measles virus	Recurrent ovarian epithelial cancer;primary peritoneal cancer	Phase 1	NCT00408590	Mayo Clinic
TMV-018 [6]	Oncolytic measles virus	Gastrointestinal cancer	Phase 1	NCT04195373	Themas Bioscience
FOR46 [7]	Antibody-drug conjugate	Multiple myeloma, relapsed or refractory	Phase 1	NCT03650491	Fortis
FOR 46	Antibody-drug conjugate	Metastatic prostate cancer	Phase 1	NCT03575819	Fortis

[1] Chimera derived from adenovirus group BAd11p/Ad3. [2] Transgene-modified variant of Enadenotucirev expressing a bi-specific T-cell activator molecule (FAP-TAc) recognizing fibroblast activating protein (FAP) on cancer associated fibroblasts (CAFs) and CD3 on T-cells. Production of FAP-TAc by virus-infected tumor cells should lead to T cell-mediated killing of CAFs and, thus, modification of the tumor microenvironment to drive effective anti-tumor immunity. [3] LOAd, the virus is a hybrid derived from adenovirus serotypes 5 and 35. It expresses immune-activating genes (trimerized membrane-bound isoleucine zipper TMZ-CD40L and 4-1BB ligand) under control of a cytomegalovirus (CMV) promoter. [4] MV-NIS, an oncolytic measles virus (MV) encoding the thyroidal sodium iodide symporter (NIS) that facilitates viral gene expression and offers a tool for radiovirotherapy. [5] MV-CEA, an oncolytic measles virus encoding the carcinoembryonic antigen (CEA). [6] Oncolytic measles virus, TMV-018-101, engineered with cytosine deaminase. [7] A monoclonal antibody to a conformationally-specific epitope of CD46 expressed only on tumor cells that is conjugated to an anti-cancer drug.

Other oncolytic strategies utilize measles virus that also targets CD46. For example, the Edmonston lineage (vaccine) strain of measles virus has been modified to express carcinoembryonic antigen or the human sodium iodide symporter (NIS) for noninvasive monitoring. These are being tested in a variety of tumor types (reviewed in [71] and see Table 1). Notably, treatment of an MM patient with an engineered oncolytic measles virus containing the NIS (termed MV-NIS) resulted in durable remission in a case report [72] and demonstrated activity in phase 1 trials for patients with ovarian cancer [73,74] and MM [75].

Another CD46-targeted therapy employs an antibody-drug conjugate (ADC) [20]. In this case, the CD46-targeting specificity is mediated by an Ab instead of a virus. As noted above, the region on chromosome 1q carrying CD46 commonly undergoes genomic amplification in relapsed myeloma patients. This amplification correlates with markedly increased expression of CD46 by the tumor [20]. The potential of the CD46-ADC approach was demonstrated in MM in which potent inhibition of myeloma cell proliferation was achieved in an orthostatic xenograft (mouse) model [20]. The CD46-ADC approach has also shown efficacy in metastatic castration-resistant prostate cancer, utilizing a tubulin inhibitor conjugated as the ADC added to a macropinocytosing anti-CD46 antibody (Ab) [65]. These studies support CD46 as a promising target for antibody-based therapeutics for certain tumor types. Two phase 1 trials using an anti-CD46 ADC are being conducted against MM and metastatic prostate cancer (Table 1).

Factors affecting the expression of CD46 and loss from the cell surface also need to be taken into consideration relative to targeting of CD46 as a therapeutic strategy. For example, a recent report demonstrated that p53, which is a frequently deleted or modified gene in human cancers, impacts CD46 expression and, thus, MM susceptibility to oncolytic measles virus [76]. Further, CD46 is known to be internalized by two mechanisms. CD46 can be constitutively internalized via clathrin-dependent endocytosis and recycled to the surface. In addition, crosslinking of CD46 on the cell surface by multivalent anti-CD46 Ab or measles virus induces ligand-engulfing pseudopodia (a process similar to macropinocytosis) and subsequently leads to CD46 degradation and downregulation on the cell surface [77]. This was demonstrated in vitro, as well as in in vivo murine and non-human primate (NHP) models. In NHPs, CD46 depletion enhanced the depletion of $CD20^+$ B cells by a low dose of rituximab [78].

4. CD46 as a Metabolic Driver

New understandings of the complement system as well as CD46 are expanding their roles beyond that traditionally appreciated. It has become increasingly recognized that most cells contain an intracellular complement system, ICS or complosome, that not only provides immune defense but also assists in key interactions for host cell functions [79]. For example, autocrine activation of CD46 via C3b plays a critical role in nutrient uptake and enhances cellular metabolism [14]. While the arsenal of complement components and specific cell types constituting the complosome continues to be elucidated, the finding of CD46 as a metabolic driver suggests a possible role in malignant transformation and/or cell proliferation.

Cancer cells are highly glycolytic and preferentially metabolize glucose anaerobically ([80] reviewed in [81]). Interestingly, new connections have been discovered between glucose metabolism and the ICS that indicate that this metabolic pathway may be driven by intracellular C3 signaling [81]. In the ICS of human $CD4^+$ T cells, C3a generated intracellularly interacts with its receptor, C3aR, expressed on lysosomes and thus provides tonic low-level activation of the mammalian target of rapamycin (mTOR) signaling pathway [16] (Figure 4). This interaction is an essential survival signal for $CD4^+$ T cells. Intracellular complement activity also drives anti-apoptotic activity through intracellularly generated C3b engagement of CD46 on the surface of T cells that subsequently enhances glycolysis [14] (Figure 4). Analogously, $CD8^+$ T cells rely on CD46 stimulation of fatty acid metabolism for optimal cytotoxic function [82]. King et al. demonstrated that intracellular C3 in pancreatic islet β cells regulates autophagy to protect β cells from death [83]. Further, CD46 has been shown to interact with Jagged1, a Notch family member, to regulate Th1 cell activation [10]. Notch is known to regulate oxidative phosphorylation and glycolysis in cancer cells [14]. Thus, a new view is emerging that intracellular complement activation regulates cell survival pathways (reviewed in [81]). Future studies addressing CD46-driven metabolic reprogramming are warranted to address its oncologic implications in cancer.

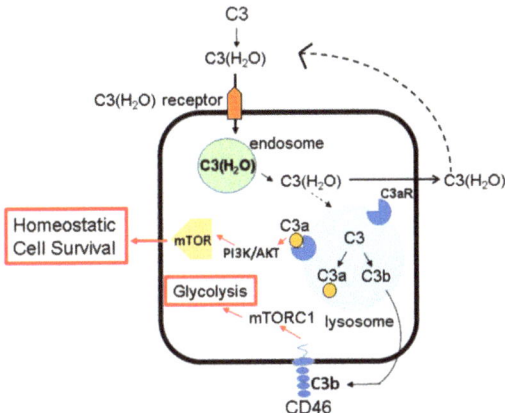

Figure 4. Intracellular C3 and CD46 drive cell metabolism and survival. Intracellular C3 is biosynthetically derived or can be loaded from the plasma. Generation of C3a and C3b from intracellular C3 can induce metabolic pathways through the PI3K-AKT-mTOR axis, enhancing glycolysis and homeostatic cell survival.

Given the importance of the CD46-C3 axis for cell survival, the source of intracellular C3 has been examined. We have shown that intracellular C3 arises via two distinct routes: either being synthesized in situ [16] or taken up from the extracellular milieu [84]. Specifically, the form taken up from the extracellular fluid is $C3(H_2O)$. Thus, $C3(H_2O)$ has two main functions—in the extracellular space, it is a trigger for the AP, and in the intracellular space, it provides a source of C3 for the complosome. In the context of cancer, $C3(H_2O)$ has not been evaluated, although, notably, dysregulation of the alternative pathway of complement activation, which can be initiated by $C3(H_2O)$, has been demonstrated in several hematological cancers [85].

Oncogenesis also may be driven by aberrant signaling processes. Buettner et al. correlated overexpression of CD46 mRNA and protein with the binding of activated signal transducers and activators of transcription 3 (STAT3) to two sites in the CD46 promoter [86]. Since STAT3 is persistently activated in a wide variety of tumors and IL-6 is increased with co-stimulation of CD46 in the presence of $C3(H_2O)$ [84], the CD46-STAT3-C3 axis may play a key role in regulating metabolic and regenerative processes. We hypothesize that CD46 isoform cytoplasmic tail switching (as occurs in activated versus quiescent T cells [87]) may be altered in cancers, such as MM. The potential for CD46-targeting to modulate this axis deserves further investigation.

5. Conclusions

Since the discovery of CD46 more than 30 years ago, much knowledge has been gleaned about this multifaceted protein [7]. The surprising finding of its alternative splicing to produce four common isoforms that co-exist on most cells has proven significant in both its function and importance to biology. Much remains to be leveraged about these roles. Because of its widespread expression, it is not surprising that at least ten human-specific pathogens have targeted CD46. Beyond its role in complement regulation, we now also appreciate CD46 as a driver of cellular metabolism and an important player in the newly described intracellular complement system. Collectively, these studies provide a strong rationale for further characterization of these interconnected players in oncology.

The success of pre-clinical studies utilizing CD46 as a therapeutic target have now led more than 20 clinical trials being conducted for cancer treatments. Thus, 'friendly fire' aimed at CD46 utilizing approaches such as oncolytic viruses or antibody-drug conjugates (alone or in combination with other therapeutics) offers promising new modalities for the treatment of malignancies.

Author Contributions: Writing, reviewing and editing: M.E., M.K.L., J.P.A.; References: M.E.; Graphics: M.E. (Figure 4), M.K.L. (Figures 1–3); Table: M.K.L.; Funding J.P.A. All authors have read and agreed to the published version of the manuscript.

Funding: This research was funded by the National Institutes of Health/National Institute of General Medical Sciences (R35-GM136352-01 and 1R01-GM99111-23) to J.P.A.

Conflicts of Interest: M.E. and M.K.L. report no competing interest. J.P.A. reports serving as a current consultant for Celldex Therapeutics; Clinical Pharmacy Services; Kypha, Inc.; Achillion Pharmaceuticals, Inc.; BioMarin Pharmaceutical Inc.; stock or equity options for Compliment Corporation; Kypha, Inc.; Gemini Therapeutics, Inc.; AdMiRx, Inc.

References

1. Cole, J.L.; Housley, G.A., Jr.; Dykman, T.R.; MacDermott, R.P.; Atkinson, J.P. Identification of an additional class of C3-binding membrane proteins of human peripheral blood leukocytes and cell lines. *Proc. Natl. Acad. Sci. USA* **1985**, *82*, 859–863. [CrossRef]
2. Seya, T.; Turner, J.R.; Atkinson, J.P. Purification and characterization of a membrane protein (gp45-70) that is a cofactor for cleavage of C3b and C4b. *J. Exp. Med.* **1986**, *163*, 837–855. [CrossRef]
3. Liszewski, M.K.; Post, T.W.; Atkinson, J.P. Membrane cofactor protein (MCP or CD46): Newest member of the regulators of complement activation gene cluster. *Annu. Rev. Immunol.* **1991**, *9*, 431–455. [CrossRef] [PubMed]
4. McNearney, T.; Ballard, L.; Seya, T.; Atkinson, J.P. Membrane cofactor protein of complement is present on human fibroblast, epithelial, and endothelial cells. *J. Clin. Investig.* **1989**, *84*, 538–545. [CrossRef] [PubMed]
5. Bora, N.S.; Lublin, D.M.; Kumar, B.V.; Hockett, R.D.; Holers, V.M.; Atkinson, J.P. Structural gene for human membrane cofactor protein (MCP) of complement maps to within 100 kb of the 3' end of the C3b/C4b receptor gene. *J. Exp. Med.* **1989**, *169*, 597–602. [CrossRef] [PubMed]
6. Yamamoto, H.; Fara, A.F.; Dasgupta, P.; Kemper, C. CD46: The 'multitasker' of complement proteins. *Int. J. Biochem. Cell Biol.* **2013**, *45*, 2808–2820. [CrossRef]
7. Liszewski, M.K.; Kemper, C. Complement in Motion: The Evolution of CD46 from a Complement Regulator to an Orchestrator of Normal Cell Physiology. *J. Immunol.* **2019**, *203*, 3–5. [CrossRef]
8. Kemper, C.; Atkinson, J.P. T-cell regulation: With complements from innate immunity. *Nat. Rev. Immunol.* **2007**, *7*, 9–18. [CrossRef]
9. Cope, A.; Le Friec, G.; Cardone, J.; Kemper, C. The Th1 life cycle: Molecular control of IFN-gamma to IL-10 switching. *Trends Immunol.* **2011**, *32*, 278–286. [CrossRef]
10. Le Friec, G.; Sheppard, D.; Whiteman, P.; Karsten, C.M.; Shamoun, S.A.; Laing, A.; Bugeon, L.; Dallman, M.J.; Melchionna, T.; Chillakuri, C.; et al. The CD46-Jagged1 interaction is critical for human TH1 immunity. *Nat. Immunol.* **2012**, *13*, 1213–1221. [CrossRef]
11. Fremeaux-Bacchi, V.; Moulton, E.A.; Kavanagh, D.; Dragon-Durey, M.A.; Blouin, J.; Caudy, A.; Arzouk, N.; Cleper, R.; Francois, M.; Guest, G.; et al. Genetic and functional analyses of membrane cofactor protein (CD46) mutations in atypical hemolytic uremic syndrome. *J. Am. Soc. Nephrol.* **2006**, *17*, 2017–2025. [CrossRef]
12. Kemper, C.; Chan, A.C.; Green, J.M.; Brett, K.A.; Murphy, K.M.; Atkinson, J.P. Activation of human CD4+ cells with CD3 and CD46 induces a T-regulatory cell 1 phenotype. *Nature* **2003**, *421*, 388–392. [CrossRef] [PubMed]
13. Cardone, J.; Le Friec, G.; Vantourout, P.; Roberts, A.; Fuchs, A.; Jackson, I.; Suddason, T.; Lord, G.; Atkinson, J.P.; Cope, A.; et al. Complement regulator CD46 temporally regulates cytokine production by conventional and unconventional T cells. *Nat. Immunol.* **2010**, *11*, 862–871. [CrossRef] [PubMed]
14. Kolev, M.; Dimeloe, S.; Le Friec, G.; Navarini, A.; Arbore, G.; Povoleri, G.A.; Fischer, M.; Belle, R.; Loeliger, J.; Develioglu, L.; et al. Complement regulates nutrient influx and metabolic reprogramming during Th1 cell responses. *Immunity* **2015**, *42*, 1033–1047. [CrossRef] [PubMed]
15. Cardone, J.; Le Friec, G.; Kemper, C. CD46 in innate and adaptive immunity: An update. *Clin. Exp. Immunol.* **2011**, *164*, 301–311. [CrossRef]

16. Liszewski, M.K.; Kolev, M.; Le Friec, G.; Leung, M.; Bertram, P.G.; Fara, A.F.; Subias, M.; Pickering, M.C.; Drouet, C.; Meri, S.; et al. Intracellular complement activation sustains T cell homeostasis and mediates effector differentiation. *Immunity* **2013**, *39*, 1143–1157. [CrossRef]
17. Gancz, D.; Fishelson, Z. Cancer resistance to complement-dependent cytotoxicity (CDC): Problem-oriented research and development. *Mol. Immunol.* **2009**, *46*, 2794–2800. [CrossRef]
18. Geller, A.; Yan, J. The Role of Membrane Bound Complement Regulatory Proteins in Tumor Development and Cancer Immunotherapy. *Front. Immunol.* **2019**, *10*, 1074. [CrossRef]
19. Roumenina, L.T.; Daugan, M.V.; Petitprez, F.; Sautes-Fridman, C.; Fridman, W.H. Context-dependent roles of complement in cancer. *Nat. Rev. Cancer* **2019**, *19*, 698–715. [CrossRef]
20. Sherbenou, D.W.; Aftab, B.T.; Su, Y.; Behrens, C.R.; Wiita, A.; Logan, A.C.; Acosta-Alvear, D.; Hann, B.C.; Walter, P.; Shuman, M.A.; et al. Antibody-drug conjugate targeting CD46 eliminates multiple myeloma cells. *J. Clin. Investig.* **2016**, *126*, 4640–4653. [CrossRef]
21. Kinugasa, N.; Higashi, T.; Nouso, K.; Nakatsukasa, H.; Kobayashi, Y.; Ishizaki, M.; Toshikuni, N.; Yoshida, K.; Uematsu, S.; Tsuji, T. Expression of membrane cofactor protein (MCP, CD46) in human liver diseases. *Br. J. Cancer* **1999**, *80*, 1820–1825. [CrossRef] [PubMed]
22. Berraondo, P.; Minute, L.; Ajona, D.; Corrales, L.; Melero, I.; Pio, R. Innate immune mediators in cancer: Between defense and resistance. *Immunol. Rev.* **2016**, *274*, 290–306. [CrossRef] [PubMed]
23. Ajona, D.; Pajares, M.J.; Corrales, L.; Perez-Gracia, J.L.; Agorreta, J.; Lozano, M.D.; Torre, W.; Massion, P.P.; de-Torres, J.P.; Jantus-Lewintre, E.; et al. Investigation of complement activation product c4d as a diagnostic and prognostic biomarker for lung cancer. *J. Natl. Cancer Inst.* **2013**, *105*, 1385–1393. [CrossRef] [PubMed]
24. Seya, T.; Hara, T.; Iwata, K.; Kuriyama, S.; Hasegawa, T.; Nagase, Y.; Miyagawa, S.; Matsumoto, M.; Hatanaka, M.; Atkinson, J.P.; et al. Purification and functional properties of soluble forms of membrane cofactor protein (CD46) of complement: Identification of forms increased in cancer patients' sera. *Int. Immunol.* **1995**, *7*, 727–736. [CrossRef]
25. Surowiak, P.; Materna, V.; Maciejczyk, A.; Kaplenko, I.; Spaczynski, M.; Dietel, M.; Lage, H.; Zabel, M. CD46 expression is indicative of shorter revival-free survival for ovarian cancer patients. *Anticancer Res.* **2006**, *26*, 4943–4948.
26. Maciejczyk, A.; Szelachowska, J.; Szynglarewicz, B.; Szulc, R.; Szulc, A.; Wysocka, T.; Jagoda, E.; Lage, H.; Surowiak, P. CD46 Expression is an unfavorable prognostic factor in breast cancer cases. *Appl. Immunohistochem. Mol. Morphol.* **2011**, *19*, 540–546. [CrossRef]
27. Ong, H.T.; Timm, M.M.; Greipp, P.R.; Witzig, T.E.; Dispenzieri, A.; Russell, S.J.; Peng, K.W. Oncolytic measles virus targets high CD46 expression on multiple myeloma cells. *Exp. Hematol.* **2006**, *34*, 713–720. [CrossRef]
28. Lu, Z.; Zhang, C.; Cui, J.; Song, Q.; Wang, L.; Kang, J.; Li, P.; Hu, X.; Song, H.; Yang, J.; et al. Bioinformatic analysis of the membrane cofactor protein CD46 and microRNA expression in hepatocellular carcinoma. *Oncol. Rep.* **2014**, *31*, 557–564. [CrossRef]
29. Taylor, R.P.; Lindorfer, M.A. Cytotoxic mechanisms of immunotherapy: Harnessing complement in the action of anti-tumor monoclonal antibodies. *Semin. Immunol.* **2016**, *28*, 309–316. [CrossRef]
30. Elvington, M.; Huang, Y.; Morgan, B.P.; Qiao, F.; van Rooijen, N.; Atkinson, C.; Tomlinson, S. A targeted complement-dependent strategy to improve the outcome of mAb therapy, and characterization in a murine model of metastatic cancer. *Blood* **2012**, *119*, 6043–6051. [CrossRef]
31. Derer, S.; Beurskens, F.J.; Rosner, T.; Peipp, M.; Valerius, T. Complement in antibody-based tumor therapy. *Crit. Rev. Immunol.* **2014**, *34*, 199–214. [CrossRef]
32. Gelderman, K.A.; Hakulinen, J.; Hagenaars, M.; Kuppen, P.J.; Meri, S.; Gorter, A. Membrane-bound complement regulatory proteins inhibit complement activation by an immunotherapeutic mAb in a syngeneic rat colorectal cancer model. *Mol. Immunol.* **2003**, *40*, 13–23. [CrossRef]
33. Fishelson, Z.; Donin, N.; Zell, S.; Schultz, S.; Kirschfink, M. Obstacles to cancer immunotherapy: Expression of membrane complement regulatory proteins (mCRPs) in tumors. *Mol. Immunol.* **2003**, *40*, 109–123. [CrossRef]
34. Gelderman, K.A.; Tomlinson, S.; Ross, G.D.; Gorter, A. Complement function in mAb-mediated cancer immunotherapy. *Trends Immunol.* **2004**, *25*, 158–164. [CrossRef] [PubMed]
35. Geis, N.; Zell, S.; Rutz, R.; Li, W.; Giese, T.; Mamidi, S.; Schultz, S.; Kirschfink, M. Inhibition of membrane complement inhibitor expression (CD46, CD55, CD59) by siRNA sensitizes tumor cells to complement attack in vitro. *Curr. Cancer Drug Targets* **2010**, *10*, 922–931. [CrossRef] [PubMed]

36. Bellone, S.; Roque, D.; Cocco, E.; Gasparrini, S.; Bortolomai, I.; Buza, N.; Abu-Khalaf, M.; Silasi, D.A.; Ratner, E.; Azodi, M.; et al. Downregulation of membrane complement inhibitors CD55 and CD59 by siRNA sensitises uterine serous carcinoma overexpressing Her2/neu to complement and antibody-dependent cell cytotoxicity in vitro: Implications for trastuzumab-based immunotherapy. *Br. J. Cancer* **2012**, *106*, 1543–1550. [CrossRef]
37. Varela, J.C.; Imai, M.; Atkinson, C.; Ohta, R.; Rapisardo, M.; Tomlinson, S. Modulation of protective T cell immunity by complement inhibitor expression on tumor cells. *Cancer Res.* **2008**, *68*, 6734–6742. [CrossRef] [PubMed]
38. Ohta, R.; Kondor, N.; Dohi, N.; Tomlinson, S.; Imai, M.; Holers, V.M.; Okada, H.; Okada, N. Mouse complement receptor-related gene y/p65-neutralized tumor vaccine induces antitumor activity in vivo. *J. Immunol.* **2004**, *173*, 205–213. [CrossRef]
39. Imai, M.; Ohta, R.; Okada, N.; Tomlinson, S. Inhibition of a complement regulator in vivo enhances antibody therapy in a model of mammary adenocarcinoma. *Int. J. Cancer* **2004**, *110*, 875–881. [CrossRef]
40. Gelderman, K.A.; Blok, V.T.; Fleuren, G.J.; Gorter, A. The inhibitory effect of CD46, CD55, and CD59 on complement activation after immunotherapeutic treatment of cervical carcinoma cells with monoclonal antibodies or bispecific monoclonal antibodies. *Lab. Investig.* **2002**, *82*, 483–493. [CrossRef]
41. Gelderman, K.A.; Kuppen, P.J.; Bruin, W.; Fleuren, G.J.; Gorter, A. Enhancement of the complement activating capacity of 17-1A mAb to overcome the effect of membrane-bound complement regulatory proteins on colorectal carcinoma. *Eur. J. Immunol.* **2002**, *32*, 128–135. [CrossRef]
42. Gelderman, K.A.; Kuppen, P.J.; Okada, N.; Fleuren, G.J.; Gorter, A. Tumor-specific inhibition of membrane-bound complement regulatory protein Crry with bispecific monoclonal antibodies prevents tumor outgrowth in a rat colorectal cancer lung metastases model. *Cancer Res.* **2004**, *64*, 4366–4372. [CrossRef] [PubMed]
43. Gelderman, K.A.; Lam, S.; Gorter, A. Inhibiting complement regulators in cancer immunotherapy with bispecific mAbs. *Expert Opin. Biol. Ther.* **2005**, *5*, 1593–1601. [CrossRef]
44. Imai, M.; Ohta, R.; Varela, J.C.; Song, H.; Tomlinson, S. Enhancement of antibody-dependent mechanisms of tumor cell lysis by a targeted activator of complement. *Cancer Res.* **2007**, *67*, 9535–9541. [CrossRef]
45. Markiewski, M.M.; Lambris, J.D. Is complement good or bad for cancer patients? A new perspective on an old dilemma. *Trends Immunol.* **2009**, *30*, 286–292. [CrossRef] [PubMed]
46. Shearer, W.T.; Atkinson, J.P.; Parker, C.W. Humoral immunostimulation. VI. Increased calcium uptake by cells treated with antibody and complement. *J. Immunol.* **1976**, *117*, 973–980.
47. Markiewski, M.M.; DeAngelis, R.A.; Benencia, F.; Ricklin-Lichtsteiner, S.K.; Koutoulaki, A.; Gerard, C.; Coukos, G.; Lambris, J.D. Modulation of the antitumor immune response by complement. *Nat. Immunol.* **2008**, *9*, 1225–1235. [CrossRef] [PubMed]
48. Corrales, L.; Ajona, D.; Rafail, S.; Lasarte, J.J.; Riezu-Boj, J.I.; Lambris, J.D.; Rouzaut, A.; Pajares, M.J.; Montuenga, L.M.; Pio, R. Anaphylatoxin C5a creates a favorable microenvironment for lung cancer progression. *J. Immunol.* **2012**, *189*, 4674–4683. [CrossRef]
49. Pio, R.; Corrales, L.; Lambris, J.D. The role of complement in tumor growth. *Adv. Exp. Med. Biol.* **2014**, *772*, 229–262.
50. Mevorach, D.; Mascarenhas, J.O.; Gershov, D.; Elkon, K.B. Complement-dependent clearance of apoptotic cells by human macrophages. *J. Exp. Med.* **1998**, *188*, 2313–2320. [CrossRef]
51. Gershov, D.; Kim, S.; Brot, N.; Elkon, K.B. C-Reactive protein binds to apoptotic cells, protects the cells from assembly of the terminal complement components, and sustains an antiinflammatory innate immune response: Implications for systemic autoimmunity. *J. Exp. Med.* **2000**, *192*, 1353–1364. [CrossRef] [PubMed]
52. Kemper, C.; Mitchell, L.M.; Zhang, L.; Hourcade, D.E. The complement protein properdin binds apoptotic T cells and promotes complement activation and phagocytosis. *Proc. Natl. Acad. Sci. USA* **2008**, *105*, 9023–9028. [CrossRef]
53. Elvington, M.; Scheiber, M.; Yang, X.; Lyons, K.; Jacqmin, D.; Wadsworth, C.; Marshall, D.; Vanek, K.; Tomlinson, S. Complement-dependent modulation of antitumor immunity following radiation therapy. *Cell Rep.* **2014**, *8*, 818–830. [CrossRef]
54. Cho, Y.S.; Do, M.H.; Kwon, S.Y.; Moon, C.; Kim, K.; Lee, K.; Lee, S.J.; Hemmi, S.; Joo, Y.E.; Kim, M.S.; et al. Efficacy of CD46-targeting chimeric Ad5/35 adenoviral gene therapy for colorectal cancers. *Oncotarget* **2016**, *7*, 38210–38223. [CrossRef] [PubMed]

55. Naniche, D.; Varior-Krishnan, G.; Cervoni, F.; Wild, T.F.; Rossi, B.; Rabourdin-Combe, C.; Gerlier, D. Human membrane cofactor protein (CD46) acts as a cellular receptor for measles virus. *J. Virol.* **1993**, *67*, 6025–6032. [CrossRef]
56. Cattaneo, R. Four viruses, two bacteria, and one receptor: Membrane cofactor protein (CD46) as pathogens' magnet. *J. Virol.* **2004**, *78*, 4385–4388. [CrossRef]
57. Gaggar, A.; Shayakhmetov, D.M.; Lieber, A. CD46 is a cellular receptor for group B adenoviruses. *Nat. Med.* **2003**, *9*, 1408–1412. [CrossRef]
58. Stein, K.R.; Gardner, T.J.; Hernandez, R.E.; Kraus, T.A.; Duty, J.A.; Ubarretxena-Belandia, I.; Moran, T.M.; Tortorella, D. CD46 facilitates entry and dissemination of human cytomegalovirus. *Nat. Commun.* **2019**, *10*, 2699. [CrossRef]
59. Dorig, R.E.; Marcil, A.; Chopra, A.; Richardson, C.D. The human CD46 molecule is a receptor for measles virus (Edmonston strain). *Cell* **1993**, *75*, 295–305. [CrossRef]
60. Maurer, K.; Krey, T.; Moennig, V.; Thiel, H.J.; Rumenapf, T. CD46 is a cellular receptor for bovine viral diarrhea virus. *J. Virol.* **2004**, *78*, 1792–1799. [CrossRef]
61. Drager, C.; Beer, M.; Blome, S. Porcine complement regulatory protein CD46 and heparan sulfates are the major factors for classical swine fever virus attachment in vitro. *Arch. Virol.* **2015**, *160*, 739–746. [CrossRef]
62. Kim, W.J.; Mai, A.; Weyand, N.J.; Rendon, M.A.; Van Doorslaer, K.; So, M. Neisseria gonorrhoeae evades autophagic killing by downregulating CD46-cyt1 and remodeling lysosomes. *PLoS Pathog.* **2019**, *15*, e1007495. [CrossRef]
63. Kurita-Taniguchi, M.; Fukui, A.; Hazeki, K.; Hirano, A.; Tsuji, S.; Matsumoto, M.; Watanabe, M.; Ueda, S.; Seya, T. Functional modulation of human macrophages through CD46 (measles virus receptor): Production of IL-12 p40 and nitric oxide in association with recruitment of protein-tyrosine phosphatase SHP-1 to CD46. *J. Immunol.* **2000**, *165*, 5143–5152. [CrossRef] [PubMed]
64. Karp, C.L.; Wysocka, M.; Wahl, L.M.; Ahearn, J.M.; Cuomo, P.J.; Sherry, B.; Trinchieri, G.; Griffin, D.E. Mechanism of suppression of cell-mediated immunity by measles virus. *Science* **1996**, *273*, 228–231. [CrossRef]
65. Su, Y.; Liu, Y.; Behrens, C.R.; Bidlingmaier, S.; Lee, N.K.; Aggarwal, R.; Sherbenou, D.W.; Burlingame, A.L.; Hann, B.C.; Simko, J.P.; et al. Targeting CD46 for both adenocarcinoma and neuroendocrine prostate cancer. *JCI Insight* **2018**, *3*. [CrossRef]
66. Anderson, B.D.; Nakamura, T.; Russell, S.J.; Peng, K.W. High CD46 receptor density determines preferential killing of tumor cells by oncolytic measles virus. *Cancer Res.* **2004**, *64*, 4919–4926. [CrossRef] [PubMed]
67. Illingworth, S.; Di, Y.; Bauzon, M.; Lei, J.; Duffy, M.R.; Alvis, S.; Champion, B.; Lieber, A.; Hermiston, T.; Seymour, L.W.; et al. Preclinical Safety Studies of Enadenotucirev, a Chimeric Group B Human-Specific Oncolytic Adenovirus. *Mol. Ther. Oncolytics* **2017**, *5*, 62–74. [CrossRef]
68. Machiels, J.P.; Salazar, R.; Rottey, S.; Duran, I.; Dirix, L.; Geboes, K.; Wilkinson-Blanc, C.; Pover, G.; Alvis, S.; Champion, B.; et al. A phase 1 dose escalation study of the oncolytic adenovirus enadenotucirev, administered intravenously to patients with epithelial solid tumors (EVOLVE). *J. Immunother. Cancer* **2019**, *7*, 20. [CrossRef]
69. Do, M.H.; To, P.K.; Cho, Y.S.; Kwon, S.Y.; Hwang, E.C.; Choi, C.; Cho, S.H.; Lee, S.J.; Hemmi, S.; Jung, C. Targeting CD46 Enhances Anti-Tumoral Activity of Adenovirus Type 5 for Bladder Cancer. *Int. J. Mol. Sci.* **2018**, *19*. [CrossRef]
70. Hulin-Curtis, S.L.; Uusi-Kerttula, H.; Jones, R.; Hanna, L.; Chester, J.D.; Parker, A.L. Evaluation of CD46 re-targeted adenoviral vectors for clinical ovarian cancer intraperitoneal therapy. *Cancer Gene Ther.* **2016**, *23*, 229–234. [CrossRef] [PubMed]
71. Msaouel, P.; Opyrchal, M.; Dispenzieri, A.; Peng, K.W.; Federspiel, M.J.; Russell, S.J.; Galanis, E. Clinical Trials with Oncolytic Measles Virus: Current Status and Future Prospects. *Curr. Cancer Drug Targets* **2018**, *18*, 177–187. [CrossRef] [PubMed]
72. Russell, S.J.; Federspiel, M.J.; Peng, K.W.; Tong, C.; Dingli, D.; Morice, W.G.; Lowe, V.; O'Connor, M.K.; Kyle, R.A.; Leung, N.; et al. Remission of disseminated cancer after systemic oncolytic virotherapy. *Mayo Clin. Proc.* **2014**, *89*, 926–933. [CrossRef]
73. Galanis, E.; Hartmann, L.C.; Cliby, W.A.; Long, H.J.; Peethambaram, P.P.; Barrette, B.A.; Kaur, J.S.; Haluska, P.J., Jr.; Aderca, I.; Zollman, P.J.; et al. Phase I trial of intraperitoneal administration of an oncolytic measles virus strain engineered to express carcinoembryonic antigen for recurrent ovarian cancer. *Cancer Res.* **2010**, *70*, 875–882. [CrossRef]

74. Galanis, E.; Atherton, P.J.; Maurer, M.J.; Knutson, K.L.; Dowdy, S.C.; Cliby, W.A.; Haluska, P., Jr.; Long, H.J.; Oberg, A.; Aderca, I.; et al. Oncolytic measles virus expressing the sodium iodide symporter to treat drug-resistant ovarian cancer. *Cancer Res.* **2015**, *75*, 22–30. [CrossRef] [PubMed]
75. Dispenzieri, A.; Tong, C.; LaPlant, B.; Lacy, M.Q.; Laumann, K.; Dingli, D.; Zhou, Y.; Federspiel, M.J.; Gertz, M.A.; Hayman, S.; et al. Phase I trial of systemic administration of Edmonston strain of measles virus genetically engineered to express the sodium iodide symporter in patients with recurrent or refractory multiple myeloma. *Leukemia* **2017**, *31*, 2791–2798. [CrossRef]
76. Lok, A.; Descamps, G.; Tessoulin, B.; Chiron, D.; Eveillard, M.; Godon, C.; Le Bris, Y.; Vabret, A.; Bellanger, C.; Maillet, L.; et al. p53 regulates CD46 expression and measles virus infection in myeloma cells. *Blood Adv.* **2018**, *2*, 3492–3505. [CrossRef]
77. Crimeen-Irwin, B.; Ellis, S.; Christiansen, D.; Ludford-Menting, M.J.; Milland, J.; Lanteri, M.; Loveland, B.E.; Gerlier, D.; Russell, S.M. Ligand binding determines whether CD46 is internalized by clathrin-coated pits or macropinocytosis. *J. Biol. Chem.* **2003**, *278*, 46927–46937. [CrossRef]
78. Beyer, I.; Cao, H.; Persson, J.; Wang, H.; Liu, Y.; Yumul, R.; Li, Z.; Woodle, D.; Manger, R.; Gough, M.; et al. Transient removal of CD46 is safe and increases B-cell depletion by rituximab in CD46 transgenic mice and macaques. *Mol. Ther.* **2013**, *21*, 291–299. [CrossRef]
79. Liszewski, M.K.; Elvington, M.; Kulkarni, H.S.; Atkinson, J.P. Complement's hidden arsenal: New insights and novel functions inside the cell. *Mol. Immunol.* **2017**, *84*, 2–9. [CrossRef]
80. Warburg, O. On respiratory impairment in cancer cells. *Science* **1956**, *124*, 269–270. [PubMed]
81. Hess, C.; Kemper, C. Complement-Mediated Regulation of Metabolism and Basic Cellular Processes. *Immunity* **2016**, *45*, 240–254. [CrossRef]
82. Arbore, G.; West, E.E.; Rahman, J.; Le Friec, G.; Niyonzima, N.; Pirooznia, M.; Tunc, I.; Pavlidis, P.; Powell, N.; Li, Y.; et al. Complement receptor CD46 co-stimulates optimal human CD8(+) T cell effector function via fatty acid metabolism. *Nat. Commun.* **2018**, *9*, 4186. [CrossRef]
83. King, B.C.; Kulak, K.; Krus, U.; Rosberg, R.; Golec, E.; Wozniak, K.; Gomez, M.F.; Zhang, E.; O'Connell, D.J.; Renstrom, E.; et al. Complement Component C3 Is Highly Expressed in Human Pancreatic Islets and Prevents beta Cell Death via ATG16L1 Interaction and Autophagy Regulation. *Cell Metab.* **2019**, *29*, 202–210.e6. [CrossRef] [PubMed]
84. Elvington, M.; Liszewski, M.K.; Bertram, P.; Kulkarni, H.S.; Atkinson, J.P. A C3(H20) recycling pathway is a component of the intracellular complement system. *J. Clin. Investig.* **2017**, *127*, 970–981. [CrossRef] [PubMed]
85. Kraut, E.H.; Sagone, A.L., Jr. Alternative pathway of complement in multiple myeloma. *Am. J. Hematol.* **1981**, *11*, 335–345. [CrossRef]
86. Buettner, R.; Huang, M.; Gritsko, T.; Karras, J.; Enkemann, S.; Mesa, T.; Nam, S.; Yu, H.; Jove, R. Activated signal transducers and activators of transcription 3 signaling induces CD46 expression and protects human cancer cells from complement-dependent cytotoxicity. *Mol. Cancer Res.* **2007**, *5*, 823–832. [CrossRef]
87. Arbore, G.; Kemper, C.; Kolev, M. Intracellular complement-the complosome-in immune cell regulation. *Mol. Immunol.* **2017**, *89*, 2–9. [CrossRef]

Publisher's Note: MDPI stays neutral with regard to jurisdictional claims in published maps and institutional affiliations.

© 2020 by the authors. Licensee MDPI, Basel, Switzerland. This article is an open access article distributed under the terms and conditions of the Creative Commons Attribution (CC BY) license (http://creativecommons.org/licenses/by/4.0/).

MDPI
St. Alban-Anlage 66
4052 Basel
Switzerland
Tel. +41 61 683 77 34
Fax +41 61 302 89 18
www.mdpi.com

Antibodies Editorial Office
E-mail: antibodies@mdpi.com
www.mdpi.com/journal/antibodies

www.ingramcontent.com/pod-product-compliance
Lightning Source LLC
LaVergne TN
LVHW070657100526
838202LV00013B/989